Atlas of Clinical and Surgical Orbital Anatomy

Commissioning Editor: **Russell Gabbedy**
Development Editor: **Nani Clansey**
Editorial Assistant: **Kirsten Lowson**
Project Manager: **Glenys Norquay/Nancy Arnott**
Designer: **Charles Gray**
Illustrator: **Thomas G. Waldrup, MSMI**
Marketing Manager(s) (UK/USA): **Gaynor Jones/Helena Mutak**

Surgical Orbital Anatomy

Second Edition

Jonathan J. Dutton MD, PhD, FACS

Professor and Vice Chair of Ophthalmology
The University of North Carolina
Chapel Hill,
North Carolina
USA

Illustrations by:

Thomas G. Waldrop, MSMI

ELSEVIER
SAUNDERS

ELSEVIER
SAUNDERS

First edition 1994
Second edition 2011

Notices

Knowledge and best practice in this field are constantly changing. As new research and experience broaden our understanding, changes in research methods, professional practices, or medical treatment may become necessary.

Practitioners and researchers must always rely on their own experience and knowledge in evaluating and using any information, methods, compounds, or experiments described herein. In using such information or methods they should be mindful of their own safety and the safety of others, including parties for whom they have a professional responsibility.

With respect to any drug or pharmaceutical products identified, readers are advised to check the most current information provided (i) on procedures featured or (ii) by the manufacturer of each product to be administered, to verify the recommended dose or formula, the method and duration of administration, and contraindications. It is the responsibility of practitioners, relying on their own experience and knowledge of their patients, to make diagnoses, to determine dosages and the best treatment for each individual patient, and to take all appropriate safety precautions.

To the fullest extent of the law, neither the Publisher nor the authors, contributors, or editors, assume any liability for any injury and/or damage to persons or property as a matter of products liability, negligence or otherwise, or from any use or operation of any methods, products, instructions, or ideas contained in the material herein.

Saunders

British Library Cataloguing in Publication Data

Dutton, Jonathan J.
   Atlas of clinical and surgical orbital anatomy. – 2nd ed.
   1. Eye-sockets–Anatomy–Atlases.   2. Eye-sockets–
Surgery–Atlases.
   I. Title
   611.8'4-dc22

ISBN-13: 978-1-4377-2272-7

Library of Congress Cataloging in Publication Data
A catalog record for this book is available from the Library of Congress.

Printed in China

Last digit is the print number: 9   8   7   6   5   4   3   2   1

*"The learning and knowledge that we have is, at the most, but little compared
with that of which we are ignorant."*

Plato, 428-348 BC

*"The known is finite, the unknown infinite, intellectually we stand on an islet in the midst of an
illimitable ocean of inexplicability. Our business in every generation is to reclaim
a little more land."*

T.H. Huxley, 1887

With the second edition of this book, we continue to explore further into the realm of orbital anatomy.
We hope thereby that we are able to contribute, however slightly,
to Huxley's precious intellectual land.

About the Authors

JONATHAN J. DUTTON, M.D., Ph.D. is currently Professor and Vice Chair of Ophthalmology at The University of North Carolina at Chapel Hill. He completed his masters and doctorate degrees in zoology, evolutionary biology, and vertebrate paleontology at Harvard University in 1970, and joined the faculty of Princeton University as Sinclair Professor of Vertebrate Paleontology from 1970 to 1973. Between 1965 and 1973 he conducted ten research expeditions to East Africa and published widely on vertebrate morphology and mammalian evolution. After returning to school and receiving his M.D. degree in 1978, and going on to residency training at Washington University Medical School, he completed a research fellowship in glaucoma at Washington University, and another fellowship in oculoplastic and orbital surgery at the University of Iowa. From 1983 to 1999 he was Professor of Ophthalmology and head of the Oculoplastic and Orbital Service at Duke University Medical Center. He served as CEO and Medical Director of the Atlantic Eye and Face Center in Cary, NC from 2000-2003 and then joined the full-time faculty at the University of North Carolina at Chapel Hill, where he is currently Professor and Vice Chair. Dr Dutton is senior preceptor of an ASOPRS-approved fellowship program that has trained 15 fellows. He specializes in oculoplastic reconstructive and orbital surgery, thyroid eye disease, and periorbital and intraocular ophthalmic oncology.

THOMAS G. WALDROP, M.S.M.I. received his Master of Science degree in medical illustration from the Medical College of Georgia in 1978. He directed the ophthalmic photography and ultrasound section of the Retina Institute in St Louis before establishing his medical illustration service in Hillsborough, North Carolina in 1980. Since then, he has worked closely with the Duke University Eye Center producing ophthalmic illustrations for publication, and he has collaborated with Dr. Dutton on several major atlases of ophthalmic surgery.

Preface to the First Edition

Few areas in ophthalmology have proven to be as elusive or difficult to teach as orbital anatomy. The grasp of clinical diagnostic techniques, and the development of sophisticated surgical skills seem far removed from the mundane and often boring tasks of plowing through pages of descriptive anatomic detail. Idealized artistic drawings have often failed to accurately portray true anatomic relationships with other structures. Photographs of clinical dissections are usually so cluttered with extraneous structures as to make interpretation of individual anatomic systems impossible. The result has been a poor understanding of orbital anatomy, not only among ophthalmologists, but also among neurosurgeons and otolaryngologists who frequently pursue lesions into the orbit.

During the past decade there has been a renewed interest in clinical eyelid and orbital anatomy. Detailed dissections and reinterpretations have markedly altered our concepts of functional morphology of such structures as Whitnall's ligament, the medial canthal tendon, orbital fascial septa, the lower eyelid retractors, and the levator aponeurosis. This has resulted in the development of new surgical procedures based on such concepts, and the resurrection and successful modification of older, long abandoned operations. With the growing appreciation of anatomical and functional relationships, older, non-physiologic procedures are slowly giving way to those directed at the site of pathology, and aimed at the restoration of normal anatomic structure and physiology. Without an intimate knowledge of the anatomy of these regions, the modern surgeon dealing with orbital and eyelid disorders can no longer function adequately. Nor can progress occur in the evolution of newer and even more physiologically appropriate therapeutic techniques.

Of all the subjects in medicine, the study of anatomy is perhaps the most visual. Few of us can easily commit to memory the numerous and frequently antiquated names given to anatomic structures. Even more confusing are the spatial relationships of different anatomic systems and their common variants. Often we rely on simple images, mental drawings that depict key landmarks in familiar juxtapositions that can be recalled during clinical evaluations or surgical operations. Most of us have divined various tricks to visually reconstruct complex anatomic detail from two-dimensional artistic renderings, or from confusing cadaver dissections. It is this very process of conjuring up prepackaged eidetic images that led to the concept of the present book.

The illustrations presented in the following pages combine the best features of several different techniques. Anatomic details and relationships are based on several human orbits cut into 300 histologic sections at 150 microns thickness. For each anatomic system (e.g. bones, arteries, nerves, etc.) each section was projected to 3X magnification and traced onto a transparent mylar sheet. Accurate registration was assured through the use of precut feduciary markings within the blocks, and adjustments for differential shrinkage and warpage were made visually. The mylar sheets were then stacked in layered fashion and the resulting three-dimensional reconstructed images were used to prepare the final illustrations. Translation into various orientations was performed visually from these base views, and from measurements calculated from the original histologic series. These techniques allowed us to image each anatomic system in isolation, or in combination with other structures by overlay of the appropriate Mylar transparencies. We have attempted to choose some views and angles not typical in some other atlases of orbital anatomy, but which we feel will enhance the visual concepts. Where possible, instead of cutting and reflecting structures to show deeper layers, we have kept structures intact, making them transparent to more accurately demonstrate relationships of features behind them. The result is a series of illustrations that create in the reader's mind a series of visual patterns that can more easily be recalled.

Each chapter focuses on a different anatomic system, such as extraocular muscles, arteries, or orbital nerves. In a series of reconstructions we sequentially add and silhouette adjacent structures to illustrate them in their proper three-dimensional perspective. Each chapter begins with a coronal view of the orbit as seen when facing the human head. The anatomic system of interest is pictured first in isolation to show its essential features. Additional systems are then added, beginning with the extraocular muscles, to demonstrate anatomic relationships. Finally the orbital bones are added. This series of images are then repeated in the lateral and superior aspects. Such transformations help translate morphological relationships into more familar surgical views. Other images at unique orientations and magnifications are used where necessary to illustrate specific anatomic detail.

This book is intended as a visual atlas. The text presents introductory material, embryology, discussions of variability, explanations of concepts, and descriptions of structures and functions that are difficult to display in pictures alone. The text also describes anatomic details in a logical sequence that follows regional, functional, or morphologic criteria that will help the reader create meaningful mental images. Since our goal is clinical anatomy, wherever possible, clinically relevant correlations are included to relate normal anatomic structure to pathologic states or to surgical procedures.

For each chapter we include a collection of full-color illustrations with appropriate labels. Because of the exquisite detail in the original histologic sections, we include as a separate chapter a series of photomicrographs illustrating the histologic cross-sectional anatomy of the orbit. Following a series of coronal sections through the orbit, we illustrate of each anatomic system or structure at appropriate magnification. In the final chapter we include a series of computerized tomographic scans and magnetic resonance images. These are figured in both the coronal and axial orientations, along with corresponding reconstructions for anatomic correlation.

For those students of orbital anatomy interested in details of structure, functional morphology, and clinical correlations, we suggest a careful reading of the text in conjunction with a systematic sequential review of the illustrations. For those more familiar with orbital anatomy who may wish only to review certain anatomic systems or structures for teaching or in preparation for surgery, the illustrations may be used independent of the text. While we do not intend reference citations to be encyclopedic, we do include sources for new findings or controversial interpretations.

It is sincerely hoped that this volume will enhance the teaching of orbital anatomy for the clinician, and serve as a stimulus for further investigation of anatomic and functional relationships which are so essential for progress. This volume should prove valuable for the resident and practicing physician in ophthalmology, otolaryngology, plastic surgery, neurosurgery, dermatology, neuroradiology and all others who diagnose and treat diseases of the eyelids and orbit.

Jonathan J. Dutton and Thomas G. Waldrop

Preface to the Second Edition

In 1994, we published the first edition of this book. Gratifyingly, this book was well received, and won awards for the best medical illustrations for 1994, as well as recognition as one of the 100 most important books published in ophthalmology in the 20th century (Thompson HS, Blanchard DL. Arch Ophthalmol 2001; 119:761-763). Our goal at that time was to produce a visual atlas of orbital and eyelid anatomy, describing anatomic details in a logical sequence following regional, functional, or morphologic criteria. These mental or eidetic images would help the reader create meaningful mental pictures that can be recalled from memory, like reading the pages of an open book. Since our goal was clinical anatomy, we included some clinically relevant correlations related to normal anatomic structures, and to some pathologic conditions.

Anatomy of relatively well-known regions of the body tends to be rather stable, with few significant changes in knowledge, at least with respect to major structures. However, during the 16 years since publication of the first edition, a great deal of new information has been added to the medical literature, especially as regards eyelid anatomy, the orbital fascial connective tissue structures, and extraocular muscle pulley systems. Some refinements also have been made to our understanding of other anatomic systems, including the vascular, neural, and muscular systems. All of these

findings have been updated in the current edition. We have added a section on facial anatomy to the Eyelid Anatomy chapter that is relevant to facial and SOOF lift procedures. Also, we added a new chapter on the cavernous sinus, since many orbital structures and pathologic conditions involving the orbital apex also involve the cavernous sinus and middle cranial fossa, so that knowledge of anatomic continuity between these structures is important. References have been updated throughout, and a number of new or modified illustrations have been added to several chapters based on recent anatomic findings. We also added new subheadings to most chapters, in order to more clearly delineate specific areas of information. We expanded sections on clinical correlations in all chapters, to better relate disease processes with anatomic structures.

As we stated in the first edition, for those students of orbital anatomy interested in details of structure, functional morphology, and clinical correlations, we suggest a careful reading of the text in conjunction with a systematic sequential review of the illustrations. For those more familiar with orbital anatomy who may wish only to review certain anatomic systems or structures, the illustrations can be used independent of the text.

Jonathan J. Dutton and Thomas G. Waldrop

Contents

CHAPTER 1

Cavernous Sinus

The cavernous sinus (CS) is a very important intracranial, extradural anatomic region that contains many structures vital for visual function. Numerous disease processes along the skull base and in the cavernous sinus can have a major impact on vision or on ocular motility. Yet, this anatomic structure remains quite unfamiliar to most ophthalmologists and orbital surgeons. It serves as a critical venous drainage route for both the orbit and the cranial base.[16] It also transmits arterial and neural structures from the intracranial compartment into the orbital apex.

The term cavernous sinus has been in use for 275 years, ever since Jacobus Winslow proposed it in 1734, reflecting his concept of a single trabeculated venous cavern similar to the corpus cavernosus of the penis.[42] His concept was incorrect, yet the term has persisted in the medical literature. It is clear from modern studies that the CS is neither cavernous nor is it an intradural sinus, but rather it is a plexus or network of extremely thin-walled veins associated with adipose tissue. Parkinson[27] emphasized the inappropriateness of this term on anatomical grounds. Hashimoto[12] recommended following Parkinson's lead in using the term "lateral sellar compartment" (LSC)[26] for this structure in its broader sense, and restricting the term "cavernous sinus" to the more limited venous pathways within the LSC. In 2003, Tobenas-Dujardin et al.[38] proposed the term "inter-periosto-dural space" which they believed would better reflect the real anatomic pattern. However, this has not gained widespread usage. While the term lateral sellar compartment might be anatomically more accurate, the term cavernous sinus remains in widespread use, especially outside the specialty of neurosurgery. Furthermore, the International Federation of Associations of Anatomists (IFAA) did not adopt an alternative terminology for the cavernous sinus in its most recent edition of Terminologia Anatomica 1998.[37] Therefore, for the present chapter we will use the classic terminology, using the term cavernous sinus for both the neural and venous components.

Embryology

The early development of the cavernous sinus is complex. Our current understanding is based on the seminal studies of Padget[23] as well as more recent works.[9,18] By the 3 mm (28-day) embryonic stage two longitudinal venous channels, the anterior cardinal veins, are laid down and extend along the ventrolateral surface of the developing brain, on the medial side of the cranial nerve roots. Three pairs of venous channels develop from these to form the superior cerebral, middle cerebral, and inferior cerebral veins. Most of each cardinal vein atrophies, except for a segment of each vein in the region of the trigeminal ganglion which becomes the forerunner of the cavernous sinus, and another segment more posteriorly which becomes the internal jugular vein.

By the 8 mm (36-day) embryonic stage the primitive supraorbital vein arises in the superficial tissues dorsal to the developing eye. It initially drains backward between the trigeminal and trochlear nerves into an anterior dural plexus, which will become the superior sagittal and transverse sinuses. A new anastomosis appears from the supraorbital vein that diverts blood over the incipient annulus of Zinn into the venous plexus of the future cavernous sinus. By the 11 mm (40-day) stage the initial formation of the chondrocranium is seen around the anterior notochord, surrounded by primitive mesenchyme. At the 14.5 mm (44-day) stage chondrification begins in the future greater and lesser wings of the sphenoid bone and in the dorsum sellae.[38] At the same time the trigeminal (gasserian) ganglion forms, along with its three major peripheral divisions. In the 23–25 mm (50-day) embryo the hypophysis and diaphragma sellae become differentiated in the region of the developing cavernous sinus. The lateral wall of the cavernous sinus is partially developed as a meningeal layer enclosing several cranial nerves, but the medial wall is not yet formed. By the 31 mm (56-day) embryo a well developed cavernous sinus with a definitive cavernous carotid artery and sympathetic plexus is present, containing two venous compartments, one on each side of the midline. Cranial nerves III, IV, VI, and the three branches of the trigeminal nerve are all differentiated and located in their approximate adult relationships.

In the 70–90 mm (13–15-week) fetal stage small ossification centers are seen in the body, greater wings, and lesser wings of the sphenoid bone. At the same time ossification is beginning in the cartilaginous petrous portion of the temporal bone.[12] The primordium of the dura mater and subarachnoid membrane are already seen lining the area of the cavernous sinus on either side of the body of the sphenoid. The pituitary gland is lined by an inner capsule and an outer meningeal layer, forming the definitive medial wall of the cavernous sinus. Many small irregularly shaped lumens develop within the mesenchyme of the cavernous sinus region, and these venous channels gradually enlarge with further fetal development. These channels meander and intertwine, and are lined only by an endothelial layer with no smooth muscle. These venous channels communicate with other venous channels. Posteriorly they drain to the basilar venous sinus and then to the jugular bulb; posteroinferiorly with the inferior petrosal sinus and then into the pterygoid venous plexus through the foramen lacerum; and posterosuperiorly with the superior petrosal sinus and then into the sigmoid sinus. The cavernous sinuses on each side communicate with each other through one or more intercavernous sinuses situated between the dural layers, below the pituitary gland.

The gasserian ganglion is situated posterior to the developing cavernous sinus on either side, over the tip of the petrous bone and lateral to the dorsum sellae. The three branches of the trigeminal nerve run forward from the gasserian ganglion. The ophthalmic branch (V1) and the maxillary branch (V2) run anteriorly in the lateral wall of the cavernous sinus, within the loose inner connective tissue endosteal layer. The oculomotor (III) and trochlear (IV) nerves enter the cavernous sinus near the posterior clinoid process and also run anteriorly within the lateral wall to the superior orbital fissure. The abducens nerve (VI) runs through the basilar venous plexus and then enters the cavernous sinus; it courses forward within the venous channels of the sinus just lateral to the internal carotid artery, and passes into the superior orbital fissure. Third order sympathetic nerve fibers enter the cranium through the foramen lacerum and become associated with these cranial nerves and vascular elements. The internal carotid artery (ICA) enters the skull base through the future carotid canal. It then penetrates the floor of the cavernous sinus inferolateral to the cartilaginous sphenoid bone. As the sella turcica develops, the ICA gradually assumes the S-shaped configuration seen in the adult.

During the 128–183 mm (18–23-week) stage of fetal development further ossification occurs in the sphenoid bone as it expands in the anterolateral directions. By the 230 mm (28-week) fetal stage a thick periosteum is seen over the surface of sphenoid bone. Dura is distinguishable along the lateral wall of the cavernous sinus as a definite meningeal layer separate from the overlying arachnoid membrane and the inner endosteal layer that is continuous with the periosteum of the sphenoid bone. Superiorly the meningeal layer folds to contribute to the diaphragma sellae over the pituitary gland. Within the mesenchyme of the cavernous sinus large well-defined venous lumens are now present. The mesenchymal tissue between lumens gradually thins to become membranes separating the individual vascular channels. Small arteries and autonomic nerve fascicles are now apparent within these membranous walls.

In the 150–200 mm (21–25-week) fetal stage, blood flow through the cavernous sinus rapidly increases, probably due to alterations in neighboring venous pathways. Nerve fascicles become surrounded by collagen fibers forming sheaths.

Simultaneous with formation of the cavernous sinus is development of the pituitary gland, which forms an important element adjacent to and above the bilateral cavernous sinuses. During the 2–3 mm (21-day) embryonic stage the gland originates from two distinct ectodermal tissues. A finger-like protrusion, called Rathke's pouch, grows upward as a dorsal evagination from the stomodeum, or mouth, just anterior to the bucco-pharyngeal membrane. It differentiates into glandular epithelium characteristic of endocrine glands. The infundibulum is a ventral evagination from the floor of the third ventricle of the diencephalon just caudal to the developing optic chiasm from the same tissue.[1] It differentiates into the exocrine component of the pituitary gland. During the

second month of embryonic development, Rathke's pouch wraps around the infundibulum, and differentiates into the anterior lobe, or adenohypophysis, of the pituitary gland. The infundibulum differentiates into the pituitary stalk and the posterior lobe, or neurohypophysis, of the gland. Ultimately, the two portions grow together to form the definitive pituitary gland. As the cavernous sinus continues to develop, the enclosing dural and endosteal sheaths conform to the body of the pituitary gland to form the medial walls of the sinus, as well as the roof and the diaphragma sellae that separates the gland from the optic chiasm.

Anatomy of the adult cavernous sinus

The cavernous sinus is a paired structure located near the center of the head on either side of the sella turcica and pituitary gland, and posterior to the sphenoid sinus. It is defined as the space between the superior orbital fissure anteriorly, the posterior petroclinoid fold and clivus dura mater posteriorly, and the inner surface of the middle cranial fossa inferolaterally, where the meningeal and periosteal layers of the dura meet and fuse.[12] It measures 8 to 10 mm in antero-posterior length, and 5 to 7 mm in height.[17] The lateral wall of the sinus is more complex, composed of a superficial (outer) meningeal layer of dura, and a deeper (inner) layer containing several cranial nerves. The cavernous sinus is therefore surrounded by this dural envelope, and contains a venous plexus, a short segment of the internal carotid artery, and the abducens nerve (VI). The venous plexus is fed by veins draining from the face, orbit, nasopharynx, cerebrum, cerebellum, and brainstem. It empties into the basilar venous system as well as into the petrosal venous sinuses. Within the lateral wall of the cavernous sinus run the oculomotor (III) and trochlear (IV) nerves, and the first two divisions (V1 and V2) of the trigeminal nerve. These latter structures, therefore, are not technically within the cavernous sinus, but are only associated with its lateral wall.

The bony boundaries of the cavernous sinus

The cavernous sinus lies within the middle cranial base. The latter is bounded anteriorly and laterally by the greater wing of the sphenoid bone, and posteriorly by the clivus and the anterior aspect of the petrous temporal bone. The body of the sphenoid bone makes up the floor of the middle cranial fossa and contains the sella turcica, situated between the anterior and posterior clinoid processes. The sella turcica consists of the tuberculum sellae anteriorly between the cranial openings of the optic canal. Behind it is the pituitary fossa, and the posterior extent of the sella is bounded by the dorsum sellae.

The cavernous sinus lies lateral to the body of the sphenoid bone, and over the top of the petrous apex of the temporal bone. The posterior portion of the sinus rests against the lateral edge of the dorsum sellae, and its anterior portion extends to the superior orbital fissure beneath the anterior clinoid process and the lesser wing of the sphenoid. Laterally the sinus extends to the junction of the sphenoid body and the greater wing, but does not include the foramen rotundum, foramen ovale, and the foramen spinosum. The latter three foramina are located just lateral to the lateral wall of the cavernous sinus. Inferiorly, the sinus extends to the lower border of the carotid sulcus, a groove along the lateral aspect of the sphenoid body in which lies the intracavernous portion of the internal carotid artery.

Lateral to the anterior clinoid process and extending superolaterally beneath the lesser sphenoid wing is the superior orbital fissure (SOF) which marks the anterior most extent of the cavernous sinus. It opens into the orbital apex, and transmits cranial nerves III, IV, VI, and branches of the ophthalmic division of the trigeminal nerve (V1). Just posterior and slightly inferior to the SOF, in the floor of the middle cranial fossa, is the foramen rotundum, lateral to the sphenoid sinus. It lies lateral to the cavernous sinus and transmits the maxillary division (V2) of the trigeminal nerve into the pterygopalatine fossa. The foramen ovale lies about 1 cm posterior and lateral to the foramen rotundum and carries the mandibular branch (V3) of the trigeminal nerve into the infratemporal fossa. The foramen lacerum is an irregular opening posteromedial to the f. ovale and transmits the internal jugular vein as it exits the cranium. In the petrous apex, near its junction with the sphenoid and occipital bones, lies the carotid canal which continues anteromedially to open into the f. lacerum.

Anteriorly, the anterior clinoid process is a rounded projection extending from the lesser wing of the sphenoid bone. It extends above the anterior roof of the cavernous sinus, and forms the lateral wall of the optic canal. Inferomedially, the lesser sphenoid wing and clinoid process are joined by the optic strut to the body of the sphenoid bone. The strut separates the optic canal from the superior orbital fissure. It also forms the floor of the optic canal and the anterior roof of the cavernous sinus. The posterior face of the optic strut has a depression to accommodate the anterior bend of the intracavernous carotid artery beneath the anterior clinoid process.

The dural folds

The cavernous sinus has four walls that mark its boundaries and delimit its anatomic extent. Dural folds help define boundaries of the cavernous sinus and provide important landmarks for surgery in this anatomic location. Anteriorly, dural structures extend from the upper and lower portions of the anterior clinoid process and surround the internal carotid artery, forming upper and lower rings in the region where the artery forms a sharp anterior bend. The segment of the carotid artery that lies between the upper and lower dural rings is the clinoid portion and lies within the anteriormost portion of the cavernous sinus. The floor of the sinus is composed of endosteum (periosteum) which also covers the body of the sphenoid bone, and is continuous with periosteum of the middle cranial fossa.

The medial wall of the sinus is divided into a lower sphenoidal portion and an upper sellar portion. The lower sphenoidal part of the medial wall overlies the body of the sphenoid bone and a horizontal groove for the carotid artery, the carotid sulcus. It is covered by endosteum continuous with periosteum of the floor of the middle cranial fossa. The bone separating the sphenoid sinus from the cavernous sinus is very thin in this region, less than 0.5 mm in most individuals,[17] and may even have spontaneous dehiscences so that the sphenoid sinus may be separated from the cavernous sinus only by layers of endosteum and sinus mucosa. The upper sellar portion of the medial wall is lined

by a meningeal layer continuous with the diaphragma sellae above. Controversy exists as to the existence of the endosteal layer in this region. Songtao et al.[34] recently reported a distinct inner layer (lamina propria), between the dural layer and the pituitary gland, that also contributed to the medial wall in two-thirds of specimens studied.

The roof of the cavernous sinus is formed by dural folds extending from the petrous apex to the anterior clinoid process (anterior petroclinoid ligament), from the petrous apex to the posterior clinoid process (posterior petroclinoid ligament), and between the anterior and posterior clinoid processes (interclinoid ligament). The diaphragma sellae completes the roof. The latter is composed of two layers, an outer superficial meningeal layer, and a deep layer of endosteum.[4] These layers form the dura, and are continuous anteriorly with dura that covers the planum sphenoidale over the body of the sphenoid bone, and posteriorly with the dura that covers the dorsum sellae and clivus. The meningeal layer is also continuous with the outer lateral wall of the cavernous sinus, the upper dural ring of the carotid artery, and the optic sheath. [6,15,35,39,41] The endosteal layer is continuous with the inner lateral wall of the cavernous sinus, the periosteum of the middle cranial fossa, the lower dural ring of the carotid artery, and periorbita of the orbital cavity. The junction of the superior and medial walls of the cavernous forms the medial edge of the diaphragma over the pituitary gland. In the center of the diaphragma sellae is an opening through which the pituitary stalk passes. The size of this opening varies from <4 mm to >8 mm, and Campero et al.[4] proposed the resulting differences in resistance could play a role in determining the direction of growth of pituitary adenomas.

The lateral wall of the cavernous sinus is the most complex. Posteriorly it forms the medial edge of Meckel's cave along the petrous apex, and extends anteriorly to the lateral edge of the superior orbital fissure. The vertical extent of the lateral wall is from the petroclinoid dural fold superiorly to the carotid sulcus inferiorly along the body of the sphenoid bone.[5] The lateral wall is bounded by a multilayered membrane consisting of several inner endosteal layers that are continuous with the endosteum of the sinus floor where it adheres to the sphenoid bone, and an outer meningeal layer that also covers the medial side of the temporal lobe of the brain.[43,44] From superior to inferior, cranial nerves III, IV, V1 and V2 lie within the inner endosteal layers of the lateral wall. These nerves, therefore, are anatomically separated from the venous channels that form the vascular component of the cavernous sinus. Marinkovic et al.[19] reported the inner layers of the lateral wall to consist of three layers of endosteum in the human fetus; an outer layer of dense connective tissue containing the trochlear nerve (IV), and a middle layer containing loose connective tissue in which runs the oculomotor nerve (III), as well as the ophthalmic (V1) and maxillary (V2) divisions of the trigeminal nerve. They reported an inner layer of endosteum running in the venous channels containing the abducens nerve (VI). Umansky et al.[40,41] found that in the adult the oculomotor, trochlear, and trigeminal nerves were included within a single irregular deep lateral wall layer. This possibly represents the fused second and third layers of Marinkovic et al.[19]

The broad posterior dural wall of the cavernous sinus extends from the posterior clinoid process and upper clivus medially, to the petrous apex laterally along the upper edge of the petroclival fissure. The upper edge of the posterior wall extends to the posterior petroclinoid dural fold, which passes from the petrous apex to the posterior clinoid process. The lateral edge of the posterior wall is situated just medial to the opening of Meckel's cave, which contains the trigeminal nerve and ganglion. Just lateral to the dorsum sellae, the posterior cavernous sinus opens into the basilar sinus, and communicates with the superior and inferior petrosal sinuses.

The intercavernous sinuses that connect the cavernous sinuses on each side pass between the dural and endosteal layers along the floor of the sella turcica, between the pituitary gland and the body of the sphenoid bone.

Nerves of the cavernous sinus

Five cranial nerves or branches pass through the cavernous sinus or travel in its walls *en route* from their origin in the brain stem to their orbital and extraorbital targets. The oculomotor, trochlear, and the first two divisions of the trigeminal nerve lie in the lateral wall of the sinus between the superficial dural and deep reticular endosteal layers. The abducens nerve runs within the sinus in a reticular layer that may be separate or part of that investing the ICA. In addition, a plexus of sympathetic nerve fibers accompanies the carotid artery and several nerve branches along their course through the sinus.[13]

The oculomotor nerve

The oculomotor nerve (III) exits the brain and runs in the interpeduncular fossa between the superior cerebellar and posterior cerebral arteries. It pierces the roof of the cavernous sinus posteriorly through the center of the oculomotor trigone, lateral to the posterior clinoid process. As it penetrates the lateral portion of the posterior petroclinoid ligament it acquires its own dural sheath. The nerve continues anteriorly within the deep endosteal layer of the lateral sinus wall. The oculomotor nerve continues forward, passes beneath the base of the anterior clinoid process, and branches into its superior and inferior divisions just before passing through the superior orbital fissure into the orbital apex. As it runs through the SOF, the oculomotor nerve is covered by a perineurium and a thin connective tissue sheath that blends with the superolateral margin of the annulus of Zinn. The nerve carries motor fibers to the superior rectus and levator palpebrae superioris muscles (superior division), and to the medial and inferior rectus muscles, and the inferior oblique muscles (inferior division). It also carries preganglionic parasympathetic visceral efferent fibers to the ciliary ganglion (see Chapter 4).

The trochlear nerve

The trochlear nerve (IV) exits the dorsal surface of the midbrain just below the inferior colliculus in the cerebellomesencephalic fissure. It curves anteriorly in the ambient cistern around the lateral aspect of the tectum and tegmentum, and proceeds in an anterolateral and slightly inferior direction to penetrate the tentorium. The nerve runs forward following the edge of the anterior petroclinoid ligament and pierces the lower part of the posterior wall of the cavernous sinus posterolateral to the oculomotor nerve. The trochlear nerve courses just inferior to the third nerve within the endosteal layer of the lateral sinus wall. As it passes beneath

the anterior clinoid process, the trochlear nerve moves upward along the lateral surface of the oculomotor nerve and crosses over it to enter the orbit through the superior orbital fissure above the annulus of Zinn. It continues medially in the superior orbit to provide motor innervation to the superior oblique muscle.

The abducens nerve

The abducens nerve (VI) leaves the pontomedullary sulcus and courses anterosuperiorly in the prepontine cistern. It pierces dura overlying the basilar venous plexus on the clivus and enters a dural channel called Dorello's canal. The nerve continues superiorly and medially over the clivus and passes beneath the posterior petroclinoid ligament where it enters the posterior cavernous sinus. It then passes around the lateral side of the intracavernous carotid artery, within the endosteal layer that surrounds it. As the abducens nerve passes forward it is joined by sympathetic fibers from the carotid autonomic plexus.[29] It then continues forward between and medial to the oculomotor and ophthalmic nerves (V1). Anteriorly, the abducens nerve gradually assumes a more inferior position relative to the ophthalmic nerve, so that as it enters the superior orbital fissure it lies medial and inferior to V1. Near the SOF the abducens nerve divides into as many as five separate rootlets.[11] These pass through the annulus of Zinn to provide motor innervation to the lateral rectus muscle.

The trigeminal nerve

The trigeminal nerve (V) is the largest cranial nerve, and arises from the lateral pons. It is a mixed nerve providing sensory innervation, proprioceptive, and nociceptive information from the head and face, as well as motor function to the muscles of mastication. A small motor and larger sensory root run anterolaterally, superior to the petrous apex. These roots enter a subarachnoid and dural outpouching known as Meckel's cave located in a small depression on the apex of the petrous portion of the temporal bone, just at the posterior edge of the cavernous sinus. The sensory nerve fascicles are joined by preganglionic parasympathetic fibers from the greater superficial petrosal nerve, and gradually coalesce to form the gasserian ganglion. The motor root passes beneath the ganglion and exits the cranium through the foramen ovale where it immediately joins the mandibular branch of the trigeminal nerve (V3) *en route* to muscles of mastication. The gasserian ganglion also receives sympathetic filaments from the carotid plexus, and gives off sensory fibers to the tentorium and dura of the middle cranial fossa.

Three nerve trunks emerge anteriorly from the gasserian ganglion; the ophthalmic, maxillary, and mandibular nerves, each exiting the cranium via a separate foramen or fissure. The ophthalmic nerve (V1, or first division of the trigeminal nerve) is the smallest of the three trunks and contains only sensory fibers. It carries sensory innervation from the cornea, ciliary body and iris, the lacrimal gland, the conjunctiva, and from the skin of the upper eyelid, forehead, scalp and nose. Tracing this branch forward, it arises from the upper part of the gasserian ganglion as a short flattened band. It enters the cavernous sinus posteriorly where it passes forward within the deep endosteal layer of the lateral cavernous sinus wall, below the oculomotor and abducens nerves. Near the anterior end of the cavernous sinus the ophthalmic nerve gives off a small recurrent branch which passes between the layers of the tentorium. The main trunk then divides into three branches, the frontal, lacrimal, and nasociliary nerves that pass into the orbit through the superior orbital fissure. The nasociliary nerve enters the orbit through the oculomotor foramen of the annulus of Zinn, into the intraconal compartment between the superior and inferior branches of the oculomotor nerve (see Chapter 4). The frontal and lacrimal nerves enter the orbit above the annulus into the superior extraconal orbital space. Occasionally the lacrimal nerve is absent, and sensory fibers reach the lacrimal gland and superolateral eyelid via the zygomaticotemporal branch of the maxillary nerve (V2). Sympathetic fibers from the cavernous plexus accompany the ophthalmic nerve into the orbital apex.

The maxillary nerve (V2) carries sensory information from the lower eyelid and cheek, the upper lip, the gums above the incisor and canine teeth, the nasal mucosa, palate and roof of the pharynx, and from the maxillary, ethmoid, and sphenoid sinuses. Tracing it forward, it arises from the central portion of the gasserian ganglion and enters the cavernous sinus where it runs for a short distance within the lateral wall. It exits the inferior sinus and penetrates the floor of the middle cranial fossa through the foramen rotundum, which is situated on a line between the superior orbital fissure and the foramen ovale. The nerve then crosses the pterygopalatine fossa, passes over the back of the maxillary bone, and enters the orbit though the inferior orbital fissure to become the infraorbital nerve. The maxillary nerve gives off a number of branches. The middle meningeal nerve is given off immediately after the maxillary nerve leaves the gasserian ganglion; it accompanies the middle meningeal artery and supplies the dura mater of the middle cranial fossa. Within the pterygopalatine fossa the maxillary nerve gives off two sphenopalatine branches that course to the sphenopalatine ganglion. The latter is a sympathetic ganglion receiving sensory, motor and sympathetic fibers distributed to the region of the pharynx, palate, and mouth. The alveolar branches emerge just before the maxillary nerve enters the inferior orbital fissure. They supply the upper gums and adjacent portions of the oral mucosa, nasal mucosa, and the maxillary sinus, and communicate with the alveolar nerves to supply the upper teeth.

The mandibular nerve (V3) does not pass through the cavernous sinus but exits the cranium lateral to the sinus through the foramen ovale. It carries sensory information from the lower lip, the lower gums and teeth, the chin and jaw, and parts of the external ear. The motor branches of the trigeminal nerve are distributed in the mandibular nerve and innervate the masseter, temporalis, medial and lateral pterygoid muscles, as well as the tensor veli palatini, mylohyoid, anterior belly of the digastric, and tensor tympani muscles.

Numerous small sympathetic nerve fibers surrounding the ICA coalesce within the cavernous sinus into discreet fiber bundles. These leave the ICA and join the abducens nerve for a few millimeters before crossing over to the ophthalmic nerve. They accompany the ophthalmic nerve into the orbit (see Chapter 4).

Internal carotid artery and its branches

The internal carotid artery (ICA) is the only artery in the body that travels completely through a venous structure. It runs a complex course from the bifurcation of the common carotid artery in the neck, into the cranium, and then takes a serpinginous path through the cranial base and cavernous sinus before terminating at the anterior and middle cerebral arteries. In 1938, Fischer[7] published a seminal paper in which he described five segments of the carotid artery based on its angiographic course and its displacement by various intracranial anomalies. While this nomenclature became widely used, it did not relate the segments of the ICA to specific anatomic compartments and it numbered the segments in the opposite direction of blood flow. In recent decades, many attempts have been made to correct these inaccuracies, but they often introduced unnecessary complexity. In 1996, Bouthillier et al.[3] proposed a classification that described segments of the ICA with a numerical scale following the direction of blood flow, and identified segments according to surrounding anatomy and the compartments through which the artery travels. These segments were as follows: cervical, petrous, lacerum-cavernous, clinoid, ophthalmic, and communicating segments. More recently, Ziyal et al.[46] proposed a more simplified classification by omitting the lacerum segment and combining the ophthalmic and communicating segments. While a final classification system is still a matter of debate, for the present chapter we have chosen to use a more simplified modified anatomic description.

The cervical segment (C1) of the ICA begins at the common carotid artery bifurcation in the neck. It runs superiorly within the carotid sheath, in company with the internal jugular vein, the vagus nerve, a venous plexus, and sympathetic nerves. Where the ICA enters the carotid canal, this sheath divides into an inner layer that becomes periosteum of the bony canal, and an outer layer that becomes periosteum of the external cranial surface.

The petrous segment (C2) of the ICA begins at the entrance of the exocranial osteum of the carotid canal on the ventral surface of the petrous portion of the temporal bone. It ascends vertically within the periosteum of the canal for a distance of about 10 mm and then turns anteromedially as a horizontal segment for about 20 mm anterior to the cochlea. Inside the carotid canal the ICA is surrounded by a venous plexus extension from the cavernous sinus, and a network of sympathetic fibers from the cervical sympathetic trunk. The ICA may give off one or two small inconsistent branches from these initial segments. The caroticotympanic branch arises from the vertical segment and enters the tympanic cavity through a small foramen in the canal. The vidian branch (artery of the pterygoid canal) may sometimes arise from the horizontal segment and provides an anastomotic connection with the external carotid system through the pterygopalatine fossa. The petrous segment of the ICA ends at the distal (intracranial) osteum of the carotid canal as it opens into the canalicular portion of the foramen lacerum (see Chapter 2).

The lacerum segment (C3) is not recognized in all classification schemes of the ICA. When recognized, the lacerum segment begins at the cranial end of the carotid canal on the posterior side of the cannalicular portion of the foramen lacerum. The artery passes across (over) the foramen lacerum and then turns vertically along the body of the sphenoid bone just lateral to the dorsum sellae. At this point the ICA lays inferomedial to the posterior surface of the gasserian ganglion within Meckel's cave. As it ascends onto the sphenoid bone, the vessel passes beneath a connective tissue band, the petrolingual ligament. This is an extension of periosteum bridging between the petrous apex posteriorly and the lingual process of the sphenoid bone at the anterior edge of the foramen lacerum. The transition between the lacerum and cavernous segments occurs at the upper end of this ligament. As with other segments of the ICA, the artery is accompanied by a venous plexus and sympathetic nerve fibers.

The cavernous segment (C4) of the ICA begins at the superior margin of the petroligual ligament. As it ascends onto the sphenoid body, the vessel penetrates dura to enter the posterior cavernous sinus just lateral to the posterior clonoid process. The artery makes an anterior-ward bend (the posterior bend of the ICA) and runs horizontally forward in a horizontal groove, the carotid sulcus, along the sphenoid bone. The ICA continues forward to the anterior clinoid process where it bends sharply upward as the anterior loop (anterior bend of the ICA), medial to the anterior clinoid process. Anteriorly, the two layers of the lateral cavernous sinus wall separate as they rotate into a horizontal position to envelop the anterior clinoid process and part of the anterior ICA loop. The deep fibrous layer of the lateral wall forms an incomplete dural ring around the carotid artery forming the proximal or lower ring. This marks the actual anterior roof of the cavernous sinus and the end of the cavernous segment of the ICA.

The vertical upward loop of the clinoid segment (C5) of the ICA begins at the proximal dural ring and ends a short distance above this at the distal or upper dural ring. The latter is a complete ring of dura extending from the superficial layer of the lateral wall of the cavernous sinus as it passes over the anterior clinoid process and surrounds the ICA. This upper ring is fused with the adventitia of the ICA laterally. It is continuous with the falciform ligament superiorly, with the roof of the cavernous sinus and the anterior clinoid process laterally, and with the diaphragma sellae medially.[32] The clinoid segment of the ICA between the two dural rings is not intracavernous, but a venous plexus, continuous with the anterior sinus channels, often extends through the incomplete lower dural ring and surrounds the ICA to the level of the upper ring.

Above the upper ring, the ICA becomes intradural as it enters the subarachnoid space and is situated between the anterior clinoid process laterally and the carotid sulcus of the basisphenoid bone medially, just posterior to the optic canal. The ophthalmic segment (C6) of the ICA begins at the upper dural ring and ends just before the origin of the posterior communicating artery. Two arterial branches arise from this segment, the superior hypophyseal artery and the ophthalmic artery (OA). The former supplies portions of the pituitary gland. The OA emerges from the anterior surface of the ophthalmic segment of the ICA immediately beneath the optic nerve. It runs anteriorly and slightly laterally below the optic nerve and on the upper surface of the optic strut, and then forward into the optic canal inferolateral to the nerve. As it passes through the optic canal along with the optic nerve, the ophthalmic artery pierces dura so that when it emerges at the orbital apex the artery is extradural in location, inferolateral to the optic nerve and sheath. In 10% of individuals, the ophthalmic artery may arise from the clinoid or even the cavernous segments,[31] or more rarely from the inferolateral trunk from the cavernous segment of the ICA.[46] In such cases,

the OA may enter the orbit through the superior orbital fissure instead of the optic canal.

The communicating segment (C7) of the ICA begins just before the origin of the posterior communicating artery and ends at the bifurcation into the anterior and middle cerebral arteries. In some classification schemes the ophthalmic and communicating segments are combined into a single supraclinoid segment.

Within the cavernous sinus the ICA gives origin to several arterial branches.[13] The most proximal branch is the meningohypophyseal trunk, arising lateral to the dorsum sellae close to the first bend in the ICA and just above the foramen lacerum. Although there is some variability in branching pattern,[14] this trunk usually gives rise to three further branches, the tentorial (Bernasconi Cassinari artery), inferior hypophyseal, and dorsal meningeal (or clival) arteries. In about 30% of individuals, one or another of these branches can arise directly from the ICA. These branches supply portions of the oculomotor, trochlear, and abducens nerves.[15] These vessels also supply blood to the roof of the cavernous sinus, the tentorium, the dura of the clivus, the capsule of the pituitary gland, and the floor of the sella turcica.

The inferolateral trunk (ILT) arises from the horizontal segment of the intracavernous ICA and gives rise to four branches. The tentorial branch supplies blood to the oculomotor and trochlear nerves, whereas small twigs from the ILT supply the abducens nerve. The orbital branch provides blood to the ophthalmic division of the trigeminal nerve, and to the orbital portions of cranial nerves III, IV, and VI. The maxillary branch nourishes the maxillary division of the trigeminal nerve, and the mandibular branch perfuses the mandibular division and portions of the gasserian ganglion.[19]

McConnell's capsular artery is the third, variably present branch from the ICA and supplies the capsule of the pituitary gland and walls of the sella turcica.[20] Arteriovenous fistulae may occur from rupture of the ICA or any of these intracaverous arterial branches.

Venous relationships

The cavernous sinus contains four major venous spaces,[31] with a variable amount of fatty connective tissue distributed between the channels. These serve as major venous drainage routes for the orbit and skull base. The orbital ophthalmic veins drain into the anteroinferior venous space, situated just behind the superior orbital fissure in a concavity within front of the anterior loop of the carotid artery.[11] This space extends anteriorly to the confluence of the superior and inferior ophthalmic veins just within the cavernous sinus. The posterosuperior venous space is located between the posterior half of the sinus roof and the posterior ascending part of the intracavernous carotid artery. It drains posteriorly into a confluence composed of the basilar sinus, the inferior petrosal sinus, and the superior petrosal sinus. The larger inferior petrosal sinus is the most important of these, draining blood from the cavernous sinus to the jugular bulb or to the lower sigmoid sinus. The medial venous space is situated between the carotid artery and the pituitary gland, and the very narrow lateral venous space lies between the carotid artery and the lateral wall of the cavernous sinus. The latter is often so narrow as to only accommodate the abducens (VI) nerve that runs through it. Small tributaries interconnect the lateral venous spaces with the pterygoid venous plexus via variable emissary veins that pass through foramina in the skull base (e.g. the foramen Vasalius). A venous plexus surrounds the maxillary nerve within the foramen ovale as it exits Meckel's cave and drains through the lateral space to the pterygoid plexus. The superficial middle cerebral veins also drain into the lateral venous space. A very small fifth venous space, called the clinoid space, extends upward from the anteroinferior space along the carotid artery between the lower and upper dural rings.

The cavernous sinus venous channels collect blood from the orbit via the superior and inferior ophthalmic veins. It also receives venous blood from the cerebral hemispheres via the middle and inferior cerebral veins, and from dura through tributaries of the middle meningeal veins. The cavernous sinus drains posteriorly into the basilar sinus which extends posterior to the dorsum sellae and interconnects the left and right cavernous sinuses. It also drains backward into the jugular bulb by way of the superior petrosal sinus, and into the transverse sinus via the inferior petrosal sinus. Under some circumstances, the cavernous sinus can also drain forward through the ophthalmic veins into the facial veins. In about one-third of individuals a tiny foramen Vesalius is present in the posterior part of the greater sphenoid wing, medial to the foramen ovale.[10] This opening transmits an emissary vessel, the vein of Vesalius, from the cavernous sinus to the pterygoid venous plexus. This vessel can transmit infection from the pterygoid plexus into the cavernous sinus in cases of facial cellulitis.

The cavernous sinuses on each side are commonly connected by one or more intercavernous sinuses. These connections lie within the sella turcica, anterior, posterior or beneath the pituitary gland. They are lined inferiorly by endosteum covering the sphenoid bone, and superiorly by meninges covering the pituitary gland. In some cases these channels are absent, and in others the anterior and posterior intercavernous sinuses, together with the cavernous sinuses proper, form a circular sinus around the pituitary gland.[32]

There remains some controversy as to whether the cavernous sinus is in reality a cavity of unbroken trabeculated venous caverns, or a plexus of veins that merge and divide as they pass through the cavernous sinus space.[2,24,36] However, both concepts are, in part, correct.[31] Some veins, such as the superior ophthalmic vein, maintain their integrity through part of the sinus, whereas in other areas large venous dural sinuses predominate. Here, the venous spaces are lined by a basal membrane surrounded by fibrous connective tissue, but without smooth muscle.[16]

The cavernous sinus to orbit transition

While we usually consider the orbital apex and cavernous sinus as separate anatomic entities, the anatomy of the superior orbital fissure area is important as a continuous transition zone between the two regions. Parkinson[25,27,28] considered the orbital apex, superior orbital fissure, and the cavernous sinus to be connected via a continuous venous link bridging these structures. Since that time a number of anatomic studies have reaffirmed Parkinson's concept.[21,22,35] Froelich et al.[8] proposed the term lateral sellar orbital junction (LSOJ) to define this transitional zone. However, this

has not achieved widespread usage, and here we will use the classic terms orbital apex, superior orbital fissure, and anterior cavernous sinus, since these are well entrenched in the medical literature.

The superior orbital fissure (SOF) is a bony opening between the orbital apex and the middle cranial fossa. The fissure is an apostrophe-shaped opening with a wider rounded portion inferomedially, and a narrow elongated portion superolaterally. It lies in the sphenoid bone between the body and lesser wing medially, and between the lesser and greater wings laterally. The bony fissure is divided into three anatomic regions by the annulus of Zinn.[33] The upper and lateral-most narrow portion of the fissure lies above the annulus and is lined by dura of the middle cranial fossa. This dural layer continues on the orbital side of the fissure where it blends into periorbita and fibers of the annulus of Zinn. This portion of the superior orbital fissure transmits the orbitomeningeal artery and dural veins that communicate between the middle cranial fossa and the orbital venous network. It also transmits the superior ophthalmic vein in its lower portion.[30] Neural elements passing through this segment of the SOF include the trochlear nerve, and the frontal and lacrimal branches of the ophthalmic nerve.[8] The trochlear and frontal nerves ascend as they pass through the SOF, and move medially so as to enter the orbit into the superior extraconal space. The lacrimal nerve runs just above the superior ophthalmic vein and passes above the superolateral portion of the annulus.

The inferior portion of the SOF lies beneath the annulus and is continuous inferiorly with the inferior orbital fissure (IOF), which separates the orbital apex from the pterygopalatine fossa. The inferior orbital fissure is bridged by the inferior smooth orbital muscle of Müller, and its lateral wall is covered by dura of the middle cranial fossa. This compartment transmits the inferior ophthalmic vein into the lower portion of the cavernous sinus.

The larger central portion of the SOF is situated just lateral to the sphenoid body, below the optic strut, and above the posterior maxillary strut. It is surrounded on the orbital side by the central opening of the annulus of Zinn (also known as the common annular tendon). All structures passing through this segment will enter the intraconal orbital space, and therefore mostly serve extraocular muscle or ocular functions. These structures include the superior and inferior divisions of the oculomotor nerve, the nasociliary branch of the ophthalmic nerve, and the abducens nerve. Each of these neural elements is covered by a perineurium and is wrapped in a layer of connective tissue. These fuse to the superolateral margin of the central annulus as they pass through it.

Clinical correlations: orbital apex/cavernous sinus syndromes

Lesions occurring at the cavernous sinus—orbital apex transition zone frequently result in ocular or orbital dysfunction. Symptoms are useful in defining the precise anatomic localization of such lesions, and this can be valuable for diagnosis and therapeutic planning. Several syndromes have been used to characterize the symptom complex associated with lesions in this area.[45] The term superior orbital fissure syndrome is often associated with lesions located just anterior to the orbital apex, and involves structures passing through the central annulus of Zinn, as well as those above the annulus. Symptoms involve multiple cranial nerve palsies involving the oculomotor, trochlear, and abducens nerves, as well as the ophthalmic division of the trigeminal nerve, but not the optic nerve. *Orbital apex syndrome* is associated with lesions at the apex involving both the superior orbital fissure and the optic canal. It involves dysfunctions of cranial nerves as seen in the SOF syndrome, as well as the optic nerve. More posterior lesions can produce a *cavernous sinus syndrome*, and may include features of the orbital apex syndrome, as well as Horner's syndrome, and possible involvement of the maxillary division of the trigeminal nerve. While these various syndromes differ in their exact anatomic locations, the pathologies causing them are similar. Therefore, we will follow Yeh and Foroozan[45] in applying the term orbital apex syndrome to all of these syndromes for convenience of discussion.

Orbital apex syndrome can result from diseases involving the cavernous sinus and/or the orbital apex. Typical signs and symptoms depend upon the specific anatomic structures involved, but frequently include ophthalmoplegia, trigeminal sensory loss, Horner's syndrome, proptosis, chemosis, and facial pain. Etiologies are numerous and may be infectious and non-infectious inflammatory conditions, vascular anomalies, neoplastic lesions, and trauma.

Inflammatory syndromes include Herpes zoster, Tolosa Hunt syndrome, sarcoidosis, Churg-Strauss syndrome, Wegener's granulomatosis, giant cell arteritis, and thyroid orbitopathy. Orbital pseudotumor is a non-specific idiopathic inflammatory process that may involve any orbital structure including those of the orbital apex, cavernous sinus, and optic nerve. With inflammatory lesions, the onset of symptoms is frequently more abrupt than with other causes, and often includes pain. Infectious etiologies include fungal infections such as Mucormycosis and Aspergillosis, bacterial infections, and tuberculosis. Cavernous sinus thrombophlebitis is a potentially lethal condition caused by bacterial or fungal invasion complicating sinusitis in immunocompromised patients.

Neoplastic tumors are a frequent cause of cavernous sinus and orbital apex syndromes, and may arise as primary lesions in the surrounding tissues or secondary to distant malignancies. Primary tumors include meningiomas, neurofibromas, gliomas, pituitary gland tumors, and tumors extending from parasellar regions such as nasopharyngeal malignancies, or from the orbit as with lacrimal gland tumors. Metastatic tumors to the cavernous sinus are most often from the breast, prostate, or lung, and lymphomas can involve the orbit or the cavernous sinus and adjacent sinuses.

Vascular lesions that can cause a cavernous sinus syndrome include aneurysms of the internal carotid artery or its intracavernous branches. Rupture of such an aneurysm or a vascular tear following trauma can result in a carotid-cavernous fistula. Such fistulas can be direct, where there is a direct communication between the carotid artery and the cavernous venous channels, or indirect where the communication is with small branches of the carotid artery. The former type has a higher blood flow, and presents with abrupt onset of proptosis, chemosis, ophthalmoplegia, and possibly loss of vision. The latter type tends to have slower blood flow, progresses more slowly, is associated with less severe symptoms, and may resolve spontaneously.

Localization of lesions affecting the cavernous sinus is important in the differential diagnosis of cavernous sinus syndrome. From the above anatomic discussions, it should be apparent that intracavernous neural structures can be affected differently in various parts of the sinus. Sensory deficits are frequently seen with cavernous sinus lesions. The maxillary nerve (V2) exits the sinus posteriorly, whereas the ophthalmic nerve (V1) courses through the sinus to the superior orbital fissure. A lesion in the anterior or middle sinus would be expected to affect V1 but not necessarily V2. Within the lateral sinus wall run from top to bottom the oculomotor nerve (III), the trochlear nerve (IV), and V1, and in the posterior cavernous sinus, V2. With expanding lesions from above, the motor nerves will be affected before any sensory deficit. The abducens nerve (VI) does not run in the lateral wall but within the sinus immediately lateral to the cavernous ICA. Being relatively unprotected, isolated sixth nerve palsies are seen earlier with ICA aneurysms or with other intracavernous lesions.

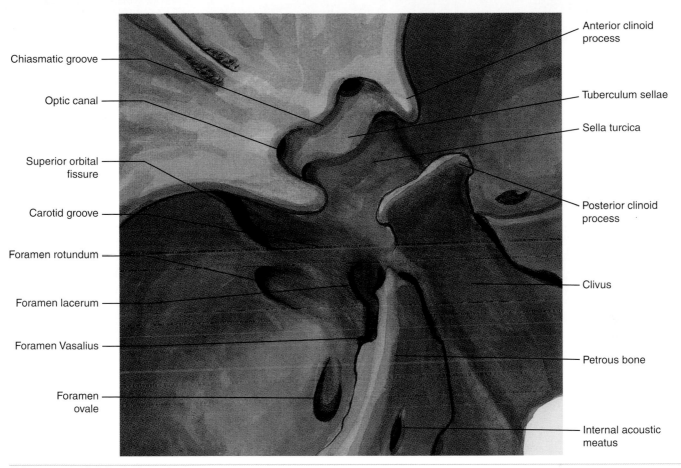

Chiasmatic groove

Optic canal

Superior orbital fissure

Carotid groove

Foramen rotundum

Foramen lacerum

Foramen Vasalius

Foramen ovale

Anterior clinoid process

Tuberculum sellae

Sella turcica

Posterior clinoid process

Clivus

Petrous bone

Internal acoustic meatus

Figure 1-1 Bony sella turcica and clinoid processes limiting the cavernous sinus.

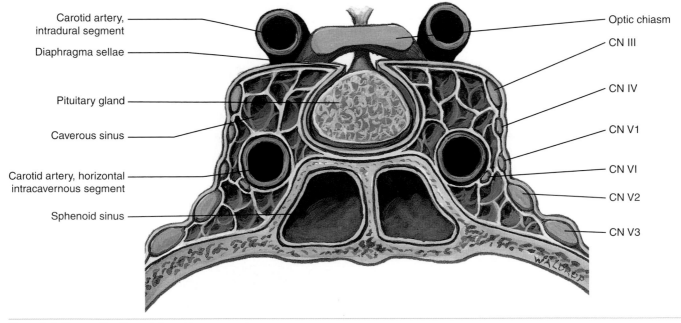

Carotid artery, intradural segment

Diaphragma sellae

Pituitary gland

Caverous sinus

Carotid artery, horizontal intracavernous segment

Sphenoid sinus

Optic chiasm

CN III

CN IV

CN V1

CN VI

CN V2

CN V3

Figure 1-2 Cross section through the mid cavernous sinus.

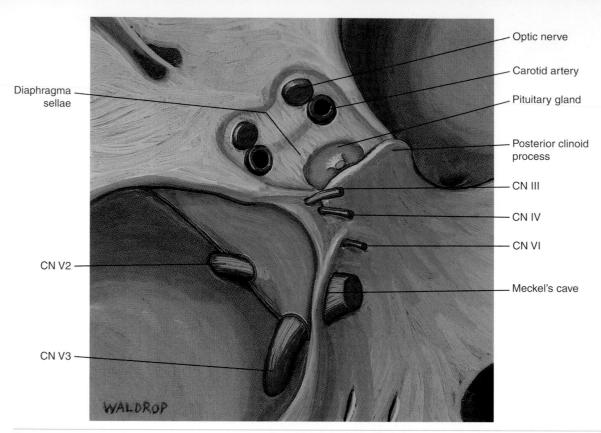

Diaphragma sellae

Optic nerve

Carotid artery

Pituitary gland

Posterior clinoid process

CN III

CN IV

CN VI

Meckel's cave

CN V2

CN V3

WALDROP

Figure 1-3 Dura mater of the cranial base and nerve roots entering the cavernous sinus.

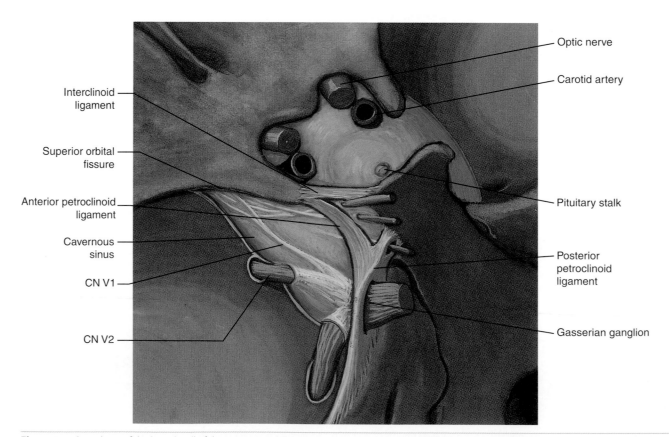

Interclinoid ligament

Superior orbital fissure

Anterior petroclinoid ligament

Cavernous sinus

CN V1

CN V2

Optic nerve

Carotid artery

Pituitary stalk

Posterior petroclinoid ligament

Gasserian ganglion

Figure 1-4 Outer layer of the lateral wall of the cavernous sinus.

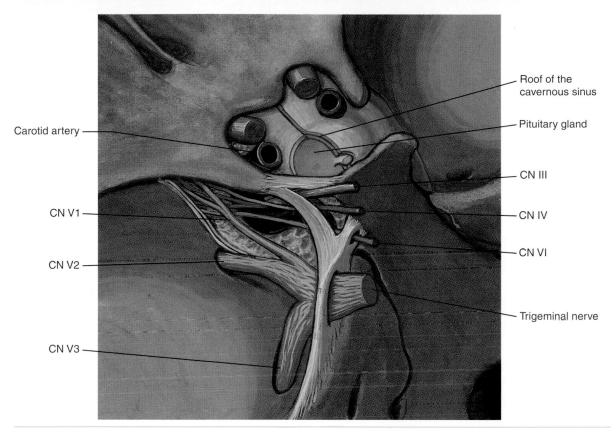

Figure 1-5 Inner layer of the lateral wall of the cavernous sinus showing cranial nerves 3, 4, and 5.

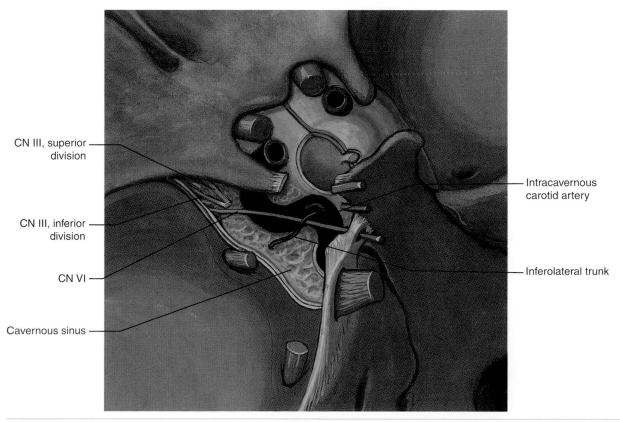

Figure 1-6 Cavernous sinus with the lateral wall removed; cranial nerves 3, 4, and 5 are cut; cranial nerve 6 and the carotid artery are shown within the sinus cavity.

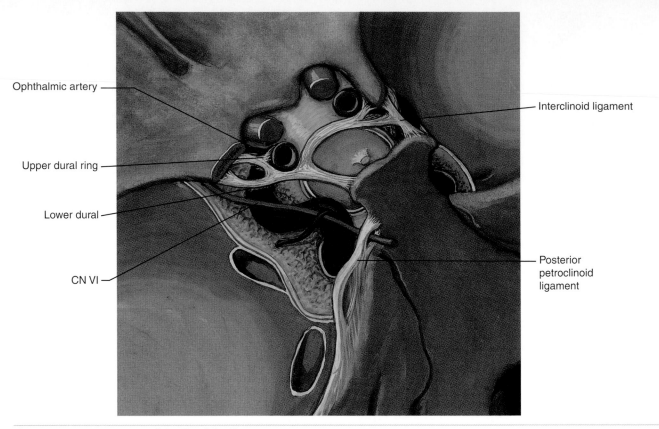

Ophthalmic artery

Upper dural ring

Lower dural

CN VI

Interclinoid ligament

Posterior petroclinoid ligament

Figure 1-7 Cavernous sinus, medial wall, and dural ligaments.

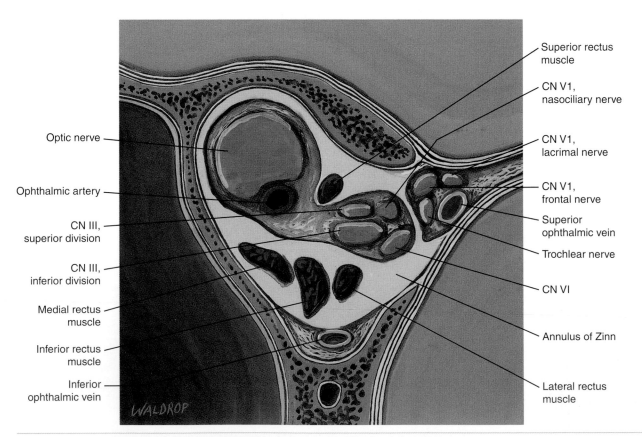

Optic nerve

Ophthalmic artery

CN III, superior division

CN III, inferior division

Medial rectus muscle

Inferior rectus muscle

Inferior ophthalmic vein

Superior rectus muscle

CN V1, nasociliary nerve

CN V1, lacrimal nerve

CN V1, frontal nerve

Superior ophthalmic vein

Trochlear nerve

CN VI

Annulus of Zinn

Lateral rectus muscle

Figure 1-8 Annulus of Zinn with major neural and vascular elements passing through to the orbital apex.

References

1. Amar AP, Weiss MH: Pituitary anatomy and physiology. *Neurosurg Clin N Am* 13:11, 2003.

2. Bedford MA: The "cavernous" sinus. *Br J Ophthalmol* 50:41, 1966.

3. Bouthillier A, van Loveren HR, Keller JT: Segments of the internal carotid artery: A new classification. *Neurosurgery* 38:425, 1996.

4. Campero A, Martins C, Yasuda, AL: Microsurgical anatomy of the diaphragma sellae and its role in directing the pattern of growth of pituitary adenomas. *Neurosurgery* 62:717, 2008.

5. Conti M, Prevedello DM, Madhok R, et al: The antero-medial triangle: The risk of cranial nerves ischemia at the cavernous sinus lateral wall. Anatomy cadaveric study. *Clin Neurol Neurosurg* 110:682, 2008.

6. Dolenc VV: *Anatomy and Surgery of the Cavernous Sinus*. Wien, Springer-Verlag, 1989, pp 3–137.

7. Fischer E: Die Lageabweichungen der vorderen hirnarterie im gefässbild. *Zentralbl Neurochir* 3:399, 1938.

8. Froelich S, Abdel KM, Aziz A, et al: The transition between the cavernous sinus and orbit. In: Dolenc VV, Rogers L (eds): *Cavernous Sinus*. New York, Springer Wien, 2009, p 27.

9. Gilmore SA: Developmental anatomy of the intracranial venous system: A review of dural venous sinus development. In: Hakuba A (ed): *Surgery of the Intracranial Venous System*. Tokyo, Springer, 1996, pp 3-13.

10. Gupta N, Ray B, Ghosh S: Anatomic characteristics of foramen vesalius. *Katmandu Univ Med J* 3:155, 2005.

11. Harris FS, Rhoton AL Jr: Anatomy of the cavernous sinus. A microscopical study. *J Neurosurg* 45:169, 1976.

12. Hashimoto M, Yokota A, Yamada H, Okudera T: Development of the cavernous sinus in the fetal period: A morphological study. *Neurol Med Chir* 40:140, 2000.

13. Inoue T, Rhoton AL Jr, Theele D, Barry ME: Surgical approaches to the cavernous sinus: A microsurgical study. *Neurosurgery* 26:903, 1990.

14. Isolan G, de Oliveira E, Mattos JP: Microsurgical anatomy of the arterial compartment of the cavernous sinus. *Arq Neuropsiquiatr* 63:259, 2005.

15. Kawase T, van Loveren H, Keller JT, Tew JM: Meningeal architecture of the cavernous sinus. Clinical and Surgical implications. *Neurosurgery* 39:527, 1996.

16. Keller JT, Leach JL, van Loveren HR, et al: Venous anatomy of the lateral sellar compartment. In: Dolenc VV, Rogers L (eds): *Cavernous sinus*. New York, Springer Wien, 2009, pp 35–52.

17. Knappe UJ, Konerding MA: Medial wall of the cavernous sinus: Microanatomcal diaphanoscopic and episcopic investigation. *Acta Neurochir* 151:961, 2009.

18. Lasjaunias P, Bernstein A, Raybaud C. Intracranial venous system. In: Lasjaunias P, Bernstein A (eds): *Functional Vascular Anatomy of the Brain, Spinal Cord and Spine*. Berlin, Springer, 1987, pp 223–266.

19. Marinkovic S, Gibo H, Vucevic R, Petrovic P: Anatomy of the cavernous sinus region. *J Clin Neurosci* 8(Suppl.):78, 2001.

20. McConnell EM: The arterial blood supply of the human hypophysis cerebri. *Anat Rec* 115:175, 1953.

21. Morard M, Tcherekayev V, de Tribolet N: The superior orbital fissure: A microanatomical study. *Neurosurgery* 35:1087, 1994.

22. Natori Y, Rhoton AL Jr: Microsurgical anatomy of the superior orbital fissure. *Neurosurgery* 36:762, 1995.

23. Padget DH: The development of the cranial venous system in man from the viewpoint of comparative anatomy. *Contrib Embryol* 247:79, 1956.

24. Parkinson D: Carotid cavernous fistula: Direct repair with preservation of the carotid artery. Technical note. *J Neurosurg* 38:99, 1973.

25. Parkinson D: Surgical anatomy of the lateral sellar compartment (cavernous sinus). *Clin Neurosurg* 36:219, 1990.

26. Parkinson D: Lateral sellar compartment. History and anatomy. *J Craniofac Surg* 5:55, 1995.

27. Parkinson D: Lateral sellar compartment O.T. (cavernous sinus): History, anatomy, terminology. *Anat Rec* 251:486, 1998.

28. Parkinson D: Extradural neural axis compartment. *J Neurosurg* 92:585, 2000.

29. Parkinson D, Johnston J, Chaudhuri A: Sympathetic connections to the fifth and sixth cranial nerves. *Anat Rec* 191:221, 1978.

30. Reymond J, Kwiatkowski J, Wysocki J: Clinical anatomy of the superior orbital fissure and the orbltal apex. *J Cranio-Maxilofac Surg* 36:346, 2008.

31. Rhoton AL, Jr: The middle cranial base and cavernous sinus. In: Dolenc VV, Rogers L (eds): *Cavernous Sinus*. New York, Springer Wien, 2009, pp 3–25.

32. Seoane E, Rhoton AL Jr, de Oliveira EP: Microsurgical anatomy of the dural collar (carotid collar) and rings around the clinoid segment of the internal carotid artery. *Neurosurgery* 42:869, 1998.

33. Shi X, Han H, Zhao J, Zhou C: Microsurgical anatomy of the superior orbital fissure. *Clin Anat* 20:362, 2007.

34. Songtao Q, Yuntao L, Jun P, et al: *Neurosurgery* 64:1, 2009.

35. Spektor S, Piontek E, Umansky F: Orbital venous drainage into the anterior cavernous sinus space: Microanatomic relationships. *Neurosurgery* 40:532, 1997.

36. Taptas JN: The so-called cavernous sinus: A review of the controversy and its implications for neurosurgeons. *Neurosurgery* 11:712, 1982.

37. Terminologia Anatomica. *Federative Committee on Anatomical Terminology*. Stuttgart, Thieme, 1998, p 292.

38. Tobenas-Dujardin AC, Dupare F, Laquerriere A, et al: Embryology of the walls of the lateral sellar compartment: Apropos of a continuous series of 39 embryos and fetuses representing the first six months of intrauterine life. *Surg Radiol Anat* 25:252, 2003.

39. Umansky F, Nathan H: The lateral wall of the cavernous sinus. With special reference to the nerves to it. *J Neurosurg* 56:228, 1982.

40. Umansky F, Valarezo A, Elidan J: The superior wall of the cavernous sinus. A microanatomical study. *J Neurosurg* 81:914, 1994.

41. Umansky F, Valarezo A, Piontek E, Spektor S: Surgical anatomy of the cavernous sinus and dural folds of the parasellar region. In: Kobayashi S, Goel A, Hongo K (eds): *Neurosurgery of Complex Tumors and Vascular Lesions*. Edinburgh, Churchill Livingstone, 1997, p 156.

42. Winslow JB: *Exposition Anatomique de la Structure du Corps Humain*. Vol. II. London, N. Prevast, 1734, p 29.

43. Yasuda A, Campero A, Martins C, et al: Microsurgical anatomy and approaches to the cavernous sinus. *Operat Neurosurg* 56:4, 2005.

44. Yasuda A, Campero A, Martins C, et al: The medial wall of the cavernous sinus: Microsurgical anatomy. *Neurosurgery* 55:179, 2004.

45. Yeh S, Foroozan R: Orbital apex syndrome. *Curr Opin Ophthalmol* 15:490, 2004.

46. Ziyal IM, Özgen T, Skhar LN, et al: Proposed classification of segments of the internal carotid artery: Anatomical study with angiographical interpretation. *Neurol Med Chir (Tokyo)* 45:184, 2005.

CHAPTER 2

Osteology of the Orbit

Embryology

The bony orbit develops from mesenchyme that encircles the optic vesicle in early embryonic development. Individual bones develop from a complex series of ossifications of two types. Endochondral bones ossify secondarily after they are preformed in cartilage. Membranous, or dermal bones, ossify directly from connective tissue without a cartilaginous precursor. The first cranial bone to appear embryologically is the maxillary bone, first recognizable at the 16 mm (6-week) embryonic stage. It is not preformed in cartilage, but arises from dermal elements as an intramembranous ossification in the region of the canine tooth. This is followed shortly by secondary ossification centers in the orbitonasal area and premaxilla.[8] The primordial maxillary sinus does not appear until the 320 mm (32-week) fetal stage. At the 30 mm (7-week) stage additional intramembranous ossifications mark the first appearance of the frontal, zygomatic, and palatine bones. As these centers enlarge, they make contact with adjacent ossifications, forming suture lines. The zygomatic and maxillary bones establish contact during the 70 mm (13-week) stage, and the zygomaticofrontal fissure is established at the 145 mm (20-week) stage. The zygomaticosphenoid fissure closes at about the time of birth.

The sphenoid bone arises from both endochondral and intramembranous ossifications. The lesser wing of the sphenoid and the optic canal begin as cartilaginous structures at the 25 mm (7-week) stage. Ossification begins at the region of the future optic strut in the 75 mm (13-week) fetus, and along the superior rim of the optic canal at the 118 mm (16-week) stage. The greater wing of the sphenoid bone is preformed in cartilage during the 52 mm (12-week) stage, and begins to ossify by the 67 mm (13-week) stage. All the elements of the sphenoid bone, both endochondral and intramembranous, finally join to form a single element in the 125 mm (18-week) fetus. The sphenoid bone enlarges and makes contact with the frontal bone, closing the lateral and superior orbital walls by the 220 mm (26-week) stage.[8]

The ethmoid bone begins as part of the cartilaginous chondrocranium in the 25 mm (7-week) embryo. Ossification begins in the 220 mm (26-week) stage on the lateral portion, at what will become the lamina papyracea. By the 320 mm (32-week) stage ossification is nearly complete, except for the nasal septum, which remains cartilaginous. The ethmoid air cells develop between the 220 and 320 mm (26–32-week) stages. The lacrimal bone develops as a thin intramembranous ossification beginning in the 75 mm (13-week) fetus.

The orbital bones form around the developing optic cup and stalk. Initially, the optic vesicles are positioned 170–180° apart, on opposite sides of the forebrain, reflecting their earlier phylogenetic vertebrate configuration. During the 4- to 8-week embryonic stages the optic cups begin to rotate anteriorly as the primordial orbital bones are laid down around them. By 3 months of fetal development, the orbital axes form an angle of about 105° between them and at birth, this angle is reduced to 45°. Only relatively slight additional remolding occurs during childhood. Failure of complete rotation results in the clinical condition of hypertelorism, whereas over rotation causes hypotelorism.[22] Malpositions in ossification of orbital bones may result in reduced orbital volume and proptosis, as seen in Crouzon disease.

The adult bony orbit

In the adult, the bony orbit is roughly pyramidal in shape. Its volume in the average individual is approximately 25 cm³, but published measurements of volume vary considerably using either direct filling or CT imaging techniques from a mean of 17.05 cm³ to 29.30 cm³.[1,9,19,34,42,50] Within the orbit the eye contributes about 7.2 cm³ based on the average diameter of about 24 mm. However, a myopic eye will be larger and a hyperopic eye will be smaller. Each change of 0.5 mm in diameter will result in a volumetric change of about 0.45 cm³. Thaller[56] measured the volume of enucleated eyes by a volume displacement technique and found the average volume to be 8.15 cm³.

The anterior entrance of the orbit forms a rough rectangle measuring approximately 43 mm (36–47 mm) wide by 34 mm (26–42 mm) high.[42] The orbit attains its widest dimensions at about 15 mm behind the bony rim. As in all other higher primates, the human orbit is completely closed behind by the sphenoid bone, except for the superior and inferior orbital fissures. The orbits are directed more forward than in other mammals, and their anterior-posterior central axes form a 45° angle between them. The two lateral orbital walls subtend a 90° angle between them. The four walls of each orbit converge posteriorly toward the orbital apex where the optic canal and superior orbital fissure pass into the middle cranial fossa.

The overall dimensions of the orbit are quite variable, especially its depth. Thus, the surgeon cannot rely on precise measurements as a guide to the exact location of the optic canal or superior orbital fissure. Nor can the position of the ethmoidal foramina, the bridging over of the infraorbital canal, or of soft tissue structures within the orbit be accurately determined preoperatively. Therefore, extreme caution must be exercised in posterior orbital dissections in any orbital surgery. During exploration of the orbital floor for entrapment of the inferior rectus muscle following trauma or in orbital decompression, the inferior orbital fissure may be encountered inferolaterally as little as 10–15 mm behind the rim. Dissection along the floor should not extend more than 40 mm posterior to the orbital rim, since the floor ends at the posterior wall of the maxillary sinus, and therefore does not extend to the apex.

The orbital rim

The orbital rim is rounded and thickened, and serves to protect the eye from facial impacts. The superior rim is the most prominent due to expansion of the underlying frontal sinus. It is more protuberant in adult males. Its significance has been a matter of debate for over 100 years,[48] but the most often cited explanation for it is that it developed to counter biomechanical stress associated with mastication.[15] Experimental data have demonstrated mastication-related strain in the interorbital and supraorbital regions. However, the degree is very small compared to other parts of the facial skeleton, and therefore does not support masticatory stress as a major evolutionary force in development of the supraorbital ridge.[25]

The medial third of the superior orbital rim is interrupted by a notch or foramen for passage of the supraorbital neurovascular bundle. One or both sides will have an open notch in 75% of all orbits. In 50% of individuals at least one side may be closed to form a foramen.[39,59] The notch is situated about 25–30 mm from the facial midline.[5,7,59] The location of this notch is an important guide in avoiding injury to the supraorbital nerve during brow and forehead surgery.

The orbital rim is flatter and less prominent between the supraorbital notch and the medial canthal ligament. A number of important neurovascular structures emerge here, including the supratrochlear and infratrochlear nerves, and the dorsal nasal artery. Just inside the rim at the superomedial corner of the orbit is the cartilaginous trochlea of the superior oblique tendon. Surgical access to the medial wall through a fronto-ethmoidal incision may interrupt these neural structures with resultant glabellar and forehead anesthesia. If necessary for orbital access, the trochlea can be disinserted by elevating the periosteum.

Medially, the orbital rim extends downward to the posterior lacrimal crest and ends at the inferior entrance to the nasolacrimal canal. The anterior lacrimal crest begins just above the medial canthal ligament, and passes downward into the inferior orbital rim. The medial rim is, therefore, discontinuous at the lacrimal sac fossa. Between the anterior and posterior lacrimal crests is the lacrimal sac fossa formed at the junction of the maxillary and lacrimal bones. The fossa measures about 16 mm in vertical length, 4–9 mm in width, and 2 mm in depth.[4] Just in front of and parallel to the anterior lacrimal crest is a vertical groove in the frontal process of the maxillary bone for a nutrient branch of the infraorbital artery. During dacryocystorhinostomy surgery this groove may be mistaken for the medial edge of anterior lacrimal crest. Brisk bleeding may occur from rupture of this vessel, but it is easily controlled.

The inferior orbital rim is formed by the maxillary bone medially and the zygomatic bone laterally. The infraorbital foramen, conducting the infraorbital artery and nerve, is located 4–10 mm below the central portion of the inferior rim. During surgery on the orbital floor, care must be taken not to elevate periosteum anterior to the central rim for more than about 4 mm, since this may injure these neurovascular structures.

The orbital rim is thickest laterally. Here it is formed by the frontal process of the zygomatic bone and the zygomatic process of the frontal bone. These two elements meet at the frontozygomatic suture line near the superotemporal corner of the orbit. This suture line is an important landmark for removing the lateral rim during orbital surgery, because the anterior cranial fossa lies 5–15 mm above this horizontal level. This is a weak suture and is frequently the site of separation following facial trauma. About 10 mm below the frontozygomatic suture line, about 4–5 mm inside the rim is a small mound, the lateral orbital tubercle of Whitnall. It serves for insertion of the posterior crus of the lateral canthal ligament, Lockwood's inferior suspensory ligament, the lateral horn of the levator aponeurosis, the lateral check ligament and pulley system of the lateral rectus muscle, and the deep layer of the orbital septum. Proper realignment of these structures after lateral orbital surgery or repair of rim fractures is essential for normal cosmetic and functional reconstruction.

The entire orbital rim is buttressed by adjacent bones and is frequently involved in complex facial fractures. The surgeon must be alert to the normal anatomic and functional relationships between the orbital bones and the nasal cavity, paranasal sinuses, cranial vault, and the temporomandibular joint.

The medial orbital wall

The medial walls of the orbits are approximately parallel to each other and to the mid-sagittal plane. The separation between the two orbits is approximately 24 mm from the medial wall of one to the medial wall of the other. The medial wall measures an average of 42 mm (range 32–53 mm) in horizontal length from the anterior lacrimal crest to the optic canal.[38] The medial wall of each orbit is formed by four osseous elements, the maxillary, lacrimal, ethmoid, and sphenoid bones. Anteriorly, the thick frontal process of the maxillary bone lies at the inferior medial rim. It contains the anterior lacrimal crest and forms the anterior portion of the lacrimal sac fossa. The lacrimal bone is a small, thin and fragile plate situated just posterior to the maxillary process. It forms the posterior portion of the lacrimal sac fossa. Running vertically along its midpoint is the posterior lacrimal crest. The suture between the maxillary and lacrimal bones generally lies along the mid-vertical line within the lacrimal sac fossa. However, in 8% of individuals this suture lies more posteriorly, occasionally nearly to the posterior lacrimal crest.[6] In such cases the thicker maxillary bone underlies most of the lacrimal sac fossa. As a result, creation of a bony osteum during dacryocystorhinostomy surgery can be more difficult than usual, and will frequently require a burr to remove excess bone.

Behind the posterior lacrimal crest is the lamina papyracea, which forms most of the lateral wall of the ethmoid labyrinth. It contributes 4–6 cm² to the orbital wall surface. This is exceptionally fragile, measuring only 0.2–0.4 mm in thickness. However, it is made more rigid by the honeycombed bony laminae surrounding the ethmoid air cells, which usually number 3–8. Resistance of the medial wall to static loading is greater when the lamina papyracea is smaller in area, when the number of air cells is greater, or when their individual sizes are smaller.[47] Song et al.[53] showed that medial wall fractures are more frequent, compared to floor fractures, when there are fewer ethmoid air cells, or when a larger area of lamina papyracea is supported by each sinus septum. The fragility of this bone is also associated with its easy displacement into the orbit with expanding lesions in the ethmoid sinus.[26] Following trauma, a 3 mm "blow-out" medial displacement of the lamina papyracea may result in a 5% increase in orbital volume, and 1.0–1.5 mm of enophthalmos.[43] The lamina papyracea offers only a minimal barrier to the spread of infection from the ethmoid sinus into the orbit,[58] sometimes resulting in the orbital edema, cellulitis, and abscess formation that is sometimes associated with ethmoid sinusitis. Surgery along the medial wall, or probing instrumentation during enucleation surgery may easily penetrate the lamina papyracea, with the possible complication of orbital emphysema or infection.[13]

Superiorly the ethmoid bone joins the orbital roof at the fronto-ethmoid suture line. This level approximately marks the roof of the ethmoid sinus labyrinth and the floor of the anterior cranial fossa. Just medial to the labyrinth, on either side of the intracranial crista galli, is the cribriform plate. This may extend 5–10 mm below the level of the fronto-ethmoid suture line in some individuals. The root of the middle nasal turbinate separates the cribriform plate on each side from the superior ethmoid air cells. This relationship must be born in mind during surgery along the medial wall, and the fronto-ethmoid suture line is a useful landmark indicating the safe upper limit for bony dissection.

At the level of the lacrimal sac fossa the anterior cranial fossa may be as little as 1 mm, or as much as 30 mm above the upper border of the medial canthal ligament. The mean value is 8.3 mm.[33] This distance tends to correlate with the size of the frontal sinus, being larger when the sinus is more extensive. At the level of the posterior lacrimal crest this distance shortens to 0–19 mm (mean of 6.5 mm), as the floor of the anterior cranial fossa slopes downward and backward. In as many as 20% of normal individuals this distance may be 3 mm or less,[33] and this may explain the occasional occurrence of a CSF leak during creation of a bony osteum in dacryocystorhinostomy surgery. This complication is more likely when the medial canthal ligament landmark is removed.[33,41] It is, therefore, safest to leave the ligament attached, and to use this structure as a guide to placement of the upper border of the bony osteum.

The anterior and posterior ethmoidal foramina usually lie within the fronto-ethmoid suture line. These openings transmit branches from the ophthalmic artery and nasociliary nerve passing out of the orbit. There is great variability in the position of these foramina and in 10–20% of cases one or both of these canals may lie outside (usually above) the fronto-ethmoid suture line as a variant or racial difference.[61] The posterior ethmoid foramen may sometimes be absent, and both foramina may be multiple. The anterior ethmoidal foramen is located about 22 mm (range 14–30 mm) behind the anterior lacrimal crest. However, it is located within the more narrow range of 20–25 mm behind the crest in two-thirds of individuals.[11,32] The posterior ethmoidal foramen lies 33 mm (range 25–41 mm) from the anterior lacrimal crest,[36,42] approximately 4–15 mm anterior to the optic canal. The anterior and posterior ethmoid foramina transmit the ethmoidal nerves and arteries into the anterior cranial fossa and to the nasal and sinus mucosa. The positions of these foramina are clinically important since they relate to important cranial structures such as the cribriform plate, and to the optic foramen. They are key landmarks during surgery along the medial orbital wall. Injury to the ethmoidal arteries can cause excessive orbital bleeding during surgery. Subperiosteal hematoma following trauma frequently results from rupture of one of these arteries, and management requires access to the medial wall with ligation or cautery of the bleeding vessel.

Posterior to the ethmoid bone is the body of the sphenoid bone that forms the short posterior portion of the medial wall. The sphenoid body lies between the two orbital apices and contains the sphenoid sinus. The optic canal is situated in the superomedial portion of the orbital apex, enclosed by the body of the sphenoid medially, the lesser wing of the sphenoid superiorly, and the optic strut inferolaterally.

The lacrimal sac fossa is a depression in the anterior inferomedial orbit.[27] It is bounded by the anterior and posterior lacrimal crests and measures about 4–9 mm in width and 16 mm in height. The fossa is formed by the frontal process of the maxillary bone anteriorly and by the lacrimal bone posteriorly. The nasolacrimal canal is a bony tube extending from the lacrimal sac fossa to the inferior nasal meatus, and it contains the membranous nasolacrimal duct. The canal measures about 5 mm in diameter and is bordered by three bones, the maxilla, the lacrimal, and the inferior turbinate bones. The canal runs inferolateral and slightly posterior in the medial wall of the maxillary bone. It measures about 12–15 mm in length.

The orbital floor

The orbital floor is a very thin plate composed of three bones (maxillary, zygomatic, and palatine). Its surface forms a triangular segment extending from the maxillary-ethmoid buttress on the medial side, horizontally to the inferior orbital fissure on the lateral side, and from the inferior orbital rim back to the posterior wall of the maxillary sinus. The floor contributes 3–5 cm² to the overall orbital wall surface. It is strengthened by the infraorbital canal which runs anteroposteriorly through it near its midline or sometimes closer to its lateral border. One or more trabeculae in the roof of the maxillary sinus are sometimes present and they serve also to buttress the floor. Nevertheless, the orbital floor shows the greatest degree of deformation with static loading of any of the orbital walls.[47] This explains the high rate of floor fractures associated with blunt trauma. A 3 mm downward displacement of the entire floor results in an increase of about 1.5 cm³ (5%) to the orbital volume, and about 1.0–1.5 mm of enophthalmos.

The major contribution to the floor is from the orbital plate of the maxillary bone, which also forms the roof of the maxillary sinus. Anterolaterally, the zygomatic bone contributes to the orbital rim and a small portion of the floor just in front of the anterior border of the inferior orbital fissure. The palatine bone lies at the extreme posterior end of the floor, near the orbital apex. In adults, it is usually fused with the maxillary bone. The floor is bounded medially by the maxilloethmoid suture line, and anterolaterally by the zygomaticomaxillary suture. From the inferior orbital rim, the floor dips downward, where it reaches its lowest point. This is about 1.5–2.0 mm below the rim in children and young adults, but reaches 3.0 mm in older adults.[40] From here the floor slopes upward to the orbital apex at an angle of about 18–22° to the horizontal Frankfort plane (inferior orbital rim [orbitale] to the upper border of the bony ear canal [porion]).

In the mid and posterior orbit, the floor ends at the inferior orbital fissure, and the posterior extent of the maxillary sinus. It is important to keep in mind that the orbital floor does not extend all the way to the apex, but rather ends at the pterygopalatine fossa. The floor is, therefore, the shortest of the orbital walls, extending only about 35–40 mm from the inferior rim to the posterior wall of the maxillary sinus. However, the distance from the rim at the infraorbital canal to the optic canal is greater, measuring 48 mm (range 41–57 mm). During surgical exploration of orbital fractures or during floor decompressions in thyroid orbital disease, dissection need not be carried further than the posterior sinus wall. However, in cases of compressive optic neuropathy in Graves' disease, it is essential to obtain an adequate decompression closer to the orbital apex.[2,30] This can be achieved on the medial wall by opening the orbit into the posterior ethmoid sinus or even into the sphenoid sinus. On the lateral wall the thicker portion of the lateral sphenoid wing can be burred down to the inner plate or even to the dura.

The infraorbital sulcus lies within the posterior portion of the orbital floor. This fissure runs approximately in the center of the floor from posterior to anterior, and carries the maxillary division of the trigeminal nerve and the associated infraorbital branch of the maxillary artery from the pterygopalatine fossa. At about the mid portion of the floor the sulcus usually becomes bridged-over by a thin plate of the maxillary bone to form the infraorbital canal. This thin plate of bone is pierced by one or more tiny foramina that transmit anastomotic vessels from the infraorbital artery to the inferior muscular branch of the ophthalmic artery (see Chapter 5). Along its course, the infraorbital canal gives off the middle and anterior superior alveolar canals, carrying corresponding nerves and vessels.[35] The infraorbital canal continues forward to the orbital rim, where it exits as the infraorbital foramen. In 2–18% of individuals the canal can be double or even triple.[23] After elevation of periosteum, the region of the infraorbital canal can usually be identified on the floor as a slightly elevated somewhat translucent ridge. Recognition of its position is critical if injury to the infraorbital nerve is to be avoided during orbital floor surgery. Damage to this nerve results in anesthesia of the lower eyelid, cheek, and upper lip, and this is not uncommon following orbit floor blow-out fractures or orbital decompression into the maxillary sinus.

Separating the floor from the lateral orbital wall is the inferior orbital fissure (IOF). This opening is approximately 30 mm in length and runs in an anterolateral to posteromedial direction. The anteriormost edge of the IOF lies approximately 24 mm (range 17–29 mm) from the inferior orbital rim at the infraorbital foramen. At the orbital apex just below the optic canal, the inferior fissure joins the superior

orbital fissure, and is contiguous with the foramen rotundum in the floor of the middle cranial fossa. The inferior fissure transmits structures into the orbit from the pterygopalatine fossa posteriorly, and from the infratemporal fossa more anteriorly. Multiple branches from the inferior ophthalmic vein pass through this opening to communicate with the pterygoid venous plexus. The inferior fissure also transmits the maxillary division (V2) of the trigeminal nerve. The latter nerve passes out of the cranium through the foramen rotundum into the pterygopalatine fossa, and then into the infraorbital sulcus in the posterior orbital floor, where it runs in company with the infraorbital artery. Postganglionic parasympathetic secretory and vasomotor neural branches from the pterygopalatine ganglion enter the orbit through the inferior orbital fissure, where they join with the maxillary nerve for a short distance before running superiorly along the lateral orbital wall to the lacrimal gland (see Chapter 4).

The lateral orbital wall

The lateral wall of the orbit is the thickest, and is composed of the zygomatic bone anteriorly and the greater wing of the sphenoid posteriorly. It is separated from the floor by the inferior orbital fissure, and from the roof, in part, by the superior orbital fissure. The lateral walls of the two orbits form an angle of approximately 90° with each other, and lie at 45° to the mid-sagittal plane. The lengths of the lateral and medial walls, from orbital rim to apex, are about the equal. Because of the oblique orientation of the lateral wall, the lateral rim lies about 10 mm posterior to the medial rim.[18] The length of the lateral wall from the lateral rim at the frontozygomatic suture to the optic canal is about 47 mm (range 39–55 mm).

The thinnest part of the lateral wall is at the zygomatic-sphenoid suture, about 8–10 mm behind the orbital rim. During lateral orbital surgery, cuts through the bony rim must be made to this level so that the rim can easily be fractured outward. Approximately 10 mm behind the zygomatic-sphenoid suture, the sphenoid bone thickens where it divides to form the anterior corner of the middle cranial fossa. Here, compact bone passes into cancellous bone, a useful landmark when taking down the lateral wall to gain wide access to the orbit or in lateral wall decompressions. In about 40% of individuals there are one or more openings within the fronto-sphenoid suture line, about 30 mm from the orbital rim. This is the cranio-orbital foramen (foramen meningo-orbitale) which transmits an anastomotic branch between the middle meningeal artery and the ophthalmic arterial system (see Chapter 5). This vessel is a remnant of the embryological development of the orbital arterial system, and usually joins the root of the lacrimal artery. Although this is a small and sometimes inconsistent branch in humans, it represents a significant supply of orbital blood in some other mammalian orders.[60] This vessel is easily ruptured during lateral orbital surgery resulting in brisk bleeding. Compression for several minutes is usually sufficient to control it.

At the junction of the lateral wall and roof is the superior orbital fissure (SOF), lying between the greater and lesser wings of the sphenoid bone near the orbital apex. It is oriented from inferomedial at the apex to superotemporal distally. The anteriormost edge of the SOF lies 37 mm (range 34–41 mm) from the lateral orbital rim. In size and shape this fissure shows considerable individual variability.[51] However, its comma-like shape is usually wider inferiorly, but then narrows more superiorly. The fissure measures about 20–25 mm in overall length. The narrow lesser wing of the sphenoid bone separates the medial edge of the superior orbital fissure from the lateral margin of the optic canal. The spinal recti lateralis is a small bony projection situated on the lateral edge of the fissure near its middle portion, at the junction of its wide and narrow portions. This projection serves as the origin for part of the lateral rectus muscle. It is formed primarily by a small groove in the sphenoid wing which lodges the superior ophthalmic vein as it passes through the fissure.[44] The superior orbital fissure transmits most of the vascular and neural structures from the middle cranial fossa into the orbit, with the major exception of the optic nerve and ophthalmic artery, which pass through the optic canal. The central portion of the fissure is anatomically divided by the annulus of Zinn, which serves as the tendinous origin for the rectus muscles. The central opening defined by the annulus, called the oculomotor foramen, transmits structures into the intraconal orbital space. Most of these structures subserve ocular function and motility. These include the superior and inferior divisions of the oculomotor nerve, the abducens nerve, and the nasociliary nerve (see Chapter 4). Other structures passing through the superior orbital fissure but outside the annulus are mainly associated with the extraconal orbital space, or are en route to extraorbital sites. These include the trochlear nerve, the frontal and lacrimal branches of the trigeminal nerve, and the superior ophthalmic vein above the annulus, and the inferior ophthalmic vein beneath the annulus.

In 8–40% of individuals, a linear vertical groove is present lying along the greater wing of the sphenoid bone, between the superior and inferior orbital fissures. This was previously believed to house an anastomotic branch between the middle meningeal and infraorbital arteries.[37] However, investigations show that this does not contain any vascular or neural structures, but rather represents an abrupt thinning of the greater wing at the transition from cancellous to compact bone.[10]

Several small foramina perforate the lateral orbital wall just behind the rim laterally and inferiorly near the anterior end of the inferior fissure. These transmit branches of the lacrimal artery and zygomatic nerve out of the orbit as the zygomaticotemporal and zygomaticofacial neurovascular bundles.

The orbital roof

The orbital roof is triangular in shape. It is formed primarily from the orbital plate of the frontal bone, with a small contribution by the lesser wing of the sphenoid bone posteriorly. It measures about 46 mm (range 35–59 mm) from the supraorbital foramen to the optic canal.[38,42] In the anterior superolateral corner is a poorly-defined concavity for the lacrimal gland. A small depression in the superomedial corner, about 3–5 mm behind the rim, houses the fibrocartilaginous trochlea for the superior oblique tendon. This structure, along with its associated pulley system, can easily be separated from the adjacent bone along with periorbita if needed during surgery. Its precise repositioning is essential to avoid postoperative motility disturbance.

The orbital roof is very thin and may have spontaneous dehiscences. During surgery along the roof, care must be taken since the use of instrumentation may perforate this fragile structure and injure intracranial dura. The frontal sinus is located within the frontal bone in the anteromedial portion of the roof. The size of this sinus is extremely variable, and in some individuals it may extend as far laterally as the lacrimal gland fossa, and as far posteriorly as the optic canal.

The optic canal is located in the roof at the apex and communicates between the middle cranial fossa and the orbit. It is bounded by the body of the sphenoid bone medially, the lesser wing of the sphenoid superiorly, and the optic strut laterally and inferiorly. The strut arises from the body of the sphenoid and is directed slightly anteriorly, upward, and laterally at an angle of about 36° to the sagittal plane.[44] The optic canal assumes a vertically oval shape at its orbital end, where it measures about 5–6 mm in horizontal diameter, and 6–8 mm vertically. In its central portion the canal is round in cross-section, and on the cranial end it is oval in the horizontal plane.[20] The canal attains adult size by the age of three years. In about 4% of normal individuals the ophthalmic artery will notch the canal floor, forming a "keyhole" deformity.[31] The canal is 8–12 mm in length and is directed posteromedially at about 35° to the mid-sagittal plane, and upward about 38° to the horizontal. On the cranial side the optic canal measures 5–7 mm horizontally and 4–6 mm vertically. The tendinous annulus of Zinn encloses the orbital opening of the optic canal so that the optic nerve and ophthalmic artery pass into the intraconal space via the oculomotor foramen.

The relationships of the optic canal and the adjacent paranasal sinuses is somewhat variable depending upon the extent to which these sinuses invade the lesser wing and the anterolateral portion of the body of the sphenoid bone.[44] In a study of 100 sphenoid sinuses, Van Alyea[57] found that the medial wall of the optic canal projected into the sinus in 40% of cases, and in rare instances it was completely surrounded by the sinus with the canal passing through the sinus cavity. Goodyear[21] described a similar relationship between the posterior ethmoid sinus and the optic canal.

Aging phenomena

The craniofacial skeleton undergoes remodeling throughout adulthood. The face shows a progressive rotation of the frontal bone forward over the orbits, and the maxillary bone extends backward beneath the orbits.[46] This process continues the morphological process of frontation seen in the evolution of higher primates. These changes are most acute in the mid-face. Angular changes in the facial skeleton are associated with compensatory changes in the soft-tissue anatomy, with weakening and stretching of the retaining ligaments, inducing descent of the mid-facial malar cheek pads and changes in the position of the lower eyelid with increasing scleral show and prominence of the inferior orbital fat pockets.

In addition to rotational changes the orbital aperture changes, increasing in length along a line from superomedial to inferolateral.[28] The loss of volume and bony projection along with laxity of retaining ligaments contribute to lateral brow hooding, lateral canthal skin redundancy, and nasolabial fold prominence. The cranial skeleton also widens, lengthens, and shows mid-face convexity with advancing age.

Clinical correlations

The orbital floor is thinnest medial to the infraorbital canal where it may be only 0.5 mm thick. This is a convenient point for initial entrance into the maxillary sinus during orbital inferior wall decompression surgery. It is this portion of the floor that is usually involved in blow-out fractures, believed to result from rim deformation and compression of orbital contents following direct blunt trauma.[52] Kwon et al.[34] measured the volumes of orbits expanded from a blow-out injury compared to the uninjured contralateral sides and reported an average expansion of 2.8 cm³.

Fan et al.[17] calculated that each 1.0 cm³ increment of orbital volume expansion would result in 0.89 mm of relative enophthalmos. Surgical correction is aimed at restoring the integrity and normal position of the fractured walls, usually with the use of alloplastic implants or autogenous bone grafts. This is indicated for cosmetically significant enophthalmos, even in the absence of motility restriction.[12] Correction of 3 mm of enophthalmos will require replacement of a 3.4 cm³ of volume, either by repositioning prolapsed fat and muscle, or with an orbital implant, or a combination of both.

The total adult orbital volume is about 25 cm³, of which the globe occupies about 7.2 cm³. Following enucleation an alloplastic spherical implant is usually placed into the anophthalmic socket to replace lost volume. The typical 18–20 mm diameter sphere replaces 3.0–4.0 cm³, and the ocular prosthesis adds another 1.5–2.5 cm³ depending upon the design and thickness. The net loss in orbital volume, therefore, may amount to 1.0–3.0 cm³. Following trauma or repeated post-traumatic orbital surgery there may be significant atrophy of orbital fat, resulting in an additional 2–3 cm³ of volume loss. The total deficit may be as much as 6 cm³ or more, resulting in significant enophthalmos and a superior sulcus deformity. This volume deficit may be replaced with an autogenous or alloplastic orbital floor implant placed subperiosteally to add volume. This will also elevate the orbital contents to correct the superior sulcus deformity.

Deviations in shape of the optic canal, horizontal enlargement of the orbital opening to more than 6.5 mm, or asymmetry of more than 1 mm difference between the two sides are suggestive of pathology. Compression of the optic nerve within the canal may be seen with slowly expanding intrinsic lesions of the nerve, such as optic gliomas or sheath meningiomas. In such cases the bony canal is commonly enlarged, and the orbital opening frequently assumes a rounded contour on radiographs.[16,45] Other causes of canal enlargement include neurofibromas, optic nerve extension of retinoblastomas, aneurysms of the ophthalmic artery, arteriovenous malformations, and chronic increased intracranial pressure.[14]

Visual loss may be seen in 0.5–1.5% of closed head traumas.[49] Fractures through the optic canal have been reported in up to 5% of head injuries,[55] but resultant optic nerve compression is unusual. Optic canal fractures associated with visual loss may sometimes be demonstrated radiographically, but are frequently difficult to visualize.[3,18,24] Immediate loss of vision following blunt head trauma more commonly results from contusion of the nerve at the canal where the nerve sheaths are fused to periosteum, resulting in interruption of vascular supply. More gradual visual loss is generally due to edema or slowly accumulating hemorrhage, with nerve compression. Vision may be salvaged in some of these latter patients with high dose intravenous steroids or surgical decompression.[3,29]

Any increase in orbital soft-tissue volume, such as with Graves' orbitopathy, results in a forward displacement of the globe, but also in an increase in intraorbital pressure. Orbital decompression by removal of one or more orbital walls may result in marked reduction in pressure of up to 85%.[54] Reduction in proptosis by expanding total orbital volume, however, requires opening of periorbita in addition to bony decompression.

Craniofacial dysplasias are teratogenic abnormalities of the face and skull due to deficiencies in growth, ossifications, or pneumatization. Developmental arrest or premature fusion of ossification centers results in different kinds of bony abnormalities. Around the orbit this causes deformities like orbital reduction, orbital dystopia, abnormal separation of the orbits, and interruption of bony orbital walls. Craniofacial synostosis is another group of teratogenic anomalies of the face, orbits, and cranium involving premature closure of bony sutures. As growth continues along other sutures, large areas of the skull distort to show abnormal shapes. Sagittal suture fusion results in dolichocephaly where the skull is long and boat-shaped, whereas with fusion of both coronal sutures the skull becomes brachycephalic, that is tall, short from front to back, and wide from side to side.

Fibrous dysplasia is a non-hereditary benign developmental fibro-osseous anomaly of the bone-forming mesenchyme. It represents a hamartomatous malformation resulting from arrest in maturation at the woven bone stage. Progressive orbital dystopia and facial asymmetry occur from thickening of orbital bones. When the frontal bone is involved, unilateral proptosis, ptosis, and a downward displacement of the orbit and globe is seen. Progressive constriction of orbital foramina and canals of the cranial base may cause cranial nerve palsies, trigeminal neuralgia, and visual loss.

Paget's disease is a metabolic disorder characterized by abnormal remodeling of bone. It generally affects adults, and is rarely seen before the age of 30. The disease progresses through an early phase of lytic osteoclastic activity followed by an intermediate osteoblastic phase, and then a final phase where previously laid down woven bone is converted to dense lamellar bone. Symptoms of cranial nerve compression can include ophthalmoplegia and visual loss.

Osteoma is a well-differentiated benign tumor of bone. Most arise in the paranasal sinuses, with about 15% resulting in orbital symptoms, where slowly progressive proptosis is the most common sign. Anteriorly placed tumors may be palpable as a rock hard mass.

The intracranial compartment

The frontal bone of the orbital roof separates the orbit from the anterior cranial fossa which contains the frontal lobes of the cerebral hemispheres. This compartment is frequently involved in orbital pathology. The anterior cranial fossa is bounded anteriorly by the inner table of the frontal bone, and posteriorly by the lesser wing of the sphenoid bone. Medially, the lesser wings terminate at the anterior clinoid processes which lie near the roof of the optic canals. The tentorium cerebelli terminates on the anterior clinoid process. In the midline of the anterior cranial fossa is a central crest, the crista galli, onto which attaches the falx cerebri. Just on each side of the crista galli is a depression with numerous perforations. These are the cribriform plates of the ethmoid bones. They form the roof of the nasal cavity, and through them filaments of the olfactory nerve pass en route to the nasal mucosa. A small foramen, the foramen cecum, is located between the cribriform plate and the crista galli on either side. It serves for transmission of a vein from the nasal mucosa to the superior sagittal sinus. The anterior ethmoidal nerve passes into the anterior cranial fossa at the lateral edge of the cribriform plate, and then into the nasal cavity through a narrow slit or foramen adjacent to the crista galli.

The middle cranial fossa consists of a narrow midline elevation formed by the body of the sphenoid bone, and two lateral depressions that house the temporal lobes of the cerebral cortex. Within the anterior central portion of the fossa, each optic canal opens into the chiasmatic groove, which terminates posteriorly at a shallow elevation, the tuberculum sellae over which lies the optic chiasm (see Chapter 1). Immediately behind this structure is a deep depression, the sella turcica, which contains the pituitary gland. Posterior to the sella is a quadrilateral plate of bone. This is the dorsum sellae which contains the posterior clinoid processes onto which attach the tentorium cerebelli. Immediately below each process is a groove for the passage of the abducens nerve. On either side of the sella turcica is a shallow curved trough, the carotid groove, which lodges the cavernous sinus and the internal carotid artery.

Medially, the floor of the middle cranial fossa is formed by the greater wings of the sphenoid bone and the petrous portions of the temporal bone. Anteriorly, bridging over the roof of the cavernous sinus, and forming a spine of bone between the optic canal and the superior orbital fissure, is the anterior clinoid process. Just lateral to the anterior clinoid, situated vertically between the greater and lesser wings of the sphenoid, is a large, sickle-shaped opening, the superior orbital fissure, which communicates with the orbit. It transmits the superior ophthalmic vein, and the oculomotor, abducens, trochlear, frontal, nasociliary and lacrimal nerves. Just behind the medial end of the superior orbital fissure is the foramen rotundum which passes through the greater sphenoid wing and transmits the maxillary division of the trigeminal nerve to the pterygopalatine fossa. Posterior and lateral to the foramen rotundum is the foramen ovale, also perforating the greater sphenoid wing. This transmits the mandibular division of the trigeminal nerve into the infratemporal fossa. It also contains an accessory meningeal artery, and sometimes the lesser petrosal nerve. Posterior and lateral the foramen ovale, in the posterior angle of the middle cranial fossa, is the small foramen spinosum which carries the middle meningeal artery. Between the apex of the petrous portion of the temporal bone and the sphenoid bone is a large irregular opening, the foramen lacerum, which in life is filled with fibrocartilage. The internal carotid artery passes over this opening as it enters the cavernous sinus.

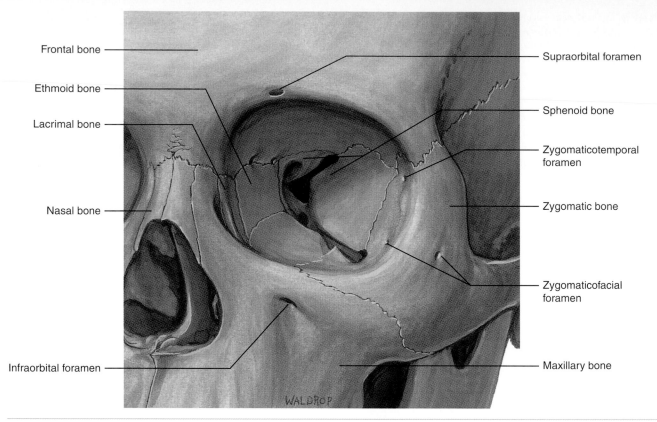

Frontal bone

Ethmoid bone

Lacrimal bone

Nasal bone

Infraorbital foramen

Supraorbital foramen

Sphenoid bone

Zygomaticotemporal foramen

Zygomatic bone

Zygomaticofacial foramen

Maxillary bone

Figure 2-1 Orbital bones, frontal view.

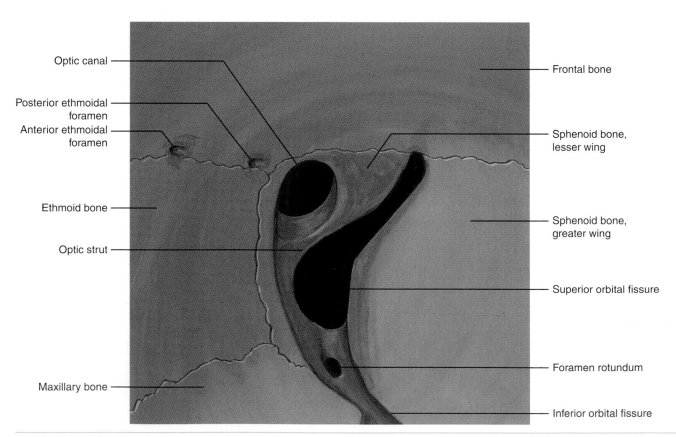

Optic canal

Posterior ethmoidal foramen

Anterior ethmoidal foramen

Ethmoid bone

Optic strut

Maxillary bone

Frontal bone

Sphenoid bone, lesser wing

Sphenoid bone, greater wing

Superior orbital fissure

Foramen rotundum

Inferior orbital fissure

Figure 2-2 Orbital bones, apex.

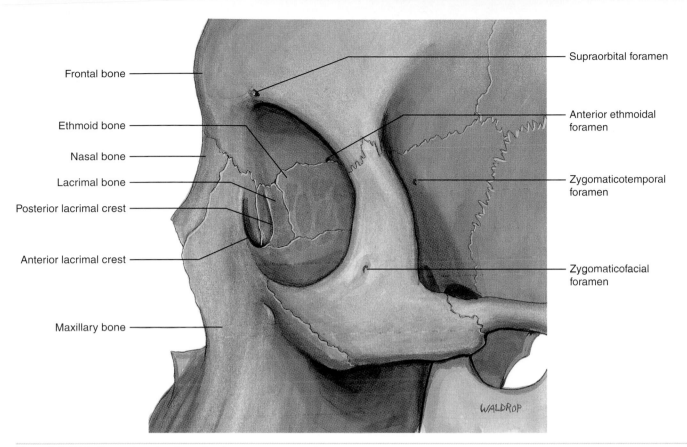

Figure 2-3 Orbital bones, lateral wall, exterior view.

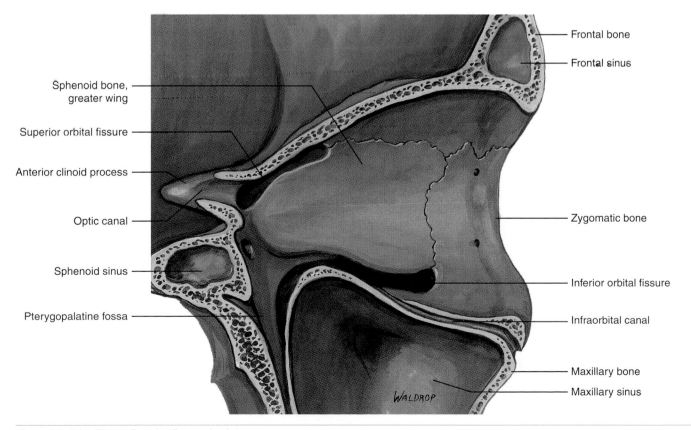

Figure 2-4 Orbital bones, lateral wall, intraorbital view.

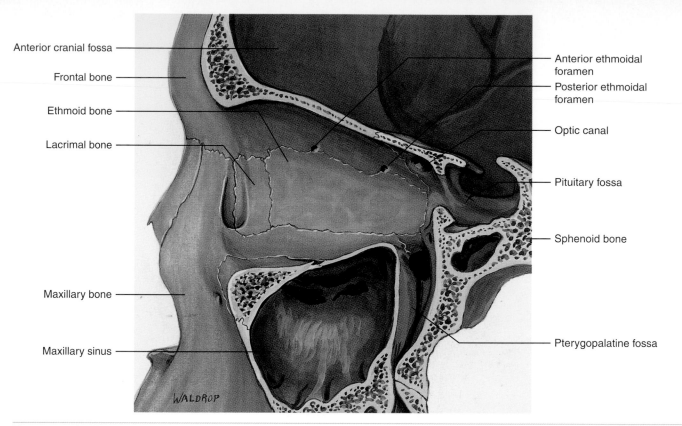

Anterior cranial fossa

Frontal bone

Ethmoid bone

Lacrimal bone

Maxillary bone

Maxillary sinus

Anterior ethmoidal foramen

Posterior ethmoidal foramen

Optic canal

Pituitary fossa

Sphenoid bone

Pterygopalatine fossa

Figure 2-5 Orbital bones, medial wall, intraorbital view.

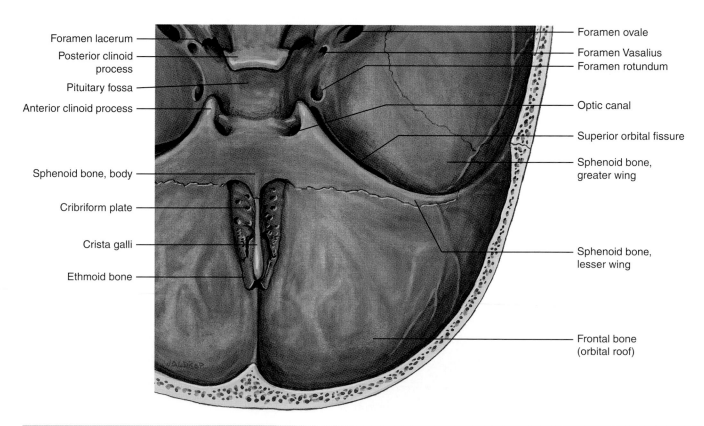

Foramen lacerum

Posterior clinoid process

Pituitary fossa

Anterior clinoid process

Sphenoid bone, body

Cribriform plate

Crista galli

Ethmoid bone

Foramen ovale

Foramen Vasalius

Foramen rotundum

Optic canal

Superior orbital fissure

Sphenoid bone, greater wing

Sphenoid bone, lesser wing

Frontal bone (orbital roof)

Figure 2-6 Orbital bones, superior wall, intracranial view.

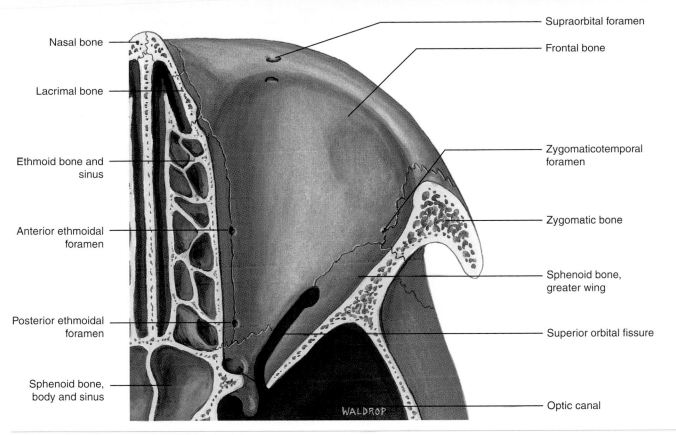

Nasal bone

Lacrimal bone

Ethmoid bone and sinus

Anterior ethmoidal foramen

Posterior ethmoidal foramen

Sphenoid bone, body and sinus

Supraorbital foramen

Frontal bone

Zygomaticotemporal foramen

Zygomatic bone

Sphenoid bone, greater wing

Superior orbital fissure

Optic canal

WALDROP

Figure 2-7 Orbital bones, superior wall, intraorbital view.

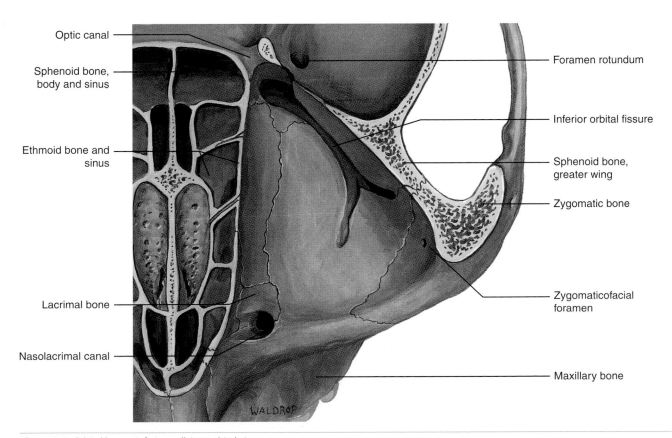

Optic canal

Sphenoid bone, body and sinus

Ethmoid bone and sinus

Lacrimal bone

Nasolacrimal canal

Foramen rotundum

Inferior orbital fissure

Sphenoid bone, greater wing

Zygomatic bone

Zygomaticofacial foramen

Maxillary bone

WALDROP

Figure 2-8 Orbital bones, inferior wall, intraorbital view.

References

1. Acer N, Sahin B, Ergür H, et al: Sterotactic estimation of the orbital volume: A criterion standard study. *J Craniofac Surg* 20:921, 2009.

2. Anderson RL, Linberg JV: Transorbital approach to decompression in Graves' disease. *Arch Ophthalmol* 99:120, 1981.

3. Anderson RL, Panje WR, Gross CE: Optic nerve blindness following blunt forehead trauma. *Ophthalmology* 89:445, 1982.

4. Bailey JH: Surgical anatomy of the lacrimal sac. *Am J Ophthalmol* 6:665, 1923.

5. Beer GM, Putz R, Mager K, et al: Variations of the exit if the supraorbital nerve: An anatomic study. *Plast Reconstr Surg* 102:334, 1998.

6. Bisaria KK, Saxena RC, Bisaria SD, et al: The lacrimal fossa in Indians. *J Anat* 166:265, 1989.

7. Burkat CN, Lemke BN: Anatomy of the orbit and its related structures. *Otolaryngol Clin N Am* 38:825, 2005.

8. de Haan AB, Willekens BL: Embryology of the orbital walls. *Mod Probl Ophthalmol* 14:57, 1975.

9. Deveci M, Oztürk S, Sengezer M, Pabuşcu Y: Measurement of orbital volume by a 3-dimensional software program: An experimental study. *J Oral Maxiofac Surg* 58:645, 2000.

10. Diamond MK: The groove in the orbital face of the greater wing of the sphenoid. A new interpretation. *J Anat* 173:97, 1990.

11. Ducasse A, Delattre JF, Segal A, et al: Anatomical basis of the surgical approach to the medial wall of the orbit. *Anat Clin* 7:15, 1985.

12. Dutton JJ: Management of blow-out fractures of the orbital floor (editorial). *Surv Ophthalmol* 35:279, 1991.

13. Dutton JJ: Orbital complications of paranasal sinus surgery. *Ophthal Plast Reconstr Surg* 2:119, 1986.

14. Dutton JJ: Radiographic evaluation of the orbit. In: Doxanas MT, Anderson RL (eds): *Clinical Orbital Anatomy*. Baltimore, Williams and Wilkins, 1984, pp 35–56.

15. Endo B: Biomechanical simulation study on the forms of the frontal bone and facial bones of the recent human facial skeleton by using a two-dimensional frame model with stepwise variable cross-section members. *Okajimas Folia Anat Jpn* 64:335, 1988.

16. Evans RA, Schwartz JF, Chutorian AM: Radiologic diagnosis in pediatric ophthalmology. *Radiol Clin N Am* 1:459, 1963.

17. Fan X, Li J, Zhu J, et al: Computer-assisted orbital volume measurement in the surgical correction of later enophthalmos caused by blowout fractures. *Ophthal Plast Reconstr Surg* 19:207, 2003.

18. Fukado Y: Results in 400 cases of surgical decompression of the optic nerve. *Mod Prob Ophthalmol* 14:474, 1975.

19. Furuta M: Measurement of orbital volume by computed tomography: Especially on the growth of the orbit. *Jpn J Ophthalmol* 45:600, 2001.

20. Goalwin HA: One thousand optic canals. Clinical, anatomic and roentgenologic study. *JAMA* 89:1745, 1922.

21. Goodyear HM: Ophthalmic considerations referable to diseases of the paranasal sinuses. *Arch Otolaryngol* 48:202, 1948.

22. Habal MB, Maniscalco JE: Surgical relationships of the orbit and optic nerve: An anatomical study under magnification. *Ann Past Surg* 4:265, 1980.

23. Harris HA: *Bone Growth in Health and Disease*. London, Oxford University Press, 1933.

24. Hughes B: Indirect injury of the optic nerves and chiasm. *Bull Johns Hopkins Hosp* 111:98, 1962.

25. Hylander WL, Picq PG, Johnson KR: Function of the supraorbital region of primates. *Arch Oral Biol* 36:273, 1991.

26. Iliff CE: Mucoceles in the orbit. *Arch Ophthalmol* 89:392, 1973.

27. Jones LT, Wobig JL: *Surgery of the Eyelids and Lacrimal System*. Birmingham, Aesculapius, 1976, p 4.

28. Katzel EB, Koltz PF, Kahn DM, et al: Aging of the facial skeleton: Aesthetic implications and rejuvenation strategies. *Plast Reconstr Surg* 125:332, 2010.

29. Kennerdell JS, Amsbaugh GA, Myers EN: Transantral-ethmoidal decompression of optic canal fracture. *Arch Ophthalmol* 94:1040, 1976.

30. Kennerdell JS, Maroon JC: An orbital decompression for severe dysthyroid exophthalmos. *Ophthalmology* 89:467, 1982.

31. Kier EL: Embryology of the normal optic canal and its anomalies. *Invest Radiol* 1:346, 1966.

32. Kirchner JA, Gisawae Y, Crelin ES: Surgical anatomy of the ethmoidal arteries. A laboratory study of 150 orbits. *Arch Otolaryngol* 74:382, 1961.

33. Kurihashi K, Yamashita A: Anatomical considerations for dacryocystorhinostomy. *Ophthalmologica* 203:1, 1991.

34. Kwon J, Barrera JE, Jung TY, Most SP: Measurement of orbital volume change using computed tomography in isolated orbital blowout fractures. *Arch Facial Plast Surg* 11:395, 2009.

35. Carsolio Diaz CM, Escudero Morere PC: Upper and medial alveolar nerves. Study of their frequency and point of origin in 100 cases. *An Fac Odontol* 25:5, 1989.

36. Lemke BN, Dells Rocca R: *Surgery of the Eyelids and Orbit: An Anatomic Approach*. East Norwalk, CT, Appleton & Lange, 1990.

37. Low FN: An anomalous middle meningeal artery. *Anat Rec* 95:347, 1946.

38. McQueen CT, DiRuggiero DC, Campbell JP, Shockley WW: Orbital Osteology: A study of the surgical landmarks. *Laryngoscope* 105:783, 1995.

39. Miller TA, Rudkin G, Honig M, et al: Lateral subcutaneous brow lift and interbrow muscle resection: Clinical experience and anatomic studies. *Plast Reconstr Surg* 105:1120, 2000.

40. Nagasao T, Hikosaka M, Morotomi T, et al: Analysis of the orbital floor morphology. *J Craniomax Surg* 35:112, 2007.

41. Neuhaus RW, Bayliss HI: Cerebrospinal fluid leakage after dacryocystorhinostomy. *Ophthalmology* 90:1091, 1983.

42. Nitek SN, Wysocki J, Reymond J, Piasecki K: Correlations between selected parameters of the human skull and orbit. *Med Sci Monit* 15:BR370, 2009.

43. Parsons GS, Mathog RH: Orbital wall and volume relationships. *Arch Otolaryngol Head Neck Surg* 114:743, 1988.

44. Patnaik VVG, Bala S, Singla RK: Anatomy of the bony orbit— Some applied aspects. *J Anat Soc India* 50:59, 2002.

45. Potter GD: Tomography of the orbit. *Radiol Clin North Am* 10:21, 1972.

46. Richard MJ, Morris CM, Deen BF, et al: Analysis of the anatomic changes of the aging facial skeleton using computer-assisted tomography. *Ophthal Plast Reconstr Surg* 25:382, 2009.

47. Jo A, Rizen V, Nikolic V, Banovic B: The role of orbital wall morphological properties and their supporting structures in the etiology of "blow-out" fractures. *Surg Radiol Anat* 11:241, 1989.

48. Russell MD: The supraorbital torus: "A most remarkable peculiarity." *Curr Anthrop* 26:337, 1985.

49. Russell WK: Injury to cranial nerves including the optic nerve and chiasm. In: Brock S (ed): *Injuries of the Skull, Brain and Spinal Cord.* London, Bailliere, 1940.

50. Scolozzi P, Momjian A, Heuberger J: Computer-aided volumetric comparison of reconstructed orbits for blow-out fractures with nonpreformed versus 3-dimensionally preformed titanium mesh plates: A preliminary study. *J Comput Assist Tomogr* 3:98, 2010.

51. Sharma PK, Malhotra VK, Tewari SP: Variation in the shape of the superior orbital fissure. *Anat Anz* 165:55, 1988.

52. Smith B, Regan WF Jr: Blow-out fracture of the orbit: Mechanism and correction of internal orbital fracture. *Am J Ophthalmol* 44:733, 1957.

53. Song WK, Lew H, Yoon JS, et al: Role of medial orbital wall morphologic properties in orbital blow-out fractures. *Invest Ophthalmol* 50:495, 2009.

54. Stanley EJ, McCaffrey TV, Offord KP, DeSanto LW: Superior and transorbital decompression procedures. *Arch Otolaryngol Head Neck Surg* 115:369, 1989.

55. Sugita S, Sugita Y, Yamada J, Kawabe Y: Die Sehstorung nach Schadeltrauma und ihre operative Behandlung. *Klin Monatsbl Augenheilk* 147:720, 1965.

56. Thaller VT: Enucleation volume measurement. *Ophthal Plast Reconstr Surg* 13:18, 1997.

57. Van Alyea OE: Sphenoid sinus: Anatomic study with consideration of the clinical significance of the structural characteristics of the sphenoid sinus. *Arch Otolaryngol* 34:225, 1941.

58. Watters EC, Waller PH, Hiles DA, Michaels RH: Acute orbital cellulitis. *Arch Ophthalmol* 94:785, 1976.

59. Webster RC, Gaunt JM, Hamdan US, et al: Supraorbital and supratrochlear notches and foramina: Anatomical variations and surgical relevance. *Laryngoscope* 96:311, 1986.

60. Wible JR: The eutherian stapedial artery: Character analysis and implications for supraordinal relationships. *Zool J Linnean Soc* 97:107, 1987.

61. Williams PL, Bannister LH, Berry MM, et al: Gray's anatomy. In: Saoemes RW (ed): *Skeletal System.* Edinburgh, Churchill Livingstone, 1999, pp 555–560.

CHAPTER 3

Extraocular Muscles

Embryology

The extrinsic muscles of the eye develop from mesenchymal condensations in the future embryonic orbital region, and can be identified as individual muscles by the 22 mm (6-week) stage.[28,60] The origin of these muscles remains a matter of some controversy. By conventional theory the extraocular muscle primordia first appear around the prechordal plate, the future site of the mouth, which appears to serve as an important organizer of the head region. The mesenchyme in this area gives rise to three preotic condensations, each supplied by its own cranial nerve (III, IV, or VI).[48] In the evolution of primitive vertebrates, these may have been anterior axial mesodermal somites continuous with those of the trunk, but separated from the latter by the expanding vertebrate braincase.[62] These muscle primordia were believed to migrate from their points of origin at the orbital apex, forward to their sites of insertion on the globe.

In higher vertebrates these primordial condensations cannot be assigned to specific mesodermal somites, and the head region does not demonstrate a clear segmental organization. In the chick embryo, however, cranial paraxial mesoderm does show vague condensations with intervening areas of less dense mesenchyme. But these somitomeres fail to transform into true somites as they do beside the hindbrain and spinal cord. These cranial somitomeres have not been identified in mammals. However, the arrangement of mesoderm in the head region of mammals is qualitatively similar to that of the chick.[50] Concomitant with development of the cranial mesoderm, neural crest cells migrate laterally and ventrally around the optic stalks and cups, and eventually form the maxillary and frontonasal processes. The periocular and orbital tissues will be derived from this complex mesenchyme, mainly of neural crests cells with some contribution from the mesoderm. The mesodermal mesenchyme gives rise to the vascular endothelium, hematopoietic tissue, and to the skeletal muscles. The neural crest mesenchyme contributes exclusively to the sensory nerves, autonomic ganglia, Schwann cells, and pigment cells, and it contributes largely to development of the cranial bones, tendons, dermis, connective tissue, and the periocular smooth muscle.

More recent observations have suggested that the extraocular muscles and their connective tissue components differentiate simultaneously along their entire lengths,[69] from mesenchyme derived from cranial neural crest cells. According to this concept the superior rectus, superior oblique, and levator muscle, and the upper portions of the medial and lateral rectus muscles develop from a superior mesenchymal complex within the developing orbit. Initially they share a common epimysium, and they insert onto the globe in a layered fashion (viz. superior oblique, superior rectus, and levator) from posterior to anterior, and from deep to superficial. The inferior rectus, inferior oblique, and the lower portions of the medial and lateral rectus muscles form from an inferior mesenchymal complex.[67,69,70] The inferior oblique and inferior rectus muscles share a common epimysium in early development, but later separate. However, in the adult, they still retain a fused sheath or conjoined fascia at their points of crossing at Lockwood's ligament.

All six extraocular muscles are distinguishable by the 22 mm (6-week) embryonic stage. By the 26 mm (7-week) stage, the origins of the rectus muscles can be seen attached to perichondrium at the orbital apex. The origin of the superior oblique is contiguous with the medial rectus muscle. The superior rectus and levator palpebrae superioris are already distinct, although they still share a common epimysium. The inferior oblique muscle originates by muscular fibers from perichondrium at the inferomedial orbital rim. Chondroblasts begin to differentiate in the region of the trochlea at this time. By the 38 mm (8-week) stage the rectus muscle tendons begin to differentiate, but the junction between them and the muscle fibers remains indistinct. Mesenchymal condensations appear in the sclera near the regions of the developing rectus muscle tendons. At this stage, the tendons insert onto the globe along a very broad zone from the equator to the future corneal limbus. The two heads of the lateral rectus muscle can be distinguished by the 54 mm (10-week) stage. By the 62 mm (12-week) stage early neuromuscular contacts are established.

Between the 38 and 210 mm (8–25-week) stages the rectus muscle insertions undergo selective degeneration, ultimately leaving only a narrow zone of attachment anterior to the equator. By the 83 mm (13-week) stage chondrocytes appear in the trochlea, and the superior oblique tendon begins to differentiate. The rectus muscle tendons mature, and are distinguished by parallel bundles of collagen by the 165 mm (22-week) fetal stage. The junctional zones between the tendon fibers and their respective muscles are clearly demarcated at this time.[69] Unlike the adult pattern, at this stage the insertions of all the rectus muscles are situated equidistant from the corneal limbus. Cytological differentiation between fiber types can be distinguished, as can the orbital and global layering structure.

Initially, the rectus muscles originate directly from the perichondrium along the cartilage precursor of the sphenoid bone at the orbital apex. Between the 40 and 210 mm (10–25-week) stages, a ring of perichondrium gradually thickens around the sites of muscle attachment. As the cartilaginous braincase ossifies beginning at the 225 mm (26-week) stage, this thickened ring of periosteum extends forward into the orbit, and partially separates from the orbital walls to form the annulus of Zinn. It remains attached to the orbital bones only at the superomedial border of the optic canal, and at the midportion of the superior orbital fissure. The levator muscle separates from the superior rectus at this time. Incomplete separation, or initiation of myopathic development prior to this stage is associated with the clinical condition of combined congenital ptosis and superior rectus muscle weakness.

At term, the superior oblique muscle separates from the annulus of Zinn, and its origin becomes restricted to the junction of the frontal and ethmoid bones, immediately above and medial to the annular origin of the medial rectus muscle. The insertions of the rectus muscle tendons on the sclera begin to migrate backward, achieving varying distances from the corneal limbus. This process continues until about 2 years of age, when adult relationships are attained, and the definitive spiral of Tillaux is finally established.

Adult anatomy

In the adult, the extraocular muscles are specialized striated skeletal muscles.[72] They differ structurally from limb muscles in showing greater variability in fiber size and shape, in having more small fibers, in containing greater vascularity, and in having a looser connective tissue envelope with greater elastic fibers. Each muscle is enclosed within a collagenous connective tissue sheath, the epimysium, which blends distally with the tendon of insertion. Extensions of this sheath divide the muscle into individual bundles or fascicles, each surrounded by a fibrous layer, the perimysium. Each of the muscle fibers is surrounded by fine collagenous fibers, the endomysium, that separates the fibers one from another.

Extraocular muscles are among the fastest muscles in mammals. The speed of muscle contraction and fatigue characteristics correlate with fiber type and structure. These types differ in myosin isoform, sarcoplasmic reticulum calcium pump type, and the quality of t-tube and sarcoplasmic reticulum elements.[57] Early studies by light microscopy recognized two fiber types by histologic appearance. The *fibrillenstruktur* fibers were described as fine, uniformly stippled fibers with small, well-organized myofibrils arranged in discrete bundles. They were thought to contract briskly to individual neurologic impulses, and to have very short contraction-relaxation cycles. These were believed to be responsible for rapid saccadic and pursuit movements. The more granular *felderstruktur* fibers were described to show a more random arrangement of irregular myofilaments that were more poorly defined and partially fused together.[19] These fibers were thought to be characterized by slower, graded contractions, the force of which is proportional to repetitive neurologic stimulation. They were believed to be responsible for coordination and maintenance of muscle tonicity. In contrast to light microscopy, histochemical classification based on characteristics

commonly used for limb muscles demonstrated at least three distinct fiber types. The fine fibers are similar to type 1 fibers of mammalian limb muscles, and are usually considered responsible for slow twitch. Granular fibers resemble type 2 fibers, and are responsible for fast twitch movements. The course fibers, equivalent to the *felderstruktur* fibers, have a unique histochemical profile, and may be equivalent to the multiple-innervated tonic fibers seen in amphibian and bird musculature.[61]

More recent studies have emphasized the distinctness of the unique extraocular muscle phenotype adapted to exploit the full range of variability in skeletal muscle.[59,72] There are now six muscle fiber types in extraocular muscles, recognized on the basis of location, color, and innervation pattern.[57] The extraocular muscles show two distinct layers characterized by different proportions of these fiber types. The outer "orbital layer" is adjacent to the orbital walls and contain about 55% of the total fibers in the muscle. The orbital layer also contains about 50% greater vascular supply compared with the global layer. 20% of the fibers in this layer are multiple innervated slow, non-twitch generating fibers. About 80% are small diameter, singly innervated fast-twitch fibers capable of rapid eye movement and saccades.[57] Most of these are red fibers that show high fatigue resistance with more developed mitochondrial content and oxidative enzyme activity.[12,72] They retain some embryonic traits such as embryonic myosin heavy chain isoforms,[5] and neural cell adhesion molecule. This orbital layer does not extend the full length of the muscle complex, but rather ends anteriorly before the muscle passes into its tendon of insertion. These fibers insert into the connective tissues of the muscle's suspensory pulley system near the equator of the globe. This layer appears to be specialized for continuous elastic loading by the pulley system.

The inner or "global" layer of each rectus muscle faces the optic nerve. About 10% if its fibers are multiply innervated slow-twitch generating fibers that are capable of slow graded pursuit movements.[12,57] 90% of its fibers are singly innervated fast-twitch generating fibers divided into red, intermediate, and white fibers distinguished by density of mitochondria and fatigue resistance. The red fibers, constituting about 33% of the total, are more highly fatigue resistant compared to the intermediate and white fibers. This global layer inserts anteriorly into the sclera through a well-defined tendon. The levator muscle does not show this layered structure.

Spindles have been described in all human extraocular muscles, although their presence in other vertebrates is variable, and does not follow any phyletic pattern. They are concentrated in the proximal and distal ends of the muscle, and are sparse in the central one-third zone, containing motor end plates. The first order afferent neurons from these structures run with their respective motor nerves, and synapse in the mesencephalic nucleus of the trigeminal nerve.[74] The function of these spindles remains uncertain, since experimental data demonstrate the absence of a stretch reflex for extraocular muscles in the monkey, and presumably also in humans.[38] Also, their anomalous and simplified structure subjects them to a greater degree of direct mechanical influences from adjacent muscle fibers,[41] throwing into question their capacity to provide useful proprioceptive information.[63] They may play a role in the unconscious maintenance of efferent signals.[22]

In addition to their function in ocular motility, the six extraocular muscles also help to suspend the eye within the axial portion of the orbit. Individually, the four rectus muscles rotate the eye into their respective fields of action. Collectively, they pull the eye posteriorly and slightly medially against the intraconal fat pockets. The two oblique muscles exert more complex vector forces, including a forward pull on the eye. The rectus muscles, together with their connective tissue sheaths and intermuscular septa, define the muscle cone which delimits the central orbital space anteriorly. More posteriorly, this cone is incomplete due to the incomplete nature of the intermuscular septum (see Chapter 7). Within this muscle cone lie structures essential to normal ocular function. These include the globe, the optic nerve, portions of the ophthalmic artery and ophthalmic veins, the oculomotor and abducens nerves, and the ciliary ganglion and nerves.

The levator palpebrae superioris muscle develops phylogenetically and embryologically from the superior rectus muscle. It has become specialized as a retractor of the upper eyelid, and is discussed in detail in Chapter 8.

The annulus of Zinn

The superior orbital fissure (SOF) is an opening between the orbit and the middle cranial fossa. It is situated between the body, greater, and lesser wings of the sphenoid bone. It is an elongated opening that slopes downward from superolateral to inferomedial at the orbital apex beneath the optic canal. The fissure is a comma-shaped opening with the narrow portion superiorly, and the wider portion inferiorly. There are three borders of the SOF.[80] The superior border is bounded by the lesser wing of the sphenoid bone, the anterior clinoid process and the optic strut. The lateral border is formed by the greater sphenoid wing. The medial border is formed by the optic strut superiorly and the body of the sphenoid bone inferiorly.

The four rectus muscles take origin from a fibrotendinous ring at the orbital apex, the annulus of Zinn or common annular tendon. The annulus begins at the orbital openings of the optic canal and superior orbital fissure as a diffuse fibrous layer. It is continuous with periorbita around the orbital apex, the dura mater of the middle cranial fossa, cavernous sinus, and the optic canal, and the fibrous component of the optic nerve sheath. Posteriorly, an extension of this fibrous layer inserts along the body of the sphenoid bone beneath the optic canal, and along the length of the optic strut. The posterior-most insertion of the annular connective tissue fibers is actually intracranial, where it originates from the lateral wall of the sphenoid bone just below the anterior clinoid process. At about 2 mm anterior to the optic strut, the annulus becomes a more well-defined circular structure. It remains firmly connected to the orbital walls medially and laterally, and a thick fibrous band anchors it inferiorly to the connective tissue and smooth muscle fibers bridging over the inferior orbital fissure.

The annulus of Zinn encloses the orbital opening of the optic canal. It does not surround the entire superior orbital fissure, but only encloses the central one-third, lateral to the optic strut and optic canal. Thus, the annulus divides the SOF into three portions, a central ring through the center of the annulus, and extra-annular portions above and below the fibrous ring.

The annulus consists of two approximate half circles, the tendon of Lockwood superiorly, and the tendon of Zinn inferiorly. Where the two meet superomedially, the annulus is firmly fused to dura and periorbita along the margin of the optic foramen. More anteriorly, attachments to the medial wall become less extensive, but the annulus maintains a broad connection to the dural sheath of the optic nerve for at least 8 mm in front of the optic strut. The annulus of Zinn encloses a central opening known as the oculomotor foramen. This opening encircles the central portion of the superior orbital fissure and the optic canal, and through it pass neurovascular elements from the middle cranial fossa into the intraconal orbital space.[49]

The tendon of Zinn is the more inferior and thicker of the two portions of the annulus of Zinn. It is attached to the greater wing of the sphenoid bone laterally through firm connections to periorbita lining the superior orbital fissure. Medially, it is attached to the body of the sphenoid bone along the medial orbital surface of the optic foramen. It serves as the origin for the inferior, medial, and lateral rectus muscles. These muscles originate as three tiny clusters of striated muscle fibers located within the fibrous annulus. They are separated from each other by wide bands of connective tissue. As these muscles extend anteriorly and thicken, the fibrous connective tissue bands between them narrow. When the muscles emerge from the anterior end of the annulus they are still separated from each other by thin laminae of fibrous tissue that finally blend into the muscular sheaths. Thus, the sheaths of the rectus muscles can be visualized as anterior sleeve-like extensions from the annulus of Zinn. As the lateral rectus muscle emerges from the annulus, it maintains strong fascial attachments to the greater wing of the sphenoid bone just below the superior orbital fissure. Medially, the medial rectus muscle also has fibrous attachments to periorbita along the body of the sphenoid bone.

From the lower edge of the tendon of Zinn, a bundle of fascial strands extends inferiorly where it joins the connective tissue and smooth orbital muscle of Müller which bridge over the inferior orbital fissure. Between the annulus and Müller's muscle are dilated venous channels derived from the inferior ophthalmic vein. The possible functional significance of this arrangement is discussed in Chapter 6.

The superior half of the annulus is formed by the much less well-developed tendon of Lockwood. Laterally, this bridges over the superior orbital fissure and inserts onto the spina recti lateralis, a small bony spur on the apical edge of the greater wing of the sphenoid bone. Here, it also attaches to periorbita around the margins of the superior orbital fissure, and blends with fibrous bands from the lateral extent of the tendon of Zinn. Immediately on either side of this attachment zone lie the neurovascular elements entering the orbit through the superior fissure. Medially, the tendon of Lockwood fuses with dura and periorbita at the lesser wing of the sphenoid along the superomedial roof of the optic foramen. The tendon of Lockwood serves as the origin for the superior rectus muscle. The medial fibers of this muscle lie in close proximity to the dural sheath of the optic nerve to which the annulus is fused in this region. The most posterior superior rectus muscle fibers may be seen originating from a fibrous central bridge between the tendons of Lockwood and Zinn. A superior head of the lateral rectus muscle may take origin from the lateral aspect of the tendon of Lockwood.

When it does, it spans across the central superior orbital fissure to join the main mass of the muscle laterally.

At their most posterior extent, the tendons of Lockwood and Zinn are connected centrally by a narrow fibrous bridge that divides the oculomotor foramen vertically, separating the optic foramen from the superior orbital fissure. This bridge is a connective-tissue forward extension of the bony optic strut. Slightly more anteriorly, where the annulus is best developed, this bridge disappears, leaving the central oculomotor foramen.

The oculomotor foramen transmits the oculomotor (III), abducens (VI), nasociliary (branch of V1) nerves, and sympathetic fibers from the cavernous sinus into the orbital apex. Just before entering the annulus, the oculomotor nerve divides into its superior and inferior divisions that course through the annular opening medial to the nasociliary nerve. The superior division enters just below the origin of the superior rectus muscle and sends branches to both the superior rectus and the levator muscles. The inferior division courses inferiorly and divides into branches to the medial and inferior rectus and the inferior oblique muscles. It also gives rise to a small motor parasympathetic root to the ciliary ganglion (see Chapter 4). The nasociliary branch of the trigeminal nerve divides from the ophthalmic nerve in the anterior cavernous sinus. It passes through the annular tendon between the two divisions of the oculomotor nerve and then crosses over the optic nerve from lateral to medial. It gives rise to a sensory root to the ciliary ganglion that arises within the annulus or in the anterior cavernous sinus.[49] The abducens nerve enters the annulus lateral to the inferior division of the oculomotor nerve and adjacent to the origin of the lateral rectus muscle that it innervates on its conal surface.

The superior sector of the SOF above the annular tendon is bounded by the lesser wing of the sphenoid superiorly and the greater wing inferiorly. It carries the frontal and lacrimal branches of the ophthalmic nerve (V1), the trochlear nerve (IV), and the superior ophthalmic vein. All structures passing through this section of the SOF are extraconal in the orbit. As the trochlear nerve runs forward in the cavernous sinus it ascends on the superomedial side of the ophthalmic nerve. It passes through the SOF above the annulus of Zinn and continues medially along the orbital roof between the levator muscle and periorbita to the superior oblique muscle.

The inferior sector of the SOF below the annulus of Zinn is bounded by the body of the sphenoid bone medially and inferiorly, the greater wing laterally, and the annular tendon superiorly. Orbital fat extends backward into this sector of the fissure, and its floor contains smooth muscle fibers continuous with that covering the inferior orbital fissure. Sympathetic nerve fibers from the intracavernous carotid plexus pass through this fat as they collect into a sympathetic root to the ciliary ganglion (see Chapter 4). The inferior ophthalmic vein also passes through this sector of the SOF.

The origin of the levator palpebrae superioris is the most anterior of all the extraocular muscles. It arises primarily from the tendon of Lockwood in the area of fusion between the latter and adjacent dura, and some fibers may also arise from adjacent periorbita over the lesser wing of the sphenoid bone. Here, the muscle has a thickened triangular shape as it is partially crowded between the origins of the superior and medial rectus muscles. However, it quickly flattens and moves upward to a position over the medial half of the superior rectus muscle.

Clinical correlations

The anatomic relationships of the rectus muscles, annulus of Zinn, superior orbital fissure, and optic canal are of some clinical significance. The contiguity of the medial and superior rectus muscles with the optic nerve sheath at the orbital apex is responsible for the painful ophthalmoplegia associated with retrobulbar optic neuritis affecting this portion of the nerve. Contraction of these muscles is transmitted directly to the inflamed dura at the entrance to the optic canal. Thickening of the medial and inferior rectus muscles associated with thyroid orbitopathy, especially when near the orbital apex, is a major cause of compression of the optic nerve as it enters the optic canal adjacent to the body of the sphenoid bone. At this point, the muscle origins are firmly embedded within the annular connective tissue, and therefore cannot be displaced by the expanding muscle mass. The annulus keeps these enlarged muscles in a rigid position resulting in compression of the optic nerve. During superior orbital surgery with unroofing of the superior orbital fissure or optic canal, the annulus of Zinn may be opened most easily between the medial edge of the superior rectus and the origin of the medial rectus muscle. Division of the annulus in this region carries the least risk to neurovascular structures, most of which are concentrated superolaterally. To gain access to this portion of the annulus, the origin of the levator must first be disinserted and reflected.[32] The annulus must then be dissected from dura covering the optic nerve, to which it is firmly adherent.

The rectus muscles

At birth, the eye muscles are about 50–60% of their final adult dimensions. During the postnatal period, corresponding to the period of visual maturation, definitive muscles characteristics become established.[57] The relative growth of muscles within the enlarging orbit, and their angular relations with the globe, then remain nearly constant from childhood into adulthood.[22]

As noted above, the rectus muscles originate within the annulus of Zinn. The zone of attachment for each muscle is cone-shaped, with central fibers located more posterior than peripheral fibers. For the first 5–6 mm of their lengths, the muscles are buried within the fibrous annulus and do not appear as individual structures. Toward the anterior surface of the annulus the medial, inferior, and lateral rectus muscles thicken within the tendon of Zinn, and abut each other along broad, flat surfaces separated only by relatively thin zones of connective tissue. The entire inferior annulus, thus, forms a single structural unit of muscle masses encased within a fibrotendinous half-ring. The medial rectus muscle arises as a single head from the annulus of Zinn and the adjacent dura around the optic nerve. The lateral rectus muscle may arise as two distinct slips. The superior rectus muscle, like the medial rectus, shows some origin from the adjacent dura of the optic nerve.[69]

By about 8 mm anterior to the optic strut the rectus muscles separate as individual structures while the fibrous tissue of the annulus thins and becomes continuous with the muscle sheaths. At this level, the medial and lateral rectus muscles lose most of their strong fascial connections to the adjacent periorbita. The four rectus muscles pass forward from the orbital apex, parallel to their respective orbital walls. Each muscle measures 40–42 mm in length, excluding its tendon of insertion, is 7–10 mm in width, and about 2.5–4.0 mm thick at its midpoint. In the orbital apex, the rectus muscles lie close to their respective bony walls, a distance generally less than 1 mm.[44] In the mid-orbit, the entire muscle cone shifts slightly medially, so that the lateral rectus lies 3–5 mm from the lateral orbital wall, whereas the other rectus muscles are located less than 1.5 mm from their respective bony walls. At the level of the ocular equator, the muscle cone becomes centered within the orbit, and the distance between the muscle insertions and the orbital walls increases to about 7–8 mm. In this region the connective tissues of the muscle suspensory and pulley systems thicken, are interconnected, and form more extensive attachments to the adjacent periorbita.

The rectus muscles continue forward where they pass through tunnels in Tenon's capsule, to enter the sub-Tenon's episcleral space. As they approach posterior Tenon's capsule numerous fine fascial bands extend from the muscle sheaths to the outer layer of Tenon's forming part of the pulley-suspensory systems. The muscles continue through Tenon's capsule where membranous extensions of the muscle sheath blend with the inner layers of Tenon's to form several prominent check ligaments associated with each muscle. These prevent the muscle from retracting into the orbit when they are disinserted during muscle or enucleation surgery. As the rectus muscles approach their insertions they arc over the globe. This zone of contact varies from 6 mm for the medial rectus muscle to 13 mm for the lateral rectus muscle. The rectus muscles finally insert onto the sclera by tendons that vary from 3.7 mm in length for the medial rectus, to 8.8 mm for the lateral rectus muscle.[1] At their insertions, the tendons measure 9–11 mm in width, except for the superior rectus muscle that only measures about 7 mm in width. Collagen fibers of the tendons blend with the superficial fibers of the sclera over an anteroposterior distance of several millimeters. The shape of the insertion zone varies from linear to oblique, to concave. Each rectus muscle is capable of rotating the eye through an arc of 75–100°.

Accessory muscles

Occasionally accessory extraocular muscles are seen in primates, and more rarely in humans.[53] These frequently represent an atavistic vestige of the retractor bulbi muscle system of lower vertebrates that disappeared in anthropoid apes and humans. This was correlated with the evolution of bifoveate fixation and the need for ocular stability.

Although there are typically four rectus muscles in humans, an accessory lateral rectus muscle is usual in cercopithecid monkeys.[33,66] It is innervated by the abducens nerve, and inserts onto the globe posterior and superior to the normal muscle. This accessory muscle may represent an evolutionary transition between the lower mammalian retractor bulbi system and the condition in higher primates, including humans, where these muscles are normally absent.[44] Although some investigators have suggested that this muscle is too small to have any significant effect on ocular motility, more recent studies have demonstrated that the accessory lateral rectus muscle does have the potential to contribute to both elevation and abduction.[4] The evolutionary loss of this muscle in humans, combined with the nasal-temporal asymmetry in movement and motion processing systems proposed by Tychsen and Lisberger,[75] has been used to explain the high incidence of esodeviations in humans and their near total absence in lower primates.[4]

The accessory lateral rectus muscle has not been described in humans, but other accessory muscles do occur. Their true incidence is probably higher than has been appreciated, and we have seen a number of examples in both cadavers and in surgical specimens. Histologic examination of accessory muscles in other mammals has shown two or three fiber types that would be expected from a muscle that is only transiently activated, as is true of the retractor bulbi system in most vertebrates and lower primates.[57] These fibers are fast and fatigable.

Accessory muscles occur most frequently in the superior orbit, associated with the superior rectus or levator muscles[35] (see Chapter 10). They are usually innervated by the oculomotor nerve. In the superomedial orbit, an accessory muscle may be seen originating from the medial edge of the levator muscle, and running along its medial side. In some cases, it may arise from the orbital fascial septa in the superomedial orbit. This muscle varies in development from only a few fibers seen histologically, to a robust muscle easily visible on gross dissection. It inserts onto the orbital fascia near the trochlea, and may additionally send some fibers to the levator aponeurosis, to the periorbita, and to the fascia surrounding the origin of the superior ophthalmic vein. Another variant is a small accessory muscle in the superolateral orbit, originating from the lateral superior rectus muscle. It runs in the superotemporal orbit near periorbita, and inserts onto the capsule of the lacrimal gland (see Figures 10-4 to 10-7). It may send some fibers to the lateral horn of the levator aponeurosis as well. Although it is highly variable in development, this muscle may serve in part to retract the lacrimal gland and lateral aponeurosis during upgaze. Accessory muscles also occur between the medial and inferior rectus muscles. Although the exact functions of these and other accessory muscles remain unclear, some probably represent developmental anomalies or retained experiments in evolutionary diversity.

Muscle sheaths and pulleys

Each of the rectus muscles is surrounded by a thin fibrous sheath that represents an anterior connective tissue extension of the annulus of Zinn. These sheaths are partially interconnected circumferentially by thin fascial sheets, which form the intermuscular septum. These layers are incomplete posteriorly, and only vaguely defined anteriorly. A complex system of fine connective tissue septa also extend between the individual muscles, the intermuscular septum, the optic nerve, Tenon's capsule, and periorbita. This system helps maintain the positional and functional relationships of these structures during ocular movement (see Chapter 7). Previous investigations suggested that, with rotation of the globe the points of tangency of the extraocular muscles in all three coordinates remain relatively constant with respect to the orbital walls, and that the unit of moment vector is also approximately fixed.[46,71] The propensity of extraocular muscles to slip sideways over the surface of the globe during excursions of gaze is related to: (1) muscle tension tending to take the shortest "great-circle" path from origin to insertion; (2) intermuscular forces created by fascial connections between muscle sheaths tending to keep the muscles from sliding over the globe; and (3) musculo-orbital forces exerted by fascial septa that fix the muscles to the orbital walls.[47] The fascial suspensory systems were, and still are generally thought of as stabilization structures. Yet, van den Bedem et al.[76] found that the pulley bands at the muscle bellies on tension showed significant slack of about 10 mm before becoming taut, and they suggested that these seemed unsuited to serve a stabilization function. Rather, they proposed that they might serve more to limit ocular excursion.

During the past decade concepts of eye movement mechanics have undergone rather dramatic change reflected in several different models.[30] The older concept where the rectus muscles pull in a straight line from their anatomic point of origin at the annulus of Zinn is no longer tenable and it is now recognized that the pull vector on the sclera is more anterior. This is associated with a complex connective tissue structure, called a pulley, that can inflect changes in the muscle paths.[15] Miller[47] was the first to advocate the "pulley" model of muscle suspension. According to this concept, the muscle sheaths and suspensory apparatus at the equator of the globe function more as pulleys through which the muscles move, and these are capable of changing the position, and therefore the direction of muscle pull with varying positions of gaze. These pulleys suspend the muscles to adjacent orbital walls by struts or "entheses" made of collagen, elastin, and smooth muscle.[9,16] More anteriorly the muscles form an encircling harness, where adjacent pulleys are coupled to each other and to the anterior hemisphere of the globe. Spencer and Porter[72] suggested that this system provides inflection points in extraocular muscle paths, thereby serving as functional origins for the muscles. Thus, both the intermuscular and musculo-orbital forces appear to play a coordinated role.

The finding of a layered compartmentalization of extraocular muscles with orbital and global layers having different insertion points led to the active pulley hypothesis. According to this concept, the outer orbital layer inserts on, and can modify movement of the pulley, whereas the inner global layer inserts onto sclera, and thereby influences movement of the globe. Movements of the globe and pulley are coordinated, but not necessarily coincident.[12,17] The active pulley system is said to use orbital layer motor units to alter pulley positions and thereby adjust muscle vector forces in different positions of gaze.[13,14,64] The various pulleys have been shown to be interconnected[40] and MRI examination shows stereotypic shifts of pulleys during gaze shifts.[10] For example, the inferior rectus pulley is coupled to the inferior oblique pulley by connective tissue bands containing heavy elastin deposits. The orbital layer of the inferior oblique muscle inserts partially on the conjoined inferior oblique-inferior rectus pulley, partially on the temporal inferior oblique muscle sheath, and partially on the pulley of the lateral rectus muscle. During downgaze, the crossing point of the inferior oblique shifts with respect to the inferior rectus muscle, related to shifting pulley positions.[18] Also, the inferior rectus pulley shifts nasally in supraduction and temporally in infraduction, thought to be related to this pulley coupling. Such gaze-related shifts can presumably change the functional origin of the muscle as far as its pull vector is concerned.

The active pulley concept proposes that this system may be a significant component of overall ocular motility.[39] During muscle contraction the orbital layer of the muscles pulls the pulleys in the anteroposterior direction against their suspensory elasticity and thereby changes force vector alignments. According to Clark et al.[10] this pulley mechanism simplifies the task of central oculomotor control by making commands independent of initial eye position.[72] Peng et al.[55] have recently shown a dual abducens nerve innervation of the lateral rectus muscle, with separate branches to the superior and inferior portions of the global layer of the muscle. While a central segregation of muscle function has not yet been determined, this anatomic finding suggests functionally distinct superior and inferior activation zones for this muscle, potentially mediating previously unappreciated torsional and vertical oculorotary actions.

Recent arguments have been put forth challenging the concept of active pulleys,[76] and Jampel et al.[34] contend that there is no physiologic evidence to support the concept of rectus muscle pulleys shifting the ocular rotation axes. Regardless of the continuing disagreement, the anatomic evidence clearly demonstrates a fascial suspensory system for each for the extraocular muscles, which in some measure can influence muscle orientation and the alignment of muscle forces. Whether this is an active or a passive system remains to be proven definitively.

The rectus muscle insertions

At the posterior surface of the globe the rectus muscles pierce the posterior portion of Tenon's capsule, where they become invested by cowl-like extensions of this fibroelastic layer. At the equator of the globe, each muscle bends to follow the curvature of the eye. As the tendons approach their points of insertion on the sclera they flatten considerably, and develop firm connections to the thickened axial surfaces of the muscle sheaths through short collagenous bundles. Thin membranes extend from the muscle sheaths and tendons to Tenon's capsule forming the check ligaments. The muscle tendons finally attach to sclera anterior to the equator, where the collagen bundles of these tendinous fibers interdigitate with superficial scleral fibers over a zone of several millimeters.[1] The terminal tendons of the rectus muscles are 9–11 mm in width. The length of these tendons varies from 3.7 mm for the medial rectus, 5.5 mm for the inferior rectus, 8.8 mm for the lateral rectus, and 5.8 mm for the superior rectus muscle. Thus, resection of the medial rectus muscle is more likely to cut across muscle fibers and result in bleeding. The average distance from the anterior corneal limbus to the insertion for each muscle is also variable, but in general progressively increases around the globe from the medial rectus muscle (5.3 mm, ±0.7 mm), to the inferior rectus (6.8 mm, ±0.8 mm), lateral rectus (6.9 mm, ±0.7 mm), to the superior rectus muscle (7.9 mm, ±0.6 mm).[31] An imaginary line drawn through these muscle insertions is known as the spiral of Tillaux.

Clinically, the rectus muscle insertions have been used as a surgical guide to the location of the ora serrata in cases where that structure cannot be directly visualized or transilluminated.[45] However, because of the progressively increasing posterior position of the muscle insertions noted above, the ora serrata more accurately defines a plane that angles through the spiral of Tillaux, intersecting it approximately at the lateral rectus muscle insertion. The medial rectus muscle inserts anterior to the ora, and the superior rectus inserts posterior to it. The midpoint of the insertion of the lateral rectus muscle lies within 1 mm of the ora in 90% of individuals, and is the most useful clinical guide to its position.[78]

The intermuscular septum

The transparent and elastic intermuscular septum is present in only fragmented form posteriorly, and becomes better-defined at about the equator of the globe. Even here, however, the septum does not exist as a single membrane, but rather as a series of fascial sheets irregularly interconnecting the muscle sheaths, their pulley systems, and periorbita. These septal sheets extend forward with the rectus muscles, where they become fused to the sleeve of Tenon's capsule investing each muscle. Beneath Tenon's the fascial sheets partially coalesce again, and the reformed intermuscular septum continues forward as a separate layer between sclera and Tenon's. This layer finally fuses to the globe 2 mm from the corneal limbus, just before Tenon's capsule merges with the superficial sclera. Fine elastic check ligaments extend between the intermuscular septum and Tenon's capsule near the muscle insertions.

The intraconal fat pocket is contained within the space defined by the rectus muscles and the intermuscular septum. It is separated anteriorly from sclera by the posterior portion of Tenon's capsule. The extraconal fat pockets lie outside the rectus muscle cone, separated from the intraconal fat by the intermuscular septum. They continue forward over the rectus muscles external to Tenon's capsule (see Chapter 7). These fat pockets extend to within 4 mm of the muscle insertions, and end about 10–15 mm behind the corneal limbus.

The superior oblique muscle

The superior oblique muscle originates from the annulus of Zinn and from the lesser wing of the sphenoid bone by a short tendon, immediately above and medial to the annulus of Zinn. It passes forward just above the frontoethmoid suture line in the superomedial orbit. As it runs forward, the superior oblique is intimately involved in a delicate connective tissue system that supports the globe and suspends the muscle from the orbital frontal bone (see Chapter 7). The muscle rapidly thickens to its maximum diameter in the mid-orbit. Like the rectus muscles, the superior oblique shows regional differentiation of fiber types with an orbital layer of smaller fibers and a global layer of larger fibers. The orbital layer adjacent to the orbital wall forms a C-shaped band that wraps around the global portion of the muscle.[40]

At about 12–15 mm behind the orbital rim the muscle becomes circumferentially invested by a layer of collagen with elastin fibers that forms a sheath. Muscle fibers of the orbital layer become embedded into this sheath. Fine connective tissue fibers join the sheath to the superomedial periorbita. At about the same level, muscle fibers from the global layer begin to pass into the thick collagenous bundles that continue forward as the rounded superior oblique

tendon. Muscle fibers extend more anteriorly in the central portion of the tendon than they do peripherally, so that the point of transition is cone-shaped. The tendon, like the muscle posterior to it, remains invested by a fibrous sheath that is supported in a complex suspensory system of fascial septa attached to the adjacent orbital wall. The narrow tendon, along with its sheath, passes through the cartilaginous trochlea.

The trochlea is a saddle-shaped cartilaginous structure measuring about 4 × 6 mm and attached to periosteum of the frontal bone at a small depression, the fovea trochlearis, just behind the superomedial orbital rim. The trochlea serves to redirect the pulling vector force of the superior oblique muscle. Initially, this vector lies parallel to the superomedial orbital wall, and the force is in a posterior direction. At the trochlea this vector is shifted, so that force is directed in an anterior and medial direction, approximately 54° to the sagittal plane. A bursa-like fibrillovascular connective tissue layer over the cartilaginous saddle allows the oblique tendon to move freely within the trochlea.[31] The tendon does not slide through the trochlea as a solid cord. Rather, the tendinous fibers slide with respect to each other and parallel to their long axes, with the central fibers demonstrating a longer excursion than the paracentral fibers. The total range of motion of the superior oblique tendon is approximately 16 mm, or 8 mm on either side of the primary position.[20] The muscle is capable of rotating the globe through an arc of 33° of infraduction, 64° of incycloduction, and about 3° of abduction.

An outer fibrous connective tissue layer attaches the trochlea to periosteum of the orbital wall. During embryological development, the perichondrium of the trochlea is attached to the frontal bone only by fine fibrous strands. These thicken into a dense suspensory system fused to periosteum beginning at the 210 mm (25-week) fetal stage. During orbital decompression, external ethmoidectomy or mucocele excision, or for drainage of subperiosteal abscess or hematoma, the trochlea can easily be separated from bone by careful elevation of periosteum. This maintains the fascial connections between the trochlea and periorbital layer. To maintain normal function of the superior oblique muscle postoperatively, it is important to reposition the trochlea by meticulously reapproximating periosteum over the medial orbital rim.

After passing through the trochlea, the superior oblique tendon turns laterally, posteriorly, and slightly inferiorly, for a distance of about 8 mm. It pierces Tenon's capsule 3–4 mm nasal to the superior rectus muscle, becomes flattened, and continues beneath the superior rectus muscle. As it passes over the globe, the tendon makes an arc of contact with the sclera of about 10–14 mm. It finally inserts onto the sclera near the superotemporal vortex vein, approximately 6.5 mm from the exit of the optic nerve. The superior oblique sheath continues laterally and horizontally where it merges with the superior rectus muscle suspensory pulley system and with posterior Tenon's capsule. Whenever possible, surgery on the superior oblique tendon should be performed on the segment between its exit beneath Tenon's capsule and its insertion into sclera. This will avoid perforation of Tenon's and exposure of extraconal fat into the wound.

A supernumerary extraocular muscle may be present in a small percentage of normal individuals. An anomalous muscle may originate from the proximal dorsal surface of the superior oblique muscle, and insert onto the trochlea or its surrounding fascia. When present it is innervated by a branch of the trochlear nerve.[79] The function of these anomalous muscles is unknown, but they do not appear to have any significant effect on the function of the normal extraocular muscles.

The inferior oblique muscle

The inferior oblique muscle arises from periosteum in a shallow depression on the maxillary bone. The site of the muscular origin is about 4 mm in horizontal width by 2.5 mm in anteroposterior extent. It is situated an average of 1.5 mm lateral to the entrance of the bony nasolacrimal canal, and less than 1 mm behind the orbital rim.[43] The origin may easily be injured during extraperiosteal dissections along the orbital floor and medial wall for blow-out fracture repair, and during orbital decompression procedures. It is important to remain behind the posterior lacrimal crest during such operations.

The inferior oblique muscle courses posteriorly and laterally at about 51° to the medial orbital wall, and 62° to the mid-sagittal plane.[43] The orbital layer of fibers in the inferior oblique muscle not only attach to its suspensory and pulley system, but also to those of the inferior and lateral rectus muscles.[17] The muscle penetrates Tenon's capsule a short distance from its origin, on the medial side of the inferior rectus muscle. Its total length is approximately 37 mm. As the inferior oblique muscle passes inferior to the inferior rectus muscle, the individual fascial sheaths and the suspensory bands of each muscle become firmly fused to each other and to Tenon's capsule. Here, they form part of Lockwood's inferior ligament of the orbit (see Chapter 7). The inferior oblique muscle continues posterolaterally, making a long 17 mm arc of contact with the globe. It inserts into the posterior sclera over the macula without a tendon. The insertion measures about 10 mm in width, and its midpoint lies about 1 mm above the horizontal meridian. The insertion is tilted so that the anterior border lies 1–2 mm lower than the posterior border, and is located about 16 mm behind the lateral corneal limbus. The posterior border of the insertion lies 5–6 mm from the exit of the optic nerve. In nearly half of normal individuals, the muscle inserts as 2–6 separate slips (usually 2 or 3) that divide 5–6 mm before fusing with sclera.[24] If not recognized, this may result in incomplete recession during strabismus surgery.

The levator palpebrae superioris muscle

The levator muscle is not involved in ocular motility, but has become specialized during vertebrate evolution as a retractor of the upper eyelid. Embryologically it differentiates from the superior rectus muscle, and throughout embryologic development these two muscles share a common thickened epimysium. They separate by the 225 mm (26-week) fetal stage.[69] Despite their common origin, the levator muscle differs from the muscles of ocular motility in fiber type, commensurate with its unique function in maintaining eyelid position and in the blink reflex.[58] This muscle lacks a distinct orbital and global layered structure, and the multiply innervated fibers types. Instead it exhibits three singly innervated fiber types similar to those seen in the global layer of the extraocular muscles. It also has a true slow-twitch fiber type not seen in these other ocular muscles.[57]

In the adult the levator muscle fibers originate as a narrow slip from the lesser wing of the sphenoid bone just above the optic foramen, with some attachments to the outer surface of the annulus of Zinn, where it blends with fibers of the superior rectus muscle. The levator courses forward in close approximation to the superior rectus muscle. About 1 cm behind the orbital septum it passes into a thin membranous expansion, the levator aponeurosis, which fans out to insert into the upper eyelid (see Chapter 8). Fine fascial septa interconnect the levator and superior rectus muscle sheaths. During super-maximal levator muscle resection procedures for ptosis repair, these fascial attachments must be divided to prevent downward traction on the superior rectus through these fascial slips. Also, large vertical superior rectus muscle resections or recessions may alter the position of the eyelid because of these septa. Therefore, in the management of Graves' orbitopathy, it is important to correct any vertical strabismus before performing ptosis or recession surgery. Significant recession of the extraocular muscles may result in further proptosis, which should be considered in estimating the desired amount of axial retrodisplacement during decompression procedures when performed before strabismus surgery.

Anomalous ectopic muscles may occasionally be seen arising in the orbital apex associated with the levator muscle and innervated by the superior branch of the oculomotor nerve. These may result embryologically from failure of fusion of discreet foci of primitive muscle cells along the differentiating muscle primordia. Anomalous slips associated with the levator muscle have been observed in up to 70% of fetuses.[56] In the adult they have been reported in 8–15% of individuals.[6,77] One such muscle appears to differentiate from the medial side of the levator near its origin, and runs forward between the levator and the superior oblique muscles.[65] This muscle (tensor trochleae) varies in development from a stout muscle band, to a imperceptible condensation of muscle fibers. Anteriorly, it becomes thinner, less well-defined, and mostly fibrous. Its major insertion is into the fascia surrounding the trochlea. Other slips are more variable and can be traced to the supratrochlear artery, the lateral intermuscular septum, and to the superior and medial rectus muscle sheaths.[27] Another occasional anomalous muscle runs forward from the lateral surface of the levator muscle in the superolateral orbit, within the upper fascial suspensory system of the lateral rectus muscle. This thin layer of muscle fibers may extend for some distance along the fascial sheets uniting the superior rectus-levator complex to the lateral rectus muscle (superolateral intermuscular septum). This anomalous structure may attain a maximum diameter of 1–2 mm in the mid-orbit. Anteriorly, it inserts onto the capsule of the lacrimal gland and the fascia of the lateral levator aponeurosis. It is innervated by a small branch from the superior division of the oculomotor nerve. The function of this muscle remains uncertain, but we have referred to it as the tensor intermuscularis.

Clinical correlations

A large variety of disorders may result in orbital myopathic dysfunction. Among the muscular dystrophies, the extraocular muscles are spared in Duchenne, limb girdle, and congenital dystrophies by some as yet unidentified protective mechanisms, whereas they are preferentially affected in oculopharyngeal dystrophy which has a different pathogenic mechanism.[72] In myotonic dystrophy and oculopharyngeal dystrophy, mild to profound ptosis is common and varying degrees of ophthalmoparesis may also be seen. Chronic progressive external ophthalmoplegia is the most common of the mitochondrial myopathies, characterized by progressive bilateral ptosis, followed months to years later by symmetric bilateral ophthalmoplegia. Ocular motility, including Bell's phenomenon, may be severely limited or absent, possibly related to EOM's high dependence on oxidative energy metabolism.[72] Because of this, in these patients extreme caution must be exercised in any repair of ptosis that could result in severe lagophthalmos.

Myasthenia gravis is a disorder of impaired neuromuscular transmission characterized by a variable decrease in strength of the affected muscles.[25] This is an autoimmune process involving the neuromuscular junction[7,23,25] in which neurotransmission is blocked by immune-mediated injury to the post-synaptic membrane. The propensity for involvement of the levator and other extraocular muscles is thought to be related to a novel acetylcholine receptor isoform in these muscles,[36] or alternatively to the low expression of a negative regulator of the complement-mediated response.[37] The extraocular muscles are among the earliest muscles involved and often they are the only muscles involved. The levator and ocular muscles are initially affected in 70% of cases, and eventually in 90%. All degrees of ocular motor dysfunction have been observed from single muscle weakness to complete external ophthalmoplegia.

Enlargement of extraocular muscles may be seen in a variety of pathologic processes. The most common cause is dysthyroid orbitopathy in which chronic lymphocytic infiltration and edema are associated with intramuscular accumulation of glycoprotein and acid mucopolysaccharide. The often massive enlargement of these muscles may be increased by as much as 400%. This process involves only the muscle fibers, not the tendons. However, muscle fibers interdigitate between the tendinous fibers at the muscle origins, so that this infiltrative process in thyroid disease may involve the muscle origins at the orbital apex right up to the annulus of Zinn. Since the muscles are fixed by this tendinous ring, and since in the orbital apex they lie against the bony walls, any significant enlargement may result in the optic nerve compression seen in some patients with dysthyroid myopathy.[69] With thickening of the muscles at their origin, even removal of the adjacent medial bony wall may not allow enough displacement to decompress the optic nerve and to improve vision.

Thyroid orbitopathy is typically a bilateral disease, although it is frequently asymmetric, and usually affects multiple muscles. The inferior and medial rectus muscles are most frequently involved. The resulting axial proptosis and forward herniation of extraconal orbital fat into the eyelids are characteristic early features of the disease. Later, inflammatory fibrotic contracture of the extraocular muscles may result in restrictive motility disturbance, usually with downward and medial deviation of the globe. Fibrosis of the levator muscle in the upper lid, and traction on the capsulopalpebral fascia of the lower lid from inferior rectus contracture, contribute to progressive eyelid retraction. In addition, fibrosis of the orbital fascial system exacerbates this process. Abnormal stimulation and hypertrophy of Müller's sympathetic muscles may also contribute to eyelid retraction, and in the case of Müller's orbital muscle, may possibly contribute to orbital venous congestion (see Chapter 6).

Idiopathic orbital myositis is another common inflammatory myopathy that presents as an acute orbital syndrome. Rapid onset of pain, proptosis, and diplopia associated with eyelid swelling, chemosis, and injection suggest an inflammatory process. This is typically a unilateral disease affecting a single muscle, usually the superior or lateral rectus muscle. Restriction is in the field of action of the affected muscle, and the globe may be abaxially displaced inferiorly or medially. The process characteristically responds dramatically to systemic corticosteroids, although in some cases very high intravenous doses will be required for control, and rarely even cytotoxic agents or radiotherapy will be needed.

Rarely, myositis may be associated with systemic disease processes, such as sarcoidosis, systemic lupus erythematosis, Crohn's disease, giant cell myocarditis, and rheumatoid arthritis, among others.[42] Traumatic myopathies of the orbital muscles frequently cause isolated extraocular muscle restriction from edema or hemorrhage. These typically resolve spontaneously. When associated with orbital wall fractures, entrapment of the muscle or its fibrous orbital septa may result in mechanical dysfunction requiring surgical release.

Extraocular muscle dysfunction has been reported following retrobulbar injection for cataract and other ocular surgery.[60] Experimental studies demonstrated myotoxicity of nearly all local anesthetics within minutes of injection into muscle, possibly due to membrane disruption and dissolution of sarcomeres at the Z-bands.[8] Regeneration is usual within 6–7 days. However, severe fibrosis and muscle contracture may occasionally be seen.[29]

Duane's retraction syndrome is a condition characterized by a horizontal motility defect in abduction, associated with some degree of restricted adduction and variable retraction of the adducted globe. Although the disorder may be bilateral, it most frequently involves the left eye, and is more common in females. Electromyographic evidence suggests that the primary cause is paradoxic innervation of the lateral rectus muscle on attempted adduction. This co-contraction of the horizontal rectus muscles on adduction causes retraction of the globe.[3]

Brown's syndrome is a congenital or acquired motility defect manifested by inability to elevate the adducted eye above the midhorizontal plane. Smaller degrees of elevation deficit are seen in the primary, and little or none in the abducted positions of gaze. An associated widening of the palpebral fissure is seen on adduction. Numerous etiologies appear to be responsible for this defect. In some patients the superior oblique tendon sheath anterior to the trochlea is unusually taut, resulting in a mechanical restriction. In others, however, the anatomic problem lies more posterior, with thickening of, or adhesions to the tendon behind the trochlea.[54] During mesenchymal maturation of the superior oblique muscle, cellular condensations of the tendon and trochlea are initially indistinguishable, and do not become discernible as separate structures until the 78 mm stage. Connective tissue adhesions remain between the tendon and trochlea, but degenerate to only fine strands by birth. Persistent thickening of these trabecular adhesions may account for the superior oblique tendon sheath syndrome in some patients.[68,69]

Extraocular muscle abnormalities associated with strabismus are unclear and inconsistent. Alterations in position of muscle pulleys have been linked to incomitant strabismus,[52] and as an aging phenomenon related to progressive inferior displacement of the inferior rectus pulley.[11]

During strabismus surgery with exposure of the muscle insertion, a cut to the level of sclera will pass through the conjunctiva, Tenon's capsule, and intermuscular septum, to enter the episcleral space. If possible, the muscle should be disinserted without cutting its sheath, to avoid bleeding and scarring. Tenon's capsule should not be opened more than 9–10 mm posterior to the limbus, since this will permit prolapse the extraconal fat pockets into the wound. Fibrofatty proliferation may result in scarring and possible motility restriction.[54] Significant recession or advancement of the muscle requires separation of the muscle sheath from the intermuscular septum for a distance of about 10 mm, and from Tenon's capsule by division of the check ligaments.

The most frequent cause of adult acquired ptosis is a defect in the mechanical linkage between the levator muscle and the eyelid. This usually results from involutional stretching of the levator aponeurosis, and less frequently from its frank disinsertion from the tarsal plate.[21] Rarely, a dehiscence may be seen at the time of surgery. Aponeurotic defects are not an uncommon sequel to ocular surgery, such as cataract extraction. In all such cases levator muscle function remains normal, despite the ptotic position of the eyelid. Surgical repair is directed at reattaching or shortening the redundant aponeurosis. Of the myogenic causes of ptosis, congenital ptosis is by far the most common etiology. Here the defect results from a developmental dysgenesis of the levator muscle, and levator muscle function is typically impaired to varying degrees.[2] A genetic basis for congenital ptosis has more recently been reported in several family lines, possibly related to neuronal maturation and development in the oculomotor nucleus.[25,51,73] For cases where good levator muscle function is present, advancement of the levator aponeurosis is usually adequate. However, when levator muscle function is minimal or absent adequate elevation of the lid can be achieved only with a frontalis suspension procedure.

In Horner's syndrome the levator muscle is anatomically and functionally normal, and the minimal ptosis results from paresis of Müller's accessory retractor muscle following sympathetic denervation. Although these lids may be repaired with aponeurotic advancement, Müller's muscle and conjunctival resection works well and is more directly related to the source of pathology.

In the neurogenic ptoses, the defect is along the route of the oculomotor nerve. Repair depends upon the residual degree of levator muscle function. In mechanical ptosis, the upper eyelid is displaced downward because of a mass lesion or other mechanical restriction. Correction is aimed at the source of the restriction.

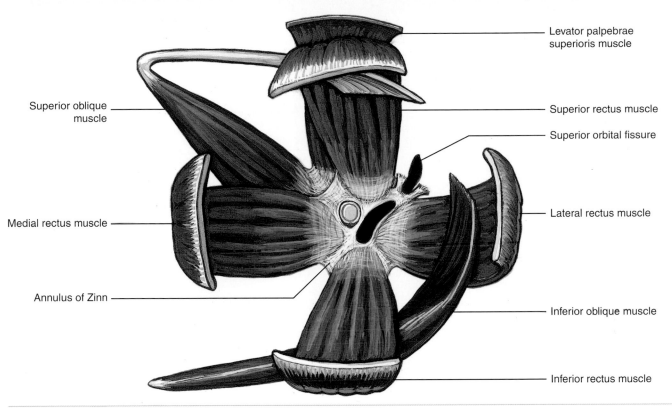

Levator palpebrae
superioris muscle

Superior oblique
muscle

Superior rectus muscle

Superior orbital fissure

Medial rectus muscle

Lateral rectus muscle

Annulus of Zinn

Inferior oblique muscle

Inferior rectus muscle

Figure 3-1 Isolated extraocular muscles, frontal view.

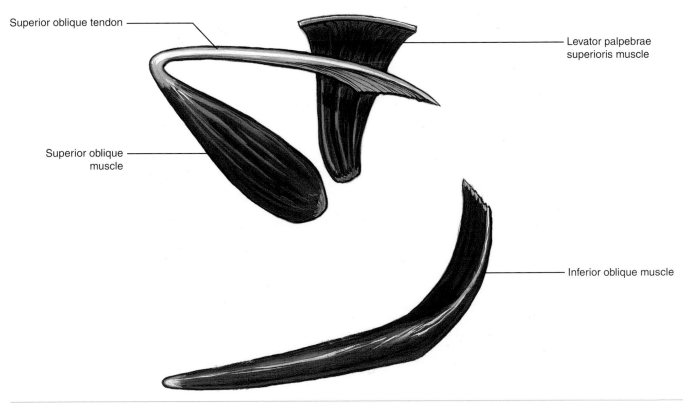

Superior oblique tendon

Levator palpebrae
superioris muscle

Superior oblique
muscle

Inferior oblique muscle

Figure 3-2 Extraocular muscles, frontal view, rectus muscles removed.

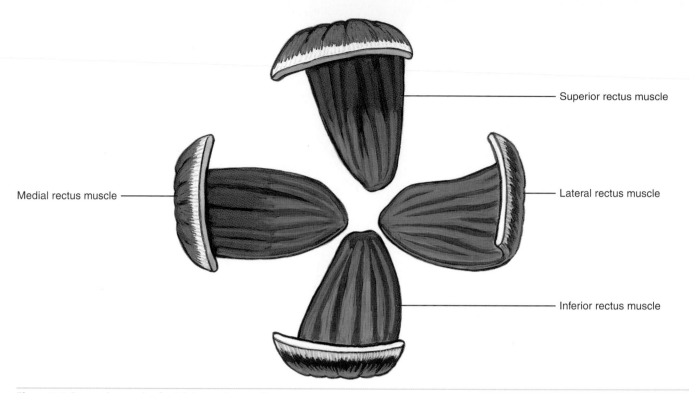

Superior rectus muscle

Medial rectus muscle

Lateral rectus muscle

Inferior rectus muscle

Figure 3-3 Extraocular muscles, frontal view, rectus muscle cone.

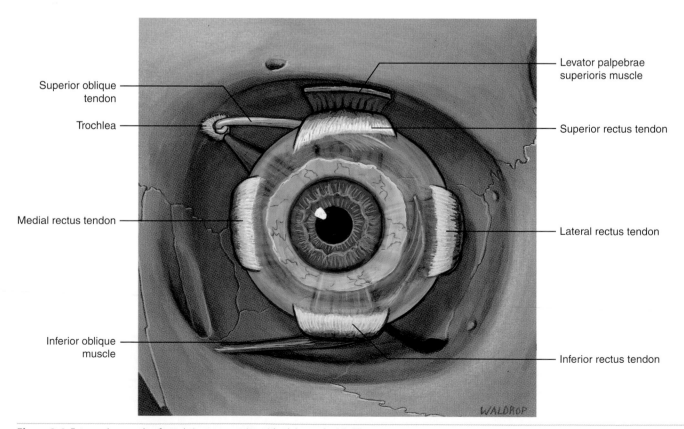

Superior oblique tendon

Trochlea

Medial rectus tendon

Inferior oblique muscle

Levator palpebrae superioris muscle

Superior rectus tendon

Lateral rectus tendon

Inferior rectus tendon

WALDROP

Figure 3-4 Extraocular muscles, frontal view, composite with globe and orbital bones.

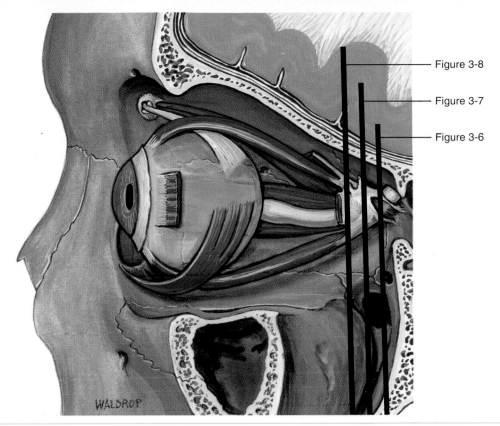

Figure 3-8

Figure 3-7

Figure 3-6

Figure 3-5 Annulus of Zinn, cross-sectional planes for Figures 3-6 through 3-8.

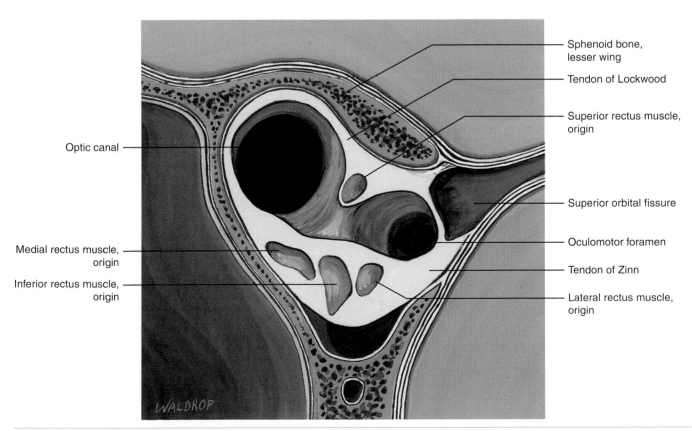

Sphenoid bone, lesser wing

Tendon of Lockwood

Superior rectus muscle, origin

Optic canal

Superior orbital fissure

Medial rectus muscle, origin

Oculomotor foramen

Inferior rectus muscle, origin

Tendon of Zinn

Lateral rectus muscle, origin

Figure 3-6 Annulus of Zinn, posterior cross-section.

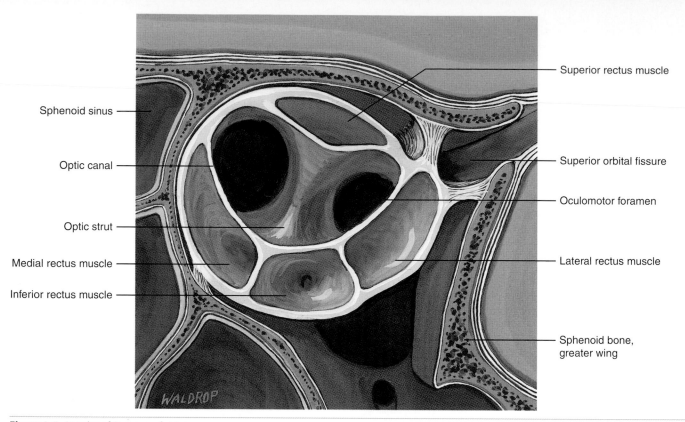

Sphenoid sinus

Optic canal

Optic strut

Medial rectus muscle

Inferior rectus muscle

Superior rectus muscle

Superior orbital fissure

Oculomotor foramen

Lateral rectus muscle

Sphenoid bone, greater wing

Figure 3-7 Annulus of Zinn, superficial view.

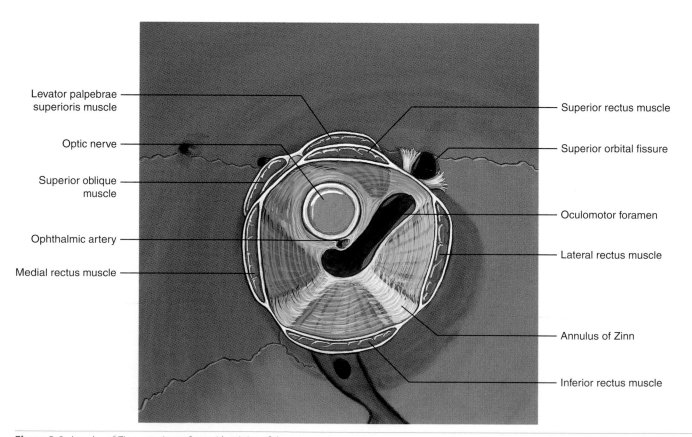

Levator palpebrae superioris muscle

Optic nerve

Superior oblique muscle

Ophthalmic artery

Medial rectus muscle

Superior rectus muscle

Superior orbital fissure

Oculomotor foramen

Lateral rectus muscle

Annulus of Zinn

Inferior rectus muscle

Figure 3-8 Annulus of Zinn, anterior surface with origins of the extraocular muscles.

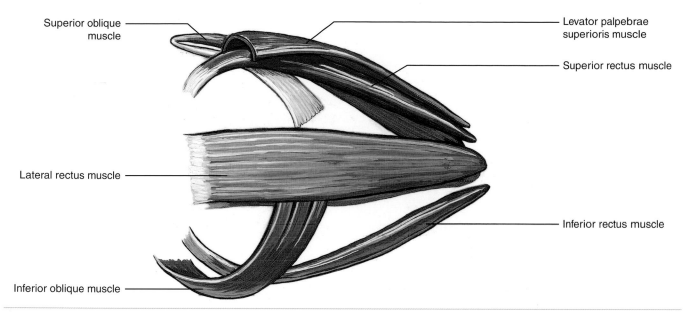

Superior oblique muscle

Levator palpebrae superioris muscle

Superior rectus muscle

Lateral rectus muscle

Inferior rectus muscle

Inferior oblique muscle

Figure 3-9 Extraocular muscles, lateral view.

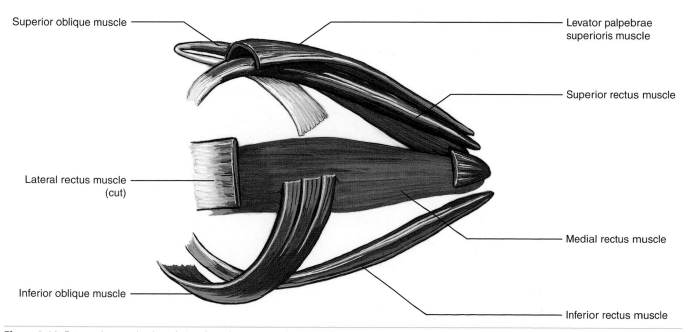

Superior oblique muscle

Levator palpebrae superioris muscle

Superior rectus muscle

Lateral rectus muscle (cut)

Medial rectus muscle

Inferior oblique muscle

Inferior rectus muscle

Figure 3-10 Extraocular muscles, lateral view, lateral rectus muscle removed.

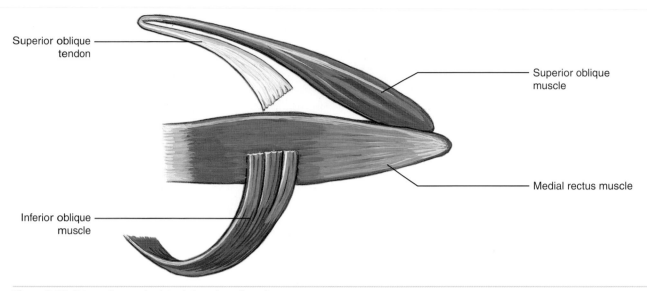

Superior oblique tendon

Superior oblique muscle

Medial rectus muscle

Inferior oblique muscle

Figure 3-11 Extraocular muscles, lateral view, deep dissection.

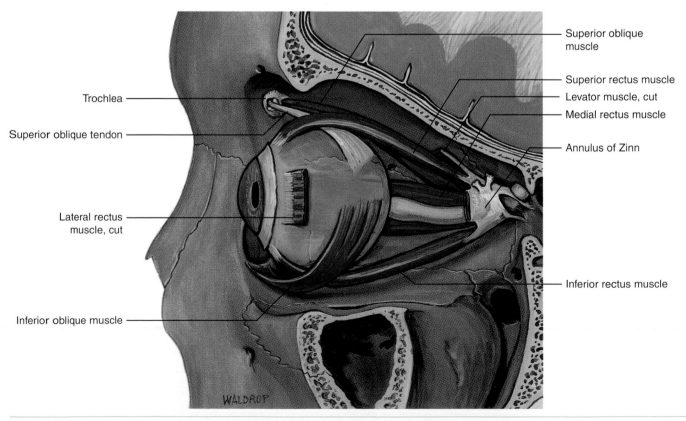

Trochlea

Superior oblique tendon

Lateral rectus muscle, cut

Inferior oblique muscle

Superior oblique muscle

Superior rectus muscle

Levator muscle, cut

Medial rectus muscle

Annulus of Zinn

Inferior rectus muscle

WALDROP

Figure 3-12 Extraocular muscles, lateral composite view with globe and orbital bones.

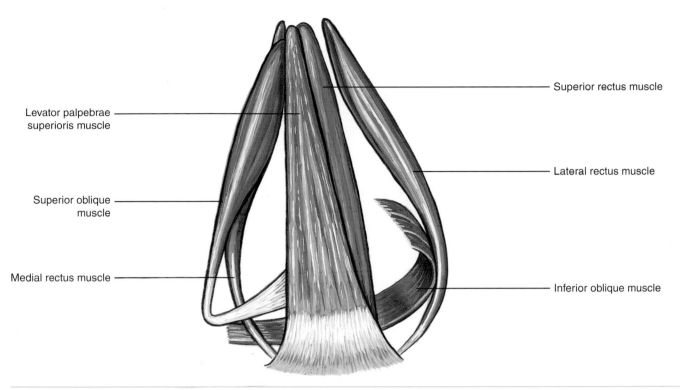

Levator palpebrae
superioris muscle

Superior oblique
muscle

Medial rectus muscle

Superior rectus muscle

Lateral rectus muscle

Inferior oblique muscle

Figure 3-13 Extraocular muscles, superior view.

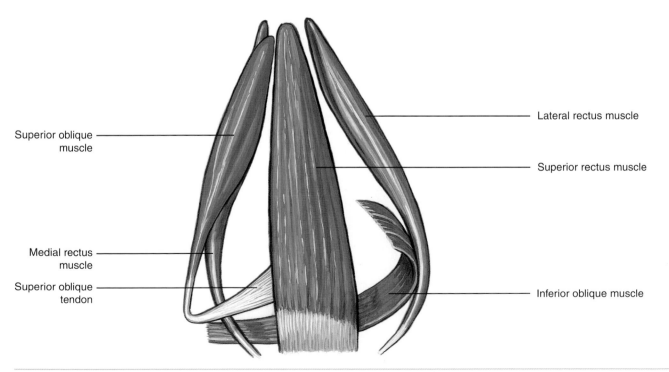

Superior oblique
muscle

Medial rectus
muscle

Superior oblique
tendon

Lateral rectus muscle

Superior rectus muscle

Inferior oblique muscle

Figure 3-14 Extraocular muscles, superior view, levator muscle removed.

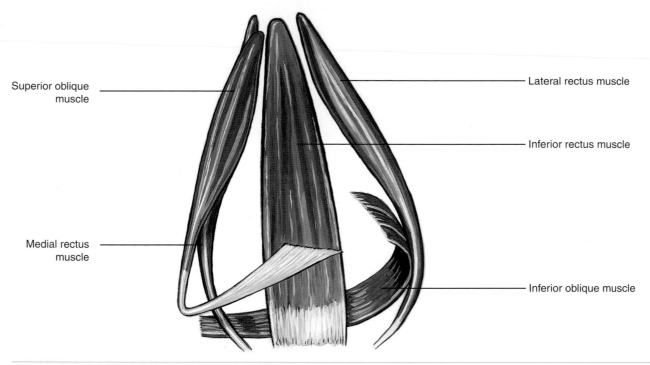

Superior oblique
muscle

Medial rectus
muscle

Lateral rectus muscle

Inferior rectus muscle

Inferior oblique muscle

Figure 3-15 Extraocular muscles, superior view, levator and superior rectus muscles removed.

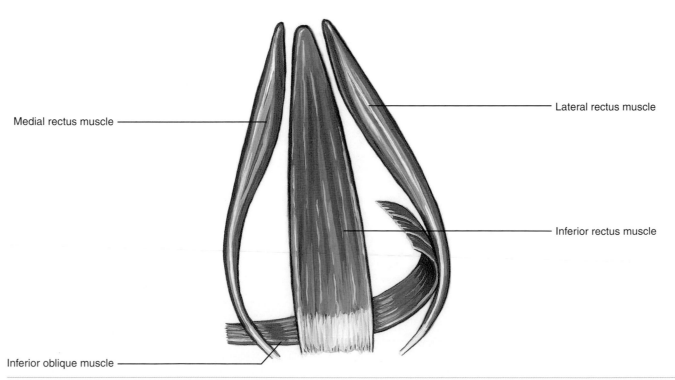

Medial rectus muscle

Lateral rectus muscle

Inferior rectus muscle

Inferior oblique muscle

Figure 3-16 Extraocular muscles, superior view, deep dissection.

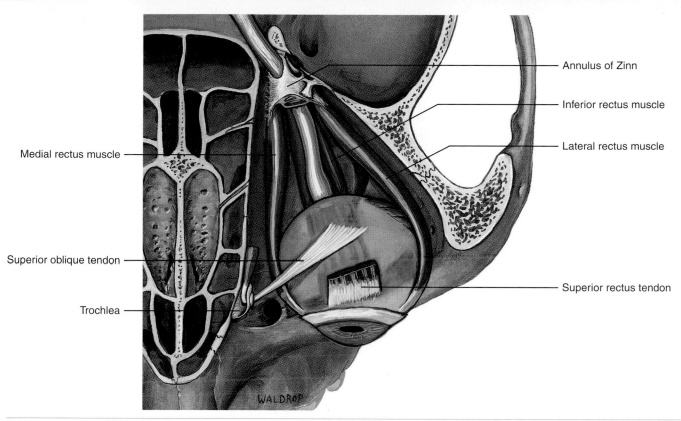

Annulus of Zinn

Inferior rectus muscle

Lateral rectus muscle

Medial rectus muscle

Superior oblique tendon

Trochlea

Superior rectus tendon

Figure 3-17 Extraocular muscles, superior view, composite view with globe and orbital bones.

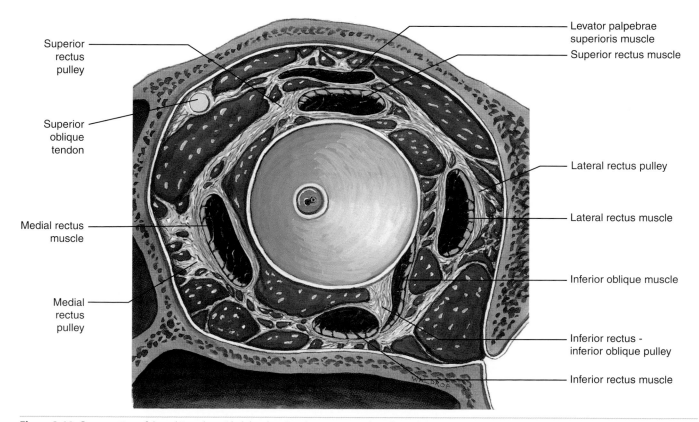

Superior rectus pulley

Superior oblique tendon

Medial rectus muscle

Medial rectus pulley

Levator palpebrae superioris muscle

Superior rectus muscle

Lateral rectus pulley

Lateral rectus muscle

Inferior oblique muscle

Inferior rectus - inferior oblique pulley

Inferior rectus muscle

Figure 3-18 Cross-section of the orbit at the mid globe showing the rectus muscle pulley systems.

References

1. Apt L: An anatomical reevaluation of rectus muscle insertions. *Trans Am Ophthalmol Soc* 78:365, 1980.

2. Baldwin HC, Manners RM: Congenital blephroptosis. *Ophthal Plast Reconstr Surg* 18:301, 2002.

3. Blodi FC, van Allen MW, Yarbrough JC: Duane's syndrome: A brain stem lesion. *Arch Ophthalmol* 72:171, 1964.

4. Boothe RG, Quick MW, Joosse MV, et al: Accessory lateral rectus muscle orbital geometry in normal and naturally strabismic monkeys. *Invest Ophthalmol* 31:1168, 1990.

5. Brueckner JK, Itkis O, Porter JD: Spatial and temporal patterns of myosin heavy chain expression in developing rat extraocular muscle. *J Muscle Res Cell Motil* 17:297, 1996.

6. Bulent Y, Hurmeric V, Loukas M, et al: Accessory levator muscle slips of the levator palpebrae superioris muscle. *Clin Exp Ophthalmol* 37:407, 2009.

7. Burde RM: Acetylcholine receptor antibodies and beyond. *J Clin Neuro Ophthalmol* 1:63, 1981.

8. Carlson BM, Emerick SE, Komorowski TE, et al: Extraocular muscle regeneration in Primates. *Ophthalmology* 99:582, 1992.

9. Clark RA, Miller JM, Demer JL: Location and stability of rectus muscle pulleys. Muscle paths as a function of gaze. *Invest Ophthalmol Vis Sci* 38:227, 1997.

10. Clark RA, Miller JM, Demer JL: Three-dimensional location of human rectus muscle pulleys by path inflections in secondary gaze positions. *Invest Ophthalmol Vis Sci* 41:3787, 2000.

11. Clark RA, Demer JL: Effect of aging on human rectus extraocular muscle paths demonstrated by magnetic resonance imaging. *Am J Ophthalmol* 134:872, 2002.

12. Demer JL: The orbital pulley system: A revolution on concepts of orbital anatomy. *Ann NY Acad Sci* 956:17, 2002.

13. Demer JL: Current concepts of mechanical and neural factors in ocular motility. *Curr Opin Neurol* 19:4, 2006.

14. Demer JL: Evidence supporting extraocular muscle pulleys: Refuting the platygean view of extraocular muscle mechanics. *J Pediatr Ophthalmol Strabismus* 43:296, 2006.

15. Demer JL: Mechanics of the orbita. *Dev Ophthalmol* 40:132, 2007.

16. Demer JL, Miller JM, Poukens V, et al: Evidence for fibromuscular pulleys of the recti extraocular muscles. *Invest Ophthalmol Vis Sci* 36: 1125, 1995.

17. Demer JL, Oh SY, Poukens V: Evidence for active control of rectus extraocular muscle pulleys. *Invest Ophthalmol Vis Sci* 41:1280, 2000.

18. Demer JL, Oh SY, Clark RA, Poukens V: Evidence for a pulley of the inferior oblique muscle. *Invest Ophthalmol Vis Sci* 44:3856, 2003.

19. Dietert SE: The demonstration of different types of muscle fibers in human extraocular muscle by electron microscopy and cholinesterase staining. *Invest Ophthalmol* 4:51, 1965.

20. Doxanas MT, Anderson RL: *Clinical Orbital Anatomy*. Baltimore, Williams and Wilkins, 1984.

21. Dutton JJ: *The Management of Ptosis. A Color Atlas and Surgical Guide*. Singapore, PG Publishing PTE LTD, 1989.

22. Eggers HM: Functional anatomy of the extraocular muscles. In: Jakobiec FA (ed): *Ocular Anatomy, Embryology, and Teratology*. Philadelphia, Harper and Row, 1982, p 827.

23. Elias SB, Apple SH: Current concepts of pathogenesis and treatment of myasthenia gravis. *Med Clin North Am* 63:745, 1979.

24. Yalcin B, Ozan H: Insertional pattern of the inferior oblique muscle. *Am J Ophthalmol* 139:504, 2005.

25. Engle AG: Morphologic and immunopathologic findings in myasthenia gravis and in congenital myasthenic syndromes. *J Neurosurg Psychiatr* 43:577, 1980.

26. Engle EC, Castro AE, Macy ME, et al: A gene for isolated congenital ptosis maps to a 3-cM region within 1p32-p34.1. *Am J Hum Genet* 60:1150, 1997.

27. Ettl A, Prilinger S, Kramer J, Koornneef L: Functional anatomy of the levator palpebrae superioris muscle and its connective tissue system. *Br J Ophthalmol* 80:702, 1996.

28. Gilbert PW: The origin and development of the human extrinsic ocular muscles. *Contr Embryol Carnegie Inst* 36:59, 1957.

29. Hamed LM, Mancuso A: Inferior rectus muscle contracture syndrome after retrobulbar anesthesia. *Ophthalmology* 98:1506, 1991.

30. Haslwanter T: Mechanics of eye movements: Implications of the "orbital revolution". *Ann NY Acad Sci* 956:33, 2002.

31. Helveston EM, Merriam WW, Ellis FD, et al: The trochlea: A study of the anatomy and physiology. *Ophthalmology* 89:124, 1982.

32. Housepian EM: Surgical treatment of unilateral optic nerve gliomas. *J Neurosurg* 31:604, 1969.

33. Isomura G: Comparative anatomy of the extrinsic ocular muscles in vertebrates. *Anat Anz* 150:498, 1981.

34. Jampel RS, Shi DX: Evidence against mobile pulleys on the rectus muscles and inferior oblique muscles: Central nervous system controls ocular kinematics. *J Pediatr Ophthalmol Strabismus* 43:289, 2006.

35. Kakizaki H, Zako M, Nakano T, et al: An anomalous muscle linking the superior and inferior rectus muscles in the orbit. *Anat Sci Int* 81:197, 2006.

36. Kaminski HJ, Kusner LL, Block CH: Expression of acetylcholine receptor isoforms at extraocular muscle endplates. *Invest Ophthal Vis Sci* 37:345, 1996.

37. Kaminski HJ, Richmonds CR, Kusner LL, Mitsumoto H: Differential susceptibility of the ocular motor system to disease. *Ann NY Acad Sci* 956:42, 2002.

38. Keller EL, Robinson DA: Absence of stretch reflex in extraocular muscle of the monkey. *J Neurophysiol* 34:908, 1971.

39. Kono R, Poukens V, Demer JL: Quantitative analysis of the structure of the huma extraocular muscle pulley system. *Invest Ophthalmol Vis Sci* 43:2923, 2002.

40. Kono R, Poukens V, Demer JL: Superior oblique muscle layers in monkeys and humans. *Invest Ophthalmol Vis Sci* 46:2790, 2005.

41. Kubota M: Ultrastructural observations on muscle spindles in extraocular muscles of pig. *Anat Anz* 165:205, 1988.

42. Lacey B, Chang W, Rootman J: Nonothyroid causes of extraocular muscle diseases. *Surv Ophthalmol* 44:1897, 1999.

43. Lang J, Kageyama I: Über die Ursprungsregion des M. obliquus bulbi inferior. *Klin Mbl Augenheilk* 196:228, 1990.

44. Lang J, Reirer W: Topographie des Orbitainhaltes. *Neurochirurgia* 33:9, 1990.

45. Machemer RA: New concept for vitreous surgery. 2. Surgical technique and complications. *Am J Ophthalmol* 74:1022, 1972.

46. Miller JM, Robins D: Extraocular muscle sideslip and orbital geometry in monkeys. *Vision Res* 27:381, 1987.

47. Miller JM: Functional anatomy of normal human rectus muscles. *Vision Res* 29:223, 1989.

48. Moore KL: *The Developing Human. Clinically Oriented Embryology*. Philadelphia, WB Saunders Co, 1973, p 36.

49. Natori Y, Rhoton AL Jr: Microsurgical anatomy of the superior orbital fissure. *Neurosurg* 36:762, 1995.

50. Noden DM: Periocular mesenchyme: Neural crest and mseodermal interactions. In: Duane TD, Jaeger EM (eds): *Biomechanical Foundations of Ophthalmology*. Philadelphia, JB Lippincott, 1988.

51. Nogami S, Ishii Y, Kawaguchi M, et al: ZFH4 protein is expressed in many neurons of developing brains. *J Comp Neurol* 482:33, 2005.

52. Oh SY, Clark RA, Velez F, et al: Incomitant strabismus associated with instability of rectus pulleys. *Invest Ophthalmol Vis Sci* 43:2169, 2002.

53. Park CY, Oh SY: Accessory lateral rectus muscle in a patient with congenital third-nerve palsy. *Am J Ophthalmol* 136:355, 2003.

54. Parks MM: *Ocular Motility and Strabismus*. Hagerstown, Harper and Row, 1975.

55. Peng M, Poukens V, da Silva Costa RM, et al: Compartmentalized innervation of primate lateral rectus muscle. *Invest Ophthalmol Vis Sci* 51:4612, 2010.

56. Plock J, Contaldo C, von Lüdinghausen M: Levator palpebrae superioris muscle in human fetuses: Anatomic findings and their clinical relevance. *Clin Anat* 18:473, 2005.

57. Porter JD, Baker RS, Ragusa RJ, Brueckner JF: Extraocular muscles: Basic and clinical aspects of structure and function. *Surv Ophthalmol* 39:451, 1995.

58. Porter JD, Burns LA, McMahon EJ: Morphological substrate for eyelid movements: Innervation and structure of primate levator palpebrae superioris and orbicularis muscles. *J Comp Neurol* 287:64, 1989.

59. Porter JD: Extraocular muscle: Cellular adaptations for diverse functional repertoire. *Ann NY Acad Sci* 956:7, 2002.

60. Rainin EA, Carlson BM: Postoperative diplopia and ptosis. A clinical hypothesis based on the myotoxicity of local anesthetics. *Arch Ophthalmol* 103:1337, 1985.

61. Ringel SP, Wilson WB, Barden MT, Kaiser KK: Histochemistry of human extraocular muscle. *Arch Ophthalmol* 96:1067, 1978.

62. Romer AS: *The Vertebrate Body*. Philadelphia, WB Saunders, 1962, p 264.

63. Ruskell GL: The fine structure of human muscle spindles and their potential proprioceptive capacity. *J Anat* 16:199, 1989.

64. Ruskell GL, Kjellevold Haugen IB, Bruenech JR, van der Werf F: Double insertions of extraocular rectus muscles in humans and the pulley theory. *J Anat* 206:295, 2005.

65. Sacks JG: The levator-trochlear muscle. *Arch Ophthalmol* 103:540, 1985.

66. Schnyder H: The innervation of the monkey accessory lateral rectus muscle. *Brain Res* 296:139, 1984.

67. Sevel D: A reappraisal of the origin of the human extraocular muscles. *Ophthalmology* 88:1330, 1981.

68. Sevel D: Brown's syndrome—A possible etiology explained embryologically. *J Pediatr Ophthalmol Stab* 18:26, 1981.

69. Sevel D: The origins and insertions of the extraocular muscles: Development, histologic features, and clinical significance. *Trans Am Ophthalmol Soc* 84:488, 1986.

70. Sevel D: Development of the connective tissue of the extraocular muscles and clinical significance. *Graefe's Arch Ophthalmol* 226:246, 1988.

71. Simonsz HJ, Harting F, deWaal BJ, Verboeter BW: Sideways displacement and curved path of recti eye muscles. *Arch Ophthalmol* 103:124, 1985.

72. Spencer RF, Porter JD: Biological organization of the extraocular muscles. *Progr Brain Res* 151:43, 2006.

73. Stackhouse JR, Escaravage GK, Dutton JJ: Monozygotic twins with incompletely concordant simple congenital ptosis in a 4-genertion pedigree. *Ophthal Plast Reconstr Surg* 25:493, 2009.

74. Taren JA: An anatomic demonstration of afferent fibers in the IV, V, and VI cranial nerves of the Macaca mulatta. *Am J Ophthalmol* 58:408, 1964.

75. Tychsen L, Lisberger S: Maldevelopment of visual motion processing in humans who had strabismus with onset in infancy. *J Neuroscience* 6:2495, 1985.

76. van den Bedem SPW, Schutte S, van der Helm FCT, Simonsz HJ: Mechanical properties and functional importance of pulley bands or "faisseaux tendineoux". *Vis Res* 45:2710, 2005.

77. von Lüdinghausen M, Miura M, Würzler N: Variations and anomalies of the human orbital muscles. *Surg Radiol Anat* 21:69, 1999.

78. White MH, Lambert HM, Kincaide MC, et al: The ora serrata and the spiral of Tillaux. *Ophthalmology* 96:508, 1989.

79. Whitnall SE: Some abnormal muscles of the orbit. *Anat Rec* 21:143, 1921.

80. Xianzhong S, Han H, Zhao J, Zhou C: Microsurgical anatomy of the superior orbital fissure. *Clin Anat* 20:362, 2007.

CHAPTER 4

Orbital Nerves

Nerves passing into the orbit represent all functions of the nervous system–motor, sensory, and autonomic. Many subserve various aspects of visual function, whereas others pass through the orbit *en route* to extraorbital sites. The complex anatomic relationships among these neural elements and other structures within the orbit are best understood if they are separated into functional groups. These are the optic nerve, the motor nerves to extraocular muscles, iris and ciliary body, the sensory branches of the trigeminal nerve, and the autonomic nervous system.

The optic nerve

Embryology

In the 1.5–2 mm (21-day) embryo with eight somites, vague optic fields can be recognized on each of the widely separated halves of the future forebrain. These optic primordia appear as thickened zones in the differentiating central nervous system that form the neural folds. Shortly thereafter a pit develops within this region. At about the 3 mm (24-day) stage the optic pits are pushed outward, away from the central nervous system and toward the surface ectoderm, as neural fold closure progresses to completion. By the 20-somite stage (25th day of development) the optic pits become pouch-shaped vesicles. These vesicles become sheathed with cells of neural crest origin which separate them from the surface ectoderm, except for a small area in the center. The structural framework of the optic nerve forms as a proximal constriction, the optic stalk, between the optic vesicle and prosencephalon at the 4 mm (28-day) embryonic stage.[98] Rapid differential marginal growth of the vesicle results in a buckling and indentation of the distal wall to form the bilaminar optic cup. The outer wall of this cup will become the pigment epithelium, whereas the inner wall is destined to become the retina.

During the 4 mm (28-day) stage the surface ectoderm over the future lips of the optic vesicle thickens. Lens induction proceeds through development of the lens pit, cup, and vesicle, and at about the 7–10 mm (36-day) stage the lens vesicle separates from the surface ectoderm. Further maturation of lens fibers occurs through the 20 mm (48-day) stage, and lens growth continues throughout life.

A partial longitudinal invagination, the optic (embryonic) fissure, develops along the ventral surface of the optic stalk, and is continuous anteriorly with a similar inferior invagination of the optic cup. Beginning in the 8–10 mm (38-day) stage, this invagination begins to close over. The process starts in the central portion of the optic cup, and is completed in this region by the 13 mm (40-day) stage. The lips of the optic stalk begin to close over the optic fissure during the 12–20 mm (40–48-day) stages as they surround the hyaloid artery that lies along the inferior side of the stalk, within the fissure (see Chapter 5). Closure of the fissure begins proximally near the forebrain, and gradually extends distally. The last portion of the fissure to close is immediately behind the future optic disc, and is complete by about the 19–20 mm (48-day) stage. When the hyaloid artery later becomes the central retinal artery, its point of entrance into the ventral optic nerve marks the posterior extent of the former optic fissure. The result of this closure is a continuity of the central cavity of the optic stalk with the interior of the optic cup, thus providing a pathway for neurosensory fibers from the retina to the brain. Incomplete closure of the fissure results clinically in a coloboma. Although this usually occurs at the iris, the last portion to fuse, it also may involve the retina, choroid, optic disc, or the more distal portions of the optic nerve.

The retina begins differentiation in the 12 mm (40-day) embryo, first near the optic stalk, and then extending peripherally.[8] The inner layer of the optic cup undergoes cellular proliferation to form a double neuroblastic layer. Initially, the innermost cells of this layer contain cilia, similar to the third ventricle to which the optic vesicle is connected via the hollow optic stalk. The inner layer of neuroblastic cells gives rise to the ganglion cells, the amacrine cells, and the bodies of the sustentacular fibers of Müller. The outer neuroblastic layer becomes the horizontal cells, the bipolar nerve cells, and the rods and cones. The macular area first appears during the fifth fetal month as an area of increased nuclear density just lateral to the developing optic disc. In the seventh month, ganglion cells begin to be displaced peripherally to form a shallow depression, the fovea centralis. This process is completed by four months of post-partum age when there are no ganglion cells overlying the fovea. The foveal cones become narrow and more closely spaced.

During the 18–25 mm (48–54-day) embryonic stages fascicles of ganglion cell axons grow from the developing retina into the optic stalk through a defect in the pigment epithelium.[45] Here they surround the hyaloid artery. *En route* to the diencephalon, these axons pick up neuroglial cells differentiated from the inner layer of the neuroectoderm that forms the stalk, as the central lumen is obliterated. The outer layer of the stalk, continuous with the pigment epithelium, begins to develop into the peripheral glial mantle.[92] At the end of the second month of gestation, the two optic nerves unite in the floor of the diencephalon, at its boundary with the telencephalon. Here, they form the optic chiasm where a partial decussation of fibers occurs. The two optic tracts diverge from the posterior aspect of the chiasm, and continue to the lateral geniculate bodies.

In a number of non-human vertebrate orders there appear to be two distinct types of fiber sorting within the retinofugal pathway. One is seen as the segregation of crossed and uncrossed fibers within the optic chiasm, and the other is the product of a chronotopic or time-related developmental process, most evident in the optic tract.[97] The oldest fibers show a marked line of decussation separating the uncrossed temporal axons from the crossed nasal axons, and lie deep in the optic tract. However, the youngest fibers cross in the chiasm regardless of their retinal origin, and lie more superficially in the tract. The nature and site of action of this chronotopic mechanism influencing the tendency of temporal fibers to follow an uncrossed path at the chiasm, remains uncertain. The significance of this process in primate and human development remains to be determined.

As neurosensory axons continue to extend into the optic stalk, the optic disc rapidly enlarges. Later development of the optic disc is related to collapse of the hyaloid system. The hyaloid artery runs in a central canal through the presumptive optic nerve. It traverses the cavity of the optic vesicle to reach the lens placode and rim of the optic cup. Here, it anastomoses with vessels of the developing chorio-capillary network (see Chapter 5). A cap of glial cells surrounds the distal hyaloid canal, beginning at the optic stalk where the hyaloid artery enters the vitreous cavity. This is Burgmeister's papilla. Starting as early as the 60 mm (12-week) stage, and continuing through nearly the remainder of fetal development, the hyaloid system and the primary vitreous involute back to the internal limiting membrane on the optic disc. During the seventh fetal month, Burgmeister's papilla finally collapses, leaving the depressed physiologic optic cup. The presence of glial remnants and the extent or depth of the physiologic cup in adults probably correlate with the degree of persistence or atrophy of this glial sheath.[98] As the hyaloid system regresses, the retinal vessels develop from vascular buds on the hyaloid artery within the base of Burgmeister's papilla, and grow into the nerve fiber layer of the retina.

Behind the optic cup the pia, arachnoid, and dura mater differentiate during the 45–80 mm (10–14-week) fetal stages. They form from neural crest mesenchymal cells surrounding the basement membrane of the developing optic nerve. Faint suggestions of these sheaths may be detected as early as the 24 mm (54-day) embryonic stage.[92] Vessels and connective tissue from the pia mater begin to enter the proximal nerve at the 65 mm (13-week) stage, and slowly enlarge the nerve septa.[73] Myelin is added to the nerve beginning at the optic chiasm in the 23rd week of gestation, and extends toward the developing eye. Myelination normally stops at the lamina cribrosa at about 1 month post-partum, although in rare instances it may continue intraocularly where it is seen clinically as myelinated nerve fibers. The nerve continues to lengthen with growth of the orbit, and to widen with an increase in myelin content and thickening of the meningeal sheaths.

The adult optic nerve

As noted above, neural fibers of the optic nerve arise from primitive neuroblasts that become the ganglion cells in the retina, and grow toward the brain. Because the retina differentiates from the wall of the forebrain, the optic nerve is not a true peripheral nerve, but is an evaginated fiber tract of the diencephalon. Nevertheless, these fibers are customarily classified as a special somatic sensory cranial nerve. The fibers are myelinated, but lack a neurolemmal sheath. The anatomic relationships of the optic nerve are complex, and are of considerable significance in the evaluation of visual function (see below).

In the adult, the optic nerve is about 50 mm in length from the optic disc to the chiasm. Each nerve contains approximately 0.7–1.4 million axons, with a mean axon diameter of 0.85 μm.[80] The highest axonal density is in the temporal inferior segment of the nerve, corresponding with the location of the major portion of the papillomacular bundle.[79] Although there is a positive correlation between axon number and optic neural cross-sectional area, there is no correlation between optic nerve diameter and scleral canal area.

Within the orbit the nerve is invested with pia, arachnoid, and dural sheaths. The subarachnoid space is continuous from the middle cranial fossa, along the nerve, and into the posterior sclera. This space is partially interrupted at the orbital apex superiorly and medially where the pia and arachnoid are loosely adherent to the dura and annulus of Zinn. Clinically, this relationship may result in optic nerve compression and papilledema from increased intracranial cerebrospinal fluid pressure. The dura of the optic nerve becomes fused to periosteum within the optic canal superomedially. Intracranially, the dura and arachnoid remain close to the bony walls of the middle cranial fossa, and the optic nerve is covered only by a pial membrane to the chiasm.

There are four anatomically important portions of the optic nerve—intraocular, intraorbital, intracanalicular, and intracranial. The center of the nerve leaves the globe 4 mm medial to, and 0.1 mm below the level of the macula.[46] The intraocular portion of the nerve lies within the limits of the posterior sclera, and measures approximately 1 mm in length. Here, it lies within the lamina cribrosa. The latter is a sieve-like connective tissue region of the posterior sclera through which pass the retinal ganglion cell axons and central retinal vessels. It preserves a pressure gradient between the intraocular and extraocular spaces. It has been thought to be a primary site of glaucomatous damage to the optic nerve.[3] The lamina cribrosa contains approximately 220–240 pores, each averaging 0.004 mm^2 in diameter.[55] Larger pore size and a higher pore area to interpore tissue occurs in the superior and inferior portions of the lamina. This distribution of larger pores correlates with the wider neuroretinal rim and the higher nerve fiber count in the superior and inferior disc regions.[56] These locations are also associated with peripheral axons, including those from the temporal raphé of the fundus, corresponding to sites of early glaucomatous damage.

As the retinal ganglion cell axons approach the lamina cribrosa they become crowded, forming the elevated papilla at the beginning of the intrascleral portion of the optic nerve. This is visible on funduscopic examination as the non-myelinated optic disc, and measures 1.5–2.0 mm in diameter. The depressed central physiologic cup is usually filled with a remnant of glial tissue originally forming Burgmeister's papilla. The subarachnoid space, which runs along the orbital portion of the optic nerve, ends blindly in the posterior one-third to one-half of the scleral thickness. Here, it is separated from the vitreous cavity only by a thin layer of scleral fibers.

Immediately behind the sclera, the intraorbital portion of the nerve axons become myelinated by oligodendrocytes. The nerve becomes surrounded by pia, arachnoid, and dura mater. The dura is continuous with superficial scleral fibers at the posterior globe, and with periosteum at the optic canal. The combination of myelination and meningeal sheaths results in an enlargement of the nerve to 3–4 mm in diameter as it exits the globe. This fact is of some clinical significance in the treatment of choroidal malignant melanomas by radioactive plaque application. Thickening of the nerve as it exits the sclera posteriorly precludes placement of any plaque closer than about 1 mm to the edges of the intraocular optic disc. Therefore, any malignancy closer than 1.5–2.0 mm to the optic disc cannot reliably be treated with an episcleral plaque.

The orbital length of the optic nerve is about 25–30 mm. It describes an S-shaped path from the globe downward, then upward to the optic canal. This redundancy provides for ocular motility without stretching of the nerve. It also allows for a considerable amount of axial proptosis without functional compromise. However, in cases of severe proptosis, or even with minimal proptosis when the optic nerve lacks this redundancy, stretching of the nerve and compression by its taut sheath may result in visual loss.[26] As the nerve passes backward from the eye it is surrounded by dura, arachnoid, and pia mater. The subarachnoid space measures about 0.4 mm in width, and may be somewhat larger immediately behind the globe. This space is further dilated in cases of ideopathic intracranial hypertension, a fact that allows for nerve sheath fenestration with a certain degree of safety.

The posterior ciliary arteries and nerves run along the orbital portion of the optic nerve. The ciliary nerves are more numerous laterally, except immediately behind the globe where some additional branches cross from the lateral to the medial side. The ciliary arteries are more evenly distributed on the medial and lateral sides of the nerve. The central retinal artery pierces the nerve sheath inferiorly, or inferomedially, about 10–15 mm behind the globe. The central retinal vein usually accompanies the artery, although its position is more variable, and it may exit the nerve some distance from the artery. Because the vein is not preformed within the embryonic optic fissure, it may penetrate the substance of the nerve anywhere in the posterior orbit, and even in the superior quadrants (see Chapter 6).

The intracanalicular portion of the nerve is about 5–6 mm in length. The ophthalmic artery also passes through the optic canal, inferior and slightly lateral to the nerve. As it passes alongside the nerve, the ophthalmic artery is contained within a longitudinal split in the dura, and thus is separated from the nerve by dural fibers. Increased cerebrospinal fluid pressure in the subarachnoid space within the optic canal can potentially compress the artery, resulting in decreased arterial flow into the orbit. Flow within the ophthalmic and posterior ciliary arteries has been seen on color doppler studies to increase following anterior optic nerve sheath fenestration (Dr. Patrick Flaherty, personal communication). Several small vessels accompany the optic nerve through the canal where they run within the dura or along the ophthalmic artery. These appear to arise from the internal carotid artery dural branches, and supply structures in the orbital apex, including the annulus of Zinn and the initial portions of the extraocular muscles. Several millimeters anterior to the optic strut, the ophthalmic artery penetrates through the outer layer of dura to enter the oculomotor foramen within the annulus of Zinn.

The canalicular portion of the optic nerve is vulnerable to compression from small mass lesions, such as optic sheath meningiomas, or from ophthalmic artery aneurysms. Because of the fusion of dura to periosteum at the superomedial canal wall, this portion of the nerve is also vulnerable to contusion injuries. With blunt trauma, the nerve may slide within its sheaths, and can result in shearing of pial vessels supplying the nerve. Also, indirect transmission of mechanical forces from the frontal bone to the bones of the canal during severe blunt frontal trauma may result in contusion and edema of the intracanalicular optic nerve, with compression and occasionally optic neuropathy from infarction.

The intracranial segment of the nerve rises upward and backward at an angle of 45° to the horizontal plane. It measures about 10 mm (3–16 mm) long, and extends from the intracranial opening of the optic canal to the optic chiasm. As the nerve passes in the suprasellar cistern above the cavernous sinus and then back to the chiasm, it lies in close approximation to a number of vascular structures. These include the internal carotid, anterior cerebral, middle cerebral, and anterior communicating arteries. Aneurysms arising from these vessels may compress the nerve in this region.

The optic chiasm is a commissure that allows crossing of the nasal retinal fibers of each optic nerve to the contralateral optic tract. It measures 13 mm (10–20 mm) in transverse diameter, 8 mm (4–13 mm) in anteroposterior extent, and is 3–5 mm thick. The chiasm normally lies above the body of the sphenoid bone, over the diaphragma sellae, but may project onto the dorsum sellae or close to the planum sphenoidale in some individuals. Its anteroposterior position is somewhat variable, and accounts for the variations in field defects associated with tumors in this region. The chiasm is separated from the diaphragma sellae and pituitary gland by the basal cistern of the subarachnoid space, an interval of up to 10 mm. Thus, expanding lesions of the pituitary gland may be quite large before resulting in chiasmal compression.

The afferent pathways diverging from the posterior aspect of the chiasm are designated as the optic tracts. They terminate in the lateral geniculate bodies of the thalamus. Here they synapse with fourth order neurons of the geniculocalcarine radiation, pass through the temporal and parietal lobes, and ultimately terminate in the medial occipital cortex surrounding the calcarine fissure.

Optic nerve clinical correlations

Lesions affecting the optic nerve in the orbit or optic canal produce characteristic, but non-localizing, field defects. Chronic nerve compression in the anterior or mid-orbit usually results in initial optic disc edema, an enlarged blind spot, and variable field defects, followed by optic atrophy, blindness, and occasionally optociliary shunt vessels. Compression within the optic canal, however, is usually associated with a normal funduscopic examination initially, but eventually results in optic atrophy. The arrangement of fibers in the optic chiasm accounts for characteristic defects in visual field with compressive or vascular lesions affecting various portions of this structure. Within the mid-portion of the optic chiasm, expanding pituitary lesions or other intracranial masses such as a craniopharyngioma may selectively damage decussating fibers. Visual impulses from the nasal halves of each retina are thus blocked, resulting in a bitemporal hemianopia. Lesions of the optic tract cause loss of vision in the corresponding halves of each retina (nasal half in one eye and temporal half in the other eye), referred to as an homonymous hemianopia.

Pupillary constriction to light is mediated by a reflex arc having both afferent and efferent limbs. Afferent pupillary fibers pass through the optic nerve, hemidecussate at the chiasm, and continue in the optic tracts. Just before reaching the lateral geniculate bodies, these fibers branch off, extend through the brachium of the superior colliculus, and synapse in several pretectal subnuclei of the mesencephalon. From here, interneurons pass to the visceral (Edinger-Westphal) nuclei of the oculomotor complex. The efferent limb of the pathway consists of parasympathetic fibers that project from the Edinger-Westphal nuclei to the iris sphincter muscle via the oculomotor nerve, ciliary ganglion, and short ciliary nerves. Unilateral impairment of optic nerve or retinal function results in diminished response to light on the affected side, and the classic relative afferent pupillary defect ("Marcus Gunn pupil").

Non-arteritic ischemic optic neuropathy (ION) is a relatively common disorder usually affecting older individuals, and resulting in painless loss of vision. Both mechanical and anatomic factors are involved in its pathophysiology. A small optic disk and physiologic cup are predisposing factors related to a small scleral canal. This may cause nerve fiber crowding and compressive ischemia from a compartment syndrome. Impaired perfusion in the paraoptic branches of the short posterior ciliary arteries has been demonstrated in some patients with ION.

Despite its redundant length in the orbit, in some individuals the optic nerve is relatively short. In the presence of significant proptosis, the nerve can be put on stretch that can be appreciated as tenting of the posterior scleral contour on neuroimaging. Tightening of the dural sheath around the nerve can cause optic nerve compression with impaired axoplasmic flow and loss of vision. Tumors or enlarged extraocular muscles can also compress the nerve in the orbital apex.

The subarachnoid space around the optic nerve is filled with cerebrospinal fluid that is continuous intracranially with the chiasmatic cistern.[70,122] Nicoll et al.[88] reported central nervous system involvement, mainly respiratory arrest, in 0.27% of 6000 retrobulbar blocks, believed to result from injection of anesthetic into the subarachnoid space around the optic nerve. Kobet[67] recovered local anesthetic from the cerebrospinal fluid by lumbar puncture following respiratory arrest after retrobulbar injection. Inadvertent injection of anesthetic into the optic nerve sheath produces pressure on the optic nerve

three to four times that of injection into the retrobulbar space (138 mmHg vs. 35 mmHg),[125] and any unusual resistance should warn the surgeon of this possibility.

The oculomotor nerve

Embryology

The oculomotor, or third cranial nerve, like all other motor nerves in the orbit, originates embryologically within the basal plate of the developing mesencephalon. In the 10 mm (5-week) embryo, neuroblasts begin to aggregate along the somatic efferent column. The caudal group will ultimately differentiate into the trochlear nucleus, and the cephalad group becomes the oculomotor nucleus. During the 13 mm (40-day) stage, cell processes from the cephalad group extend downward to emerge from the ventral surface of the mesencephalon. They aggregate to form the oculomotor nerve, and become associated with Schwann cells derived from the neural crest. Between the 19 mm (46-day) and 50 mm (10-week) stages, the subdivisions of the oculomotor nucleus begin to differentiate on the ipsilateral side to the muscles they will innervate.[19] The cell bodies constituting the subnucleus for the superior rectus muscle migrate to the contralateral side, but project their axons across the midline.[35,47] By the 26 mm (7-week) stage, the peripheral nerve fibers finally make contact with their muscles of innervation.[110] Initially, undifferentiated nerve endings divide and ramify around the early myoblasts, forming a fine net. During the 54–61 mm (11–12-week) stages many of these fine branches degenerate. Specialized nerve endings are first seen beginning in the 68 mm stage, and by the 80 mm (14-week) stage specific motor and sensory fibers can be distinguished. Myelination of the oculomotor nerve trunk commences at about the 90 mm (15-week) fetal stage,[107] but does not begin in the intramuscular component of the nerve until term.[110] Most of the myelinization here occurs after birth. Sympathetic fibers are not seen in the muscle until the 165 mm (22-week) stage, associated with the developing arterioles.

The adult oculomotor nerve

The oculomotor nerve carries somatic motor fibers to the medial, superior, and inferior rectus muscles, the inferior oblique muscle, and to the levator palpebrae superioris muscle. It also carries parasympathetic fibers to the intrinsic muscles of the eye, and sensory neurons from proprioceptive receptors in the extraocular muscles it innervates. Motor neurons arise in the somatic portion of the oculomotor nucleus of the midbrain, just ventral to the aqueduct of Sylvius. There is a topographic localization of neurons within the nucleus that can be traced to the individual ocular muscles.[34,82,96,126] The subnuclei lie in a long column and are arranged in the order MR—IR—SR—IO from rostral to caudal.[96] Subnuclei of the inferior and medial rectus and inferior oblique muscles are paired, and innervate muscles on the ipsilateral side. The superior rectus subnuclei are situated medially on each side of the midbrain. Their fascicular fibers cross the midline, passing through the subnucleus on the opposite side to join with axons from other oculomotor subnuclei on that side. The motor cells that supply the levator muscle of both sides lie in a single subnucleus in the dorsal midline.

The fascicular portion of the oculomotor nerve extends through the midbrain across the medial longitudinal fasciculus, the tegmentum, the red nucleus, and the medial margin of the substantia nigra, and finally emerge as a series of rootlets in the interpeduncular fossa on the medial aspect of the cerebral peduncle. These rootlets immediately converge to form the oculomotor nerve trunk which lies between the superior cerebellar and posterior cerebral arteries.

The nerve passes forward, downward, and laterally through the subarachnoid cistern, and runs medial to and slightly beneath the free edge of the tentorium. It continues lateral to the posterior clinoid process, and pierces the dura mater at the top of the clivus as it enters the lateral roof of the cavernous sinus, slightly above and lateral to the abducens nerve.[114] As the nerve passes through the cavernous sinus, it lies just above the trochlear nerve, within the deep layer of the lateral wall of the sinus (see Chapter 1). There is some controversy concerning the exact relationships of the oculomotor and other neural elements within the lateral wall of the sinus. Some descriptions place the nerves embedded within the wall, and others place them between split dural layers.[119]

In the cavernous sinus, the oculomotor nerve may break up into a variable number of smaller fascicles that then reunite. Within the main nerve trunk, pupillomotor fibers maintain a superomedial position,[62] where they are susceptible to early compression by aneurysms of the posterior communicating artery. Fibers destined for the superior division of the oculomotor nerve run in the dorsolateral half of the nerve,[97] while fibers destined for the inferior division are distributed throughout the nerve trunk. Anteriorly in the cavernous sinus, the oculomotor nerve apparently receives sympathetic fibers from the superior cervical sympathetic ganglion via the internal carotid artery plexus.[129]

The oculomotor nerve enters the superior orbital fissure through the oculomotor foramen of the annulus of Zinn adjacent to the lateral surface of the optic strut. As it passes through the orbital fissure, or sometimes within the anterior cavernous sinus, the oculomotor nerve divides into a superior and inferior division. The smaller superior division passes into the orbit beneath the origin of the superior rectus muscle. It extends forward within the superolateral portion of the intraconal space for a short distance, moves medially toward the lateral edge of the superior rectus muscle, and breaks up into 3–7 small branches.[106,131] Some of these branches continue forward for several millimeters, then pass upward to enter the conal surface of the posterior one-third of the superior rectus muscle 10–20 mm anterior to the annulus. As is true for the innervation of all the extraocular muscles, nerve fibers run both distally and proximally between the muscle fibers before terminating at the myoneural junctions. One to 2 other fiber bundles from the superior division pass medially around (84%) or directly through (16%) the superior rectus muscle to insert into the inferior surface of the levator muscle as 1–5 separate fascicles.[131]

The larger inferior division of the oculomotor nerve enters through the annulus of Zinn inferomedially, medial to the nasociliary and abducens nerves. At the orbital apex it divides into three or more branches as it enters the intraconal space. These run forward, lateral to the optic nerve, and further divide into 8–10 fascicles. As they continue forward, these trunks move downward and medially to a position midway between the optic nerve and the inferior rectus muscle. Several branches turn medially below the optic nerve and further ramify into 3–8 fibers along the belly of the medial rectus muscle. They enter the muscle on the posterior third of its conal surface 10–20 mm anterior to the annulus. Another branch continues forward inferolaterally and further divides into 3–10 tiny fascicles that penetrate the posterior conal surface of the inferior rectus muscle.[131] A third, slightly larger branch separates early from the nerve bundles of the inferior division. It runs anteriorly along the lateral border of the inferior rectus muscle, or sometimes passes through its substance. This branch finally breaks up into 3–7 smaller twigs that enter the inferior oblique muscle in the midportion of its posterolateral surface.

The inferior division of the oculomotor nerve gives off one or more small trunks near the orbital apex, usually from the branch destined for the inferior oblique muscle. These carry preganglionic parasympathetic fibers that course upward and forward to join with and synapse in the ciliary ganglion, located in the orbital fat inferolateral to the optic nerve.[38]

Injury to the oculomotor nerve results in weakness or paralysis of the extraocular muscles supplied by its motor fibers. The clinical signs depend upon the specific point of axonal interruption.[2] Nuclear lesions may result in unilateral third nerve palsy with contralateral superior rectus weakness and either no ptosis, or bilateral ptosis.[22] Complete dysfunction of the third nerve results in a downward and outward deviation of the globe, as well as ipsilateral upper eyelid ptosis. The pupil is dilated without reaction to light or accommodation. Adduction is absent and both elevation and depression are impaired. Partial dysfunction of the nerve or its nucleus will produce incomplete portions of the above picture. Lesions located in the cavernous sinus tend to result in partial third-nerve palsies with sparing of pupillary function, and, because of the proximity of the trochlear and abducens nerves, tend to be associated with other extraocular muscle palsies. Sympathetic paresis may accompany cavernous sinus lesions, as these fibers enter the orbit from the carotid plexus within the sinus. Oculomotor palsy may be the presenting symptom of diabetes, characterized by painful ophthalmoplegia with sparing of the pupil.[37,85]

The ciliary ganglia

The ciliary ganglion is a parasympathetic synaptic ganglion associated with the ophthalmic division of the trigeminal nerve and the inferior division of the oculomotor nerve. It is analogous to parasympathetic ganglia associated with the maxillary division (sphenopalatine ganglion) and the mandibular division (otic and submaxillary ganglia) of the trigeminal nerve. The ciliary ganglion is a small, irregular structure measuring 2 mm horizontally by 1 mm vertically. It is located in the loose fatty tissue at the orbital apex, about 10 mm anterior to the medial end of the superior orbital fissure and 3 mm from the optic nerve. The ganglion is lateral or inferolateral to the ophthalmic artery, between the optic nerve and lateral rectus muscle. Three small nerve roots enter the ganglion. A sensory root carries sensory fibers from the globe via the short posterior ciliary nerves. They pass through the ciliary ganglion without synapse, and then to the nasociliary nerve and on to the gasserian ganglion. Some of these sensory fibers also pass from the globe directly to the nasociliary nerve via the long posterior ciliary nerves. A short parasympathetic motor root enters the ciliary ganglion from the inferior division of the oculomotor nerve and runs to the globe. It may be double, and in 6% of cases may even be missing, in which case the ganglion is attached directly to the inferior branch of the oculomotor nerve.[111] A third root carries sympathetic fibers from the carotid or ophthalmic artery plexus through the ciliary ganglion without synapse, and then on to the globe.

The autonomic functions of the oculomotor nerve are carried via parasympathetic fibers that arise from cells in the most superior portion of the oculomotor nucleus (Edinger-Westphal nucleus). These fibers follow the same course as the third nerve to the superior orbital fissure, and enter the inferior division as it passes into the orbit. Preganglionic fibers leave the oculomotor nerve via the small trunk, usually from the branch running to the inferior oblique muscle, and pass to the ciliary ganglion in the motor root. This trunk may be absent and in some cases the ciliary ganglion may lie in contact with the inferior division of the oculomotor nerve. Within the ciliary ganglion preganglionic parasympathetic fibers synapse with postganglionic fibers. Synaptic ganglion cells may extend into the roots connecting the oculomotor and nasociliary nerves,[68] and accessory ciliary ganglia may be present along one or more of the short ciliary nerves.[47] They may even occur in the episclera or within the scleral canals.[9] Some experimental evidence suggests that synapses in the main ciliary ganglion may be concerned with pupillary reaction to light, whereas the those in the accessory ganglia may mediate pupillary constriction to convergence and accommodation.[34] Postganglionic parasympathetic motor fibers pass from the ciliary ganglion into 4–6 short posterior ciliary nerves which further divide into 6–10 branches,[51] and sometimes as many as 20 branches that penetrate the posterior sclera adjacent to the optic nerve. Additional short ciliary nerves may sometimes arise directly from the motor root to the ciliary ganglion.[111] Upon approaching the globe these become highly convoluted and redundant to allow for ocular movement without injury. Most of these enter the sclera on the temporal side, with usually only 2–3 entering medial to the optic nerve.[40,111] Within the globe they run anteriorly in the suprachoroidal space. About 95–97% of these fibers innervate the ciliary muscle, with 3–5% destined for the sphincter pupillae muscle of the iris.

In addition to containing parasympathetic motor synapses, the ciliary ganglion transmits sensory fibers from the eye. These enter the ganglion via the short posterior ciliary nerves and pass through the ganglion without synapse. They exit the ganglion posteriorly via the small sensory root, join the nasociliary branch of the trigeminal nerve, and travel to the gasserian ganglion where they synapse. Sympathetic nerve fibers from the cavernous carotid plexus enter the ciliary ganglion through a small sympathetic root between the motor and sensory roots and run to the choroidal vasculature through the short posterior ciliary nerves. In most cases these originate directly from the carotid artery plexus and enter the orbit through the superior orbital fissure as one or more separate filaments. Occasionally they may originate in the orbit from the perivascular plexus surrounding the ophthalmic artery.[111] Other sympathetic fibers, mainly to the dilator muscle of the iris, travel with or within the nasociliary nerve, bypass the ciliary ganglion, and reach the eye through the long posterior ciliary nerves.

Other parasympathetic fibers enter the orbit through several routes. Numerous fibers pass from the pterygopalatine ganglion through Müller's orbital muscle in the inferior orbital fissure. Ganglion cells may be distributed along these branches.[10,11] These have diffuse targets within the orbit, including the lacrimal gland. Other fibers enter along the maxillary nerve, via its zygomatic branch, and carry additional parasympathetic efferents to the lacrimal gland. In monkeys, a parasympathetic ocular pathway supplementing the oculomotor supply through the ciliary ganglion, has been described along the facial nerve.[102] Its existence in humans has not been confirmed.

Disorders of parasympathetic motor function to the eye may originate anywhere along the neuronal route from the Edinger-Westphal nucleus to the intrinsic motor targets of the eye. Lesions affecting the oculomotor nucleus or nerve trunk are often associated with paralysis of both pupillary function and ocular motility. Aneurysms of the posterior communicating artery may result in pupil-involving third nerve palsy. Within the cavernous sinus, parasympathetic fibers group together to pass into the superficial medial portion of the inferior division of the nerve as it enters the orbit. Here they are vulnerable to compression from expanding aneurysms resulting in pupillary abnormalities. However, auxiliary vascular supply from the overlying epineurium protects them from ischemic injury, resulting in pupillary sparing in diabetic oculomotor palsies. Insults to postganglionic parasympathetic fibers within the ciliary ganglion or short posterior ciliary nerves may cause isolated internal ophthalmoplegia referred to as tonic pupil.

In Adie's tonic pupil, reaction to light is sluggish or absent, and delayed constriction to accommodative stimuli is present.[117] Other features may include sectoral palsy of the pupillary sphincter, "tonic" redilation, and paresis of accommodation. This is usually associated with deep tendon hyporeflexia, probably resulting from degeneration of cell bodies in the dorsal columns of the spinal cord similar to that which occurs in the ciliary ganglion. Since 97% of postganglionic fibers leaving the ciliary ganglion are originally targeted to the ciliary muscle,[127] misdirected regeneration of these fibers to the pupillary sphincter results in recovery of brisk pupillary constriction to accommodative stimuli, a form of "light-near dissociation". Direct pupillary response to light remains impaired because most of the fibers originally targeted to the sphincter muscle regenerate misdirected to the ciliary muscle. Hypersensitivity to cholinergic stimulation suggests denervation at the level of the postganglionic parasympathetic fiber, and can be demonstrated clinically using weak-strength miotic agents.

The position of the ciliary ganglion is somewhat variable, but, in general, it lies about 10 mm anterior to the superior orbital fissure and 7 mm anterior to the annulus of Zinn. Its position in relation to the orbital rim depends upon the depth of the orbit, and is of some clinical interest. During cataract and other ocular surgeries, retrobulbar anesthesia is given into the posterior inferior orbit through a needle 31–50 mm in length. The anesthetic agent must be placed in the vicinity of the ciliary ganglion and the motor nerves to the extraocular muscles in order to achieve both sensory and motor blockade. The distance from the inferolateral orbital rim to the optic canal varies from 42–54 mm,[59] and in the shorter orbits there is a risk of inadvertent penetration of the optic nerve. This risk is greater with needles over 31.5 mm in length.[59]

The trochlear nerve

Embryology

The trochlear or fourth cranial nerve is first recognizable in the 18–24 mm (6–7-week) embryo.[110] By the end of the embryonic period (10 weeks) it has established connections between the brainstem and the superior oblique muscle.

The adult trochlear nerve

Fibers destined for the trochlear nerve originate from the trochlear nucleus at the caudal end of the oculomotor nuclear complex, ventral to the aqueduct of Sylvius, and at the level of the inferior colliculus. The fascicular axons emerge from the upper aspect of the nucleus. They pass dorsally to decussate in the anterior medullary velum immediately caudal to the inferior colliculus, and exit on the dorsal surface of the brainstem on the opposite side. This is the only crossed cranial nerve, and the only one to exit on the dorsal side of the midbrain.[124] The decussation is incomplete, however, and about 5% of the motor neurons pass to the ipsilateral trochlear nerve.[81] Also, some neurons exhibit axonal branching and may control the superior oblique muscles bilaterally.[81] For the most part, however, the axons of each trochlear nucleus innervate the contralateral superior oblique muscle.

The trochlear nerve runs ventrally around the cerebral peduncle above the pons, between the posterior cerebral and superior cerebellar arteries. It extends along the free border of the tentorium and pierces the dura into the cavernous sinus dorsal to the posterior clinoid process, and inferior and lateral to the oculomotor nerve. Within the cavernous sinus the trochlear nerve runs in the deep layer of the lateral wall, between the oculomotor nerve and the ophthalmic branch of the trigeminal nerve (see Chapter 1). As it courses forward, the trochlear nerve moves superiorly, crosses over the oculomotor nerve, and enters the orbit through the lateral superior orbital fissure, above the upper border of the annulus of Zinn,[39] in company with the frontal and lacrimal branches of the ophthalmic division of the trigeminal nerve. Here it is associated with filaments from the carotid sympathetic plexus. As the trochlear nerve extends forward, it moves medially as two individuals bundles (range 1–4),[131] crossing over the origin of the superior rectus muscle, and runs medially between the orbital roof and the levator palpebrae superioris muscle. It continues to the lateral surface of the superior oblique muscle where it breaks up into 4 to 10 fascicles that penetrate the muscle on its superolateral surface about 8–17 mm from the annulus of Zinn. In some cases the nerve may pass around the lateral side of the muscle to insert into its lateral or inferior surface.

The trochlear nerve has a long intracranial course where it is predisposed to injury from a variety of intracranial lesions.[2] For part of its intraorbital extent the nerve lies adjacent to the bony orbital wall where it is vulnerable to injury from blunt head trauma, resulting in isolated unilateral or bilateral superior oblique palsies, even following relatively trivial blows.

The abducens nerve

Embryology

The abducens or sixth cranial nerve is the last of the motor nerves to the extraocular muscles to appear in embryogenesis. It is first seen in the 31–34 mm (8–9-week) stage.[107] Failure of the abducens nerve to develop properly may result in aberrant innervation of the lateral rectus muscle by the oculomotor nerve (Duane's syndrome).

The adult abducens nerve

The abducens nerve carries somatic motor fibers to the lateral rectus muscle. These neurons arise in the paired motor nuclei which lie in the pons, immediately ventral to the floor of the fourth ventricle. Fascicular axons pass ventrally and caudally on the lateral side of the pyramidal tract, passing medial to the superior olivary nucleus. They emerge near the midline in the sulcus between the pons and medulla oblongata. In about 6% of cases, this nerve emerges as a double trunk.[93] The abducens nerve courses up the ventral surface of the pons, between the latter and the anterior inferior cerebellar artery. In up to 30% of individuals, the intracranial abducens nerve may exist as two or more separate trunks that fuse just before passing into the orbit.[25,43,96]

The abducens nerve continues to ascend through the subarachnoid space along the clivus. During this ascent, the abducens nerves from both sides lie in close proximity, and some distance from other neural structures. Thus, compressive lesions in this region, such as basilar artery aneurysms or chordomas, can result in bilateral sixth nerve palsies without other associated neurologic deficits. In about 8% of cases where the nerve trunk is single, it divides into two branches within the subarachnoid space. The nerve then pierces the dura mater and passes around or through the inferior petrosal sinus. It bends over the petrous apex, and passes through Dorello's canal (see Chapter 1). The latter is an osteofibrous conduit within a venous confluence formed by the posterior cavernous, and the inferior petrosal and basilar sinuses.[120] This cavity of venous blood is traversed by several trabeculae, the most consistent being the petroclinoid (Gruber's) ligament. The abducens nerve passes beneath this ligament, usually in company with the dorsal meningeal artery which supplies the nerve in this region. During its course through the canal, the abducens nerve changes direction rather abruptly as it passes over the petrous apex and under Gruber's ligament, sometimes to nearly 90°. This anatomic relationship and the long and tortuous intracranial path of the nerve along the cranial base contributes to its vulnerability to compressive and other injuries.[121]

As the abducens nerve emerges from Dorello's canal, it finally enters the posterior cavernous sinus just lateral to the apex of the posterior clinoid process. Within the sinus, nerves with the divided branches unite into a single nerve trunk.[43] This trunk courses forward and bends laterally around the intracavernous carotid artery to which it is fixed by connective tissue. It then runs medial and parallel to the ophthalmic division of the trigeminal nerve. Unlike the oculomotor and trochlear nerves, the abducens nerve does not lie within the lateral wall of the sinus, but rather runs within the body of the sinus just lateral to the internal carotid artery.[43] It is, therefore, usually the first nerve affected by an intracavernous carotid aneurysm. The oculosympathetic fibers from the carotid plexus to the iris dilator muscle run with the abducens nerve for a short distance before joining the ophthalmic division of the trigeminal nerve. Thus, a sixth nerve palsy associated with an ipsilateral Horner's syndrome can be localized to the cavernous sinus.

The abducens nerve enters the orbit through the superior orbital fissure and the oculomotor foramen of the annulus of Zinn, adjacent to the origin of the lateral rectus muscle. As it passes through the annulus, the abducens nerve runs inferior and medial to the frontal and trochlear nerves, and lateral to the superior and inferior divisions of the oculomotor nerve.[49] In some individuals it is separated from the oculomotor nerve by a dense collagenous septum that extends from the origin of the inferior rectus muscle to the sheath of the superior rectus muscle.[86] Within the orbital apex, the nerve may run as a single trunk, but more frequently it ramifies early into 2–7 branches. These branches course laterally and penetrate the sheath of the lateral rectus muscle shortly after leaving the annulus of Zinn. They run within clefts on the medial surface of the muscle where they further divide into about 10 filaments before finally penetrating the conal surface of the muscle at the junction of the posterior and middle thirds of its length.

The abducens nerve is predisposed to injury from head trauma and intracranial lesions because of its course along the base of the skull, and its abrupt angulation over the petrous ridge.[2] As the nerve passes through the confinement of Dorello's canal beneath the petroclinoid ligament, it may be affected by chronic mastoiditis. In the preantibiotic era, abducens nerve palsy was a common sequel to suppurative otitis media in the adjacent petrous portion of the temporal bone ("Gradenigo's syndrome": apical petrousitis, hearing loss, sixth nerve palsy, and severe ipsilateral facial pain).

The oculomotor, trochlear, and abducens nerves also carry sensory fibers from proprioceptive receptors in the extraocular muscles which they innervate. These pass backward in their respective nerves to the mesencephalic nucleus of the trigeminal nerve.

Defects affecting neuronal control of ocular movement

The ocular motor nuclei mediate contraction of individual extraocular muscles that are responsible for specific eye movements. Lesions affecting the motor pathways anywhere from the central motor nuclei to the myoneural junctions result in specific motility defects. Loss of motor control to the medial rectus muscle results in defective adduction, or medial rotation, of the eye. Lesions affecting contraction of the lateral rectus muscle produce loss of abduction, or lateral rotation, of the eye. The superior and inferior rectus muscles produce more complex ocular movements that depend upon the position of gaze. In the primary position, the eyes are directed forward, parallel to the mid-sagittal plane, but the orbital axes, and therefore the vertical rectus muscles, are oriented 23° to this plane. Thus, in primary or in adducted positions of gaze, the superior rectus muscle elevates, intorts, and slightly adducts the globe. Starting from the same position, the inferior rectus muscle

depresses, extorts, and slightly adducts the globe. When the eye is abducted 23° from the primary position, the superior rectus muscle acts as a pure elevator and the inferior rectus as a pure depressor of the globe.

The superior oblique tendon is oriented at 51° to the sagittal plane, and inserts lateral and posterior to the midpoint of ocular rotation. When the globe is in the primary position of gaze, contraction of the superior oblique muscle produces both depression and intortion of the eye. When the eye is abducted 39° to the sagittal plane, the superior oblique acts as a pure intorter of the globe. When the globe is maximally adducted to 51°, this muscle acts as a pure depressor of the eye. The inferior oblique muscle is also oriented at approximately 51° to the sagittal plane. Like its superior counterpart, it also inserts onto the globe lateral and posterior to the midpoint of ocular rotation. In the primary ocular position, this muscle acts to elevate and extort the globe. At 39° of abduction, the only action is pure extortion. At 51° of adduction, the only movement is pure elevation.

In addition to simple ductions of the globe, highly complex ocular movements are able to adjust eye positions with head and body movement, maintain alignment at various distances, smoothly pursue moving targets, and rapidly redirect foveal fixation from one object to another. These movements are coordinated and executed by a number of supranuclear pathways. These include the supranuclear frontomesencephalic and occipitomesencephalic pathways, the subthalamic pretectal areas, the mesencephalic and pontine reticular formation, the medial longitudinal fasciculus, vestibular pathways, and areas of the medulla connecting with the oculomotor system. Lesions in these areas may result in defects in rapid eye movement, deficits in smooth pursuit mechanisms, impersistence of conjugate gaze or steady fixation, paresis of vertical gaze and convergence, tonic deviations, and dysconjugate eye movements.[36]

The trigeminal nerve

The trigeminal nerve is a mixed nerve that consists of a small motor component and a larger sensory component.[69] The motor fibers arise from a superior nucleus along the lateral portion of the cerebral aqueduct, and from an inferior nucleus in the upper pons. Fibers from the two nuclei join to form the motor root. The motor neurons emerge with the sensory fibers of the trigeminal nerve, pass beneath the gasserian ganglion, and continue in the mandibular division of the nerve. These fibers supply the masseter, temporalis, and internal pterygoid muscles, the tensor tympani, tensor veli palatini, omohyoid, and the anterior belly of the digastricus muscle.

The sensory component of the trigeminal nerve carries fibers for pain, touch, temperature, and proprioception from the eye, face, sinus mucosa, and scalp. These neurons pass backward in the ophthalmic, maxillary, and mandibular divisions of the nerve to synapse in the gasserian (semilunar) ganglion over the apex of the petrous portion of the temporal bone. The ganglion is situated lateral to the posterior portion of the cavernous sinus and internal carotid artery. The second order sensory neurons then extend caudally, pass through Meckel's cave formed by a split in the dura over the petrous bone, cross to the posterior cranial fossa, and enter the pons at its junction with the middle cerebellar peduncle. Upon entering the pons, the trigeminal root divides into an ascending tract to the main sensory nucleus and the mesencephalic trigeminal subnuclei, and a descending bundle to the spinal tract of the trigeminal nerve that ends in the substania gelatinosa of Rolando. These three subnuclei represent the rostral to caudal portions of the trigeminal nucleus, respectively. Sensory information entering from cranial nerves V, VII, IX, and X is also sent to the trigeminal nucleus which then contains a complete sensory map of the face and mouth. The different parts of the trigeminal nucleus receive and process different types of sensory information—pain/temperature, touch/position, and proprioception. Information is modified at the level of the trigeminal nucleus by interneurons from the reticular formation before second order neurons pass to the thalamus via several tracts where they again synapse before being projected onto various areas of the cerebral cortex.

Of the three main divisions of the trigeminal nerve (ophthalmic, maxillary, and mandibular), the ophthalmic division (V1) carries the major sensory input from the eyelids and orbit. The maxillary division contributes a small component from the lower eyelid. Tracing the nerve forward into the orbit, the ophthalmic division arises from the anterior aspect of the gasserian ganglion, and passes forward within the lateral wall of the cavernous sinus below the trochlear nerve (see Chapter 1). Within the sinus the ophthalmic nerve receives tiny branches from the oculomotor, trochlear, and abducens nerves. These carry sensory information from the extraocular muscles supplied by these nerves. Additional recurrent branches form a rich plexus of nerves that contribute to sensory innervation from the intracranial dura. Sympathetic fibers from the carotid plexus also join the ophthalmic nerve at this point. Just before exiting from the anterior end of the cavernous sinus, the ophthalmic nerve divides into three branches, the lacrimal, frontal, and nasociliary nerves.

The lacrimal nerve is the smallest branch of the ophthalmic division. It enters the orbit through the superior orbital fissure, above the annulus of Zinn and the head of the lateral rectus muscle. It courses anteriorly in the extraconal orbital space along the superior border of the lateral rectus muscle, and enters the posterior substance of the lacrimal gland. Just before entering the lacrimal gland it is joined by one or two small communicating branches derived from the zygomaticotemporal nerve off the maxillary division. These zygomatic branches carry some of the parasympathetic secretomotor fibers from the pterygopalatine ganglion to the lacrimal gland. Several terminal twigs of the lacrimal nerve pass through or around the gland, and end in the conjunctiva and skin of the lateral upper eyelid.

The frontal nerve is the largest branch of the ophthalmic division. It enters the orbit through the superior orbital fissure above the annulus of Zinn in close association with the trochlear nerve. It passes forward and medially to a position along the mid-orbital roof, between the levator muscle and periorbita. About halfway from the orbital apex to the orbital rim, the frontal nerve usually divides into two branches, the supratrochlear and the supraorbital nerves. This point of division is variable, and occasionally the frontal nerve may remain as a single trunk until after it exits from the supraorbital notch. The supratrochlear nerve courses anteromedially where it passes above the pulley system of the superior oblique muscle. It usually gives off a communicating branch to the infratrochlear branch of the nasociliary nerve and then pierces the orbital septum at the superomedial orbital rim between the trochlea and supraorbital notch. The nerve divides into one to three branches, ascends onto the central forehead under and through the corrugator supercilii and frontalis muscles, and receives sensory input from the skin of the lower portion of the forehead, and from skin and conjunctiva of the medial one-third of the upper eyelid (see Chapter 8).

The supraorbital branch of the frontal nerve (supraorbital nerve) arises from the frontal nerve and passes forward nearly in the midline of the orbit just on the orbital side of periorbita. It exits the orbit superomedially in company with the supraorbital artery. Just prior to, or more commonly just after exiting the orbit the supraorbital nerve may divide into as many as four branches. Small palpebral filaments transmit sensory fibers from conjunctiva and skin of the central two-thirds of the upper eyelid. It also carries sympathetic fibers from the carotid plexus mediating sudomotor and vasomotor responses to the forehead.[89]

The branches of the supraorbital nerve exit the orbit in the submuscular plane, about 2–3 cm lateral to the midline of the forehead. This point of exit is marked on the orbital rim of the frontal bone by a notch, or less frequently by a foramen. In 60–70% of individuals a notch is present instead of a foramen.[17,65,128] Initially, these neural branches lie deep to the orbicularis and frontalis muscles, in close approximation to the periosteum of the supraorbital ridge. The medial branches ascend as they run superiorly on the forehead, becoming more superficial as they pass through the corrugator and frontalis muscles to reach the subcutaneous plane. It divides into multiple branches that run cephalad in the most superficial fibers of the frontalis muscle forming a wide fan pattern to enter the scalp.

The lateral or deep branch of the supraorbital nerve runs laterally along the orbital rim or sometimes up to 1.5 cm superior to the rim.[31,32] It remains in the deep galea beneath the frontalis muscle and turns cephalad at about the level of the later third of the eyebrow. The most lateral branches remain within the deep fascia until the level of the hairline[33] at which point they become more superficial as they innervate the scalp. This anatomic relationship is of surgical significance during dissections involving the forehead, such as direct brow lifts. Excision of tissue just above the brow should avoid the superficial frontalis muscle fibers in the medial eyebrow to avoid injury to the superficial supraorbital branches. More laterally, the dissection can be deeper, to the submuscular plane. The supraorbital nerve carries sensory information from the skin of the scalp as far back as the lamdoidal suture and to the pericranium.

The nasociliary branch of the ophthalmic division of the trigeminal nerve (nasociliary nerve) enters the intraconal orbital space at the superior orbital fissure. In most cases it passes through the annulus of Zinn along with the oculomotor nerve branches. Rarely, the nasociliary nerve may enter extraconally, above the oculomotor foramen. In such instances, the nasociliary nerve runs forward for 3–4 mm and then penetrates the annulus through a small canal in the region joining the tendons of Lockwood and Zinn. Shortly after entering the intraconal space, along the lateral side of the optic nerve, the nasociliary nerve gives off a small sensory branch to the ciliary ganglion. It may be joined by sympathetic filaments from the cavernous sinus carotid plexus. These sensory fibers pass through the ganglion without synapsing and continue within the short posterior ciliary nerves to the globe. Here they penetrate sclera near the optic nerve.

After giving off the sensory branch to the ciliary ganglion, the nasociliary nerve turns medially, and passes over the optic nerve 8–12 mm anterior to the orbital apex. Just medial to the optic nerve it gives off two to three long ciliary nerves. These travel alongside the short ciliary nerves, and penetrate sclera adjacent to the optic nerve, usually one medially and the others laterally. They continue in the medial and lateral suprachoroidal space to the iris, ciliary muscle, and cornea where they receive sensory input. These nerves also carry efferent autonomic fibers from the cavernous sympathetic plexus to the dilator muscles of the iris.

The main trunk of the nasociliary nerve continues medially in company with the ophthalmic artery. Its relationship to the artery is variable, and the nerve may cross over the latter several times before reaching the medial orbital wall.[27] Here it may divide into several fascicles that run together. These turn anteriorly between the superior oblique and medial rectus muscles, and extend along the medial orbital wall. In this region, the nasociliary nerve gives off one or more anterior ethmoidal branches which pass through the anterior ethmoidal foramen. The presence of a posterior ethmoidal nerve is quite variable. When present, it may run a rather circuitous route from the nasociliary nerve trunk to the posterior ethmoidal foramen. The ethmoidal nerves pass into the ethmoid sinus mucosa and then re-enter the cranial vault, cross the anterior portion of the cribriform plate beneath the dura of the anterior cranial fossa, and enter the nasal cavity through the anterior nasal canals at the side of the crista galli. They receive sensory fibers from nasal and ethmoid sinus mucosa. The terminal portion of the nasociliary nerve extends forward in the orbit as the infratrochlear nerve, where it runs along the superior border of the medial rectus muscle. It runs beneath the trochlea, where it usually remains lateral to the ophthalmic artery, and then penetrates the orbital septum above the medial canthal tendon. The infratrochlear nerve receives sensory input from the medial portion of the eyelids, the medial conjunctiva, caruncle, lacrimal sac, and the side of the nose.

The maxillary, or second division of the trigeminal nerve (V2) leaves the gasserian ganglion just posterolateral to the cavernous sinus and enters the sinus where it travels within the lateral wall below cranial nerves III, IV, and V1. It exits the cranium through the foramen rotundum in the greater wing of the sphenoid bone to enter the pterygopalatine fossa.[100] Here it gives off small palatine and nasal branches, and the zygomatic nerve. It then enters the orbit through the inferior orbital fissure terminating as the infraorbital nerve. This is the largest of the branches of the maxillary nerve. The infraorbital nerve runs in the infraorbital canal in the orbital floor, and exits at the infraorbital foramen below the central inferior orbital rim beneath the levator labii superioris muscle. It divides into four branches with some variation. The external nasal branch runs medially to the side of the nose, and the internal nasal branch supplies the nasal septum and nasal vestibule. The labial branch innervates the upper lip and mucosa. The palpebral branch turns sharply upward to innervate the skin of the lower eyelid and conjunctiva.[48]

It divides into two further branches, one to the medial and the other to the lateral eyelid. In most cases the infraorbital artery is located in the middle of the infraorbital nerve bundles.

The zygomatic nerve emerges from the maxillary division within the pterygopalatine fossa, and it enters the infraorbital canal along with the infraorbital nerve. It divides into two branches, the zygomaticotemporal and zygomticofacial nerves that exit into the orbit just before the infraorbital groove becomes bridged over with bone to form the infraorbital canal. The zygomaticotemporal nerve runs laterally and superiorly along the lateral orbital wall and passes through the zygomticotemporal foramen into the temporalis fossa where it supplies the lateral temporal skin. The zygomaticofacial nerve runs anteriorly and laterally to enter the zygomticofacial canal in the zygomatic bone near the inferolateral orbital rim. It exits onto the lateral cheek to transmit cutaneous sensory information from this region of the face.

The infraorbital canal is always present but may be a double or even triple opening in 10% of individuals.[58,60] It runs in the orbital floor within the maxillary bone. Its roof may be complete throughout its length (50%) or unbridged forming an open groove for its proximal half (50%). The roof where present is very thin, whereas the floor of the canal is thick. Within the canal the infraorbital nerve is accompanied by the infraorbital artery superomedially and the infraorbital vein inferiorly. As it courses forward, the infraorbital nerve consists of 3–8 interwoven fascicles enclosed within a loose connective tissue sheath along with the artery and vein. After exiting onto the face, these fascicles radiate into the subcutaneous tissues of the check and upper lip. Because of the extreme thinness of the orbital floor, orbital fractures frequently involve the floor and infraorbital canal. Trauma to the infraorbital nerve results in paresthesia in the skin of the lower eyelid, cheek, and the gum above the incisor and canine teeth.

Clinical correlations

The ophthalmic division of the trigeminal nerve is involved in several important clinical phenomena. When *Herpes zoster* infection affects the dorsal root or extramedullary cranial nerve ganglia, it often shows a predilection for the gasserian ganglion and ophthalmic nerve. It is ushered in by a severe, unilateral, disabling neuralgia, followed after several days by vesicular eruption and swelling in the distribution of the ophthalmic nerve. These areas include the upper eyelid, forehead, and tip of the nose. Superficial and deep corneal opacities may occur, associated with an anterior uveitis. When the vesicles rupture, hemorrhagic areas remain that heal in several weeks, leaving deep-pitted scars. Post herpetic neuralgia resistant to treatment may persist in a small number of cases.[108]

Gradenigo's syndrome has become rare in the antibiotic era. It results from suppurative otitis media associated with inflammatory edema at the apex of the petrous pyramid, and sometimes from osteomyelitis of the petrous apex. Pain in the distribution of the trigeminal nerve, and lateral rectus palsy are secondary to involvement of adjacent portions of these nerves.

The oculocardiac reflex is defined as any intraoperative bradycardia exceeding 10% of preoperative heart rate occurring during ocular manipulation.[15] It may result in clinically profound bradycardia (35–40 beats per minute), nausea, and light-headedness during ophthalmic surgery.[7] The reflex has also been associated with atrioventricular block, bigeminy, and cardiac arrest. In addition, the reflex increases vagal tone and may cause generalized vasodilatation and hypoperfusion. This phenomenon poses a significant risk for intraoperative morbidity and even death. It is most commonly associated with traction on the extraocular muscles,[83] especially the medial rectus muscle.[5] The reflex has also been described with stretching of the eyelid retractors,[3] during blepharoplasty procedures with traction on the medial fat pocket,[75] and during enucleation.[84] Sensory neurons forming the afferent limb of this reflex arc run in the ophthalmic division of the trigeminal nerve to the gasserian ganglion, and then on to the main sensory nucleus along the fourth ventricle. After descending in the spinal trigeminal tract, sensory stimuli cross via polysynaptic pathways in the reticular formation to the visceral motor nucleus of the vagus nerve. The resulting excessive vagal stimulation results in the clinical symptoms noted above, and may be blocked with atropine sulfate. This reflex may be reduced, but not completely prevented, with administration of local retrobulbar anesthetic.[77] However, the use of such blocks may itself precipitate the reflex.[107]

The oculorespiratory reflex was first described in rabbits by Aschner,[9] and later confirmed in humans by Petzetakis.[95] Blanc et al.[12] reported that this reflex was a frequent and potentially dangerous result of traction on the extraocular muscles during surgery. Although any muscle can invoke this reflex, the medial rectus muscles appears to be the most sensitive, as is true also for the oculocardiac reflex. Shallowness of respiratory movement and apnea of up to 20 seconds duration have been noted. Respiratory arrhythmia and irregular respiratory arrest have followed intraorbital stimulation.[54] Retrobulbar anesthesia can completely block this reflex. However, vagotomy, atropine sulfate, and glycopyrrolate have no effect, suggesting that the efferent pathway is different from that of the oculocardiac reflex.[63]

The cavernous sinus syndromes occur in a variety of presentations, depending upon the anatomy of the specific region of the sinus involved. Lesions of the posterior sinus involve cranial nerves III, IV, V1, V2, V3, and VI, due to the close approximation of the sinus with the trigeminal ganglion in Meckel's cave. Clinically this presents as partial or complete ophthalmoplegia, associated with ipsilateral facial anesthesia and loss of masticatory function. Injury to the central portion of the sinus usually involves cranial nerves III, IV, V1, V2, and VI, with sparing of V3, since the mandibular division exits the cranium through the foramen ovale. Ophthalmoplegia here is associated with preservation of sensation in the mandible, and with preservation of masticatory function. Damage to the anterior cavernous sinus involves cranial nerves III, IV, V1, and VI. The maxillary division is spared because it exits the sinus through the foramen rotundum. In this case, ophthalmoplegia is associated with a sensory deficit only in the ophthalmic division of the trigeminal nerve. In addition, anterior sinus syndromes are more likely to involve the optic nerve.[114]

The extraorbital branches of the trigeminal nerve can be damaged during forehead, eyebrow, and facial surgery and

reconstructions. In direct brow lift procedures care must be taken to avoid injury to the medial superficial branches of the supraorbital nerve. Endoscopic forehead elevation carries a risk of injury to the supraorbital nerve at its exit from the supraorbital notch or foramen.

Sympathetic system

The efferent sympathetic innervation to the eye and orbit is thought to arise within the hypothalamus. First-order neurons descend uncrossed in the ventrolateral portion of the brainstem to synapse in the ciliospinal center of Budge in the spinal cord. Second order neurons leave the spinal cord with the ventral roots of the last cervical to second thoracic spinal nerves. They soon leave these roots as the white rami communicantes to enter the paravertebral sympathetic chain. Those neurons destined for the eye synapse in the superior cervical ganglion. Some of the third-order postganglionic neurons extend along the external carotid artery branches and are responsible for facial vasodilatation and sweating. Others pass intracranially as a plexus that follows the internal carotid artery, through the carotid canal, to the region of the gasserian ganglion and cavernous sinus. The exact relationships if the sympathetic pathway within the sinus remains controversial. The sympathetic plexus has been variously described as following the route of the carotid and ophthalmic arteries into to the orbit, as passing directly to the ciliary ganglion through the superior orbital fissure, as passing along the ophthalmic division of the trigeminal nerve, as following the course of cranial nerves III, IV, V1 and VI, or various combinations of all four.[114] Earlier histologic studies failed to show sympathetic fibers along the oculomotor and trochlear nerves,[99] but small unmyelinated fibers have been observed associated with the abducens nerve.[61] The traditional major pathway most workers agree upon for the sympathetic plexus within the cavernous sinus is that from the ICA they run a short course with the abducens nerve, then join the ophthalmic division of the trigeminal and proceed to the superior orbital fissure to enter the orbit.[94] This explains two possible clinical syndromes that have been observed: one involving Horner's syndrome with trigeminal dysfunction, and the other involving Horner's syndrome with sixth nerve paresis. Sporadic clinical occurrences of the latter conditions have been reported.[1,44]

More recently the autonomic pathways to the orbit have been shown to be considerably more complex. Sympathetic branches from the cavernous ICA plexus have been demonstrated in close proximity to the oculomotor and trochlear nerves in addition to the abducens nerve. Bleys et al.[13] described a lateral extension of the autonomic nerve plexus associated with the ICA and the abducens nerve, mainly medial to the trochlear and ophthalmic nerves along the lateral wall of the cavernous sinus. From this plexus fibers joined the oculomotor and trochlear nerves *en route* to the orbit. The main sympathetic plexus associated with the ICA and abducens nerve continue as a separate group. Oikawa et al.[90] reported a plexus of sympathetic nerves surrounding the ophthalmic artery and all branches of V1 proximal to the annulus of Zinn. Ruskell[104] and Thakker et al.[116] have demonstrated sympathetic fibers from the cavernous sinus passing into the orbit through the optic canal. These nerve fibers are located in the adventitia of the ophthalmic artery, the surrounding adipose connective tissue, the dura of the optic nerve, and in the periosteum of the bony canal. Although some fibers course directly to the eye, most join the short posterior ciliary nerves. However, the number of fibers is small so that despite these findings the major sympathetic routes to the orbit still appear to be along the sensory nerve branches of the trigeminal nerve through the superior orbital fissure.

Rusu et al.[105] demonstrated the importance of the pterygopalatine fossa in the distribution of sympathetic fibers to the orbit. Using immunohistochemical techniques, they showed sympathetic fibers from the superior cervical ganglion (SCG) passing along the external carotid artery plexus, through the pterygopalatine fossa, and into the orbit along the maxillary artery and infraorbital nerve branches. Following injection into the SCG, labeled fibers and terminals were observed in the choroid associated with smooth muscle cells of arterioles. The choroid thus appears to have a dual autonomic innervation, parasympathetic along nerves from the pterygopalatine ganglion, and sympathetic along blood vessels from the pterygopalatine fossa. This dual innervation maintains homeostasis of vasoconstriction and vasodilatation.[66] A similar dual innervation from the pterygopalatine fossa appears to exist for the lacrimal gland.

Regardless of the specific routes into the orbit, sympathetic fibers enter the ciliary ganglion via the tiny sympathetic rootlet, between the branches from the oculomotor and nasociliary nerves. These fibers pass through the ganglion without synapsing and enter into the short ciliary nerves through which they reach the globe. They provide vasoconstrictor stimulation to uveal blood vessels. Other sympathetic branches bypass the ciliary ganglion, leave the nasociliary nerve via the long posterior ciliary nerves, and penetrate sclera near the optic nerve to supply the dilator muscle of the iris. In addition to the fibers that travel within the ciliary nerves, a diffuse nerve plexus is present in the posterior orbit consisting of both sympathetic and parasympathetic fibers. These travel to various orbital structures along neurovascular pathways, and along fascial planes unrelated to specific arteries and nerves.[11] Sympathetic fibers to the central retinal artery suggest some effect over optic disc and retinal artery perfusion.[116,130] Studies have shown sympathetic fibers along the lacrimal nerve and artery that appear to serve both vascular and secretory functions.[14,76,103]

Thakker et al.[116] noted that arteries in the orbit tend to travel in close association with sensory nerves. They suggested that a functional explanation might lie in the possibility that the sensory nerves provide a continuous supply of sympathetic nerves to the arteries. They also suggested that sympathetic fibers travel with motor nerves to provide dynamic modulation of muscle motility through smooth muscle fibers located within the extraocular muscle suspensory and pulley systems[24] (see Chapter 3).

Sympathetic innervation from the superior cervical ganglion to Müller's supratarsal muscle has been demonstrated,[18] and Thakker et al.[116] showed that the major pathway was along the infratrochlear and lacrimal branches of the ophthalmic nerve. Here, the arteries to the lids do not appear to be a major pathway.[74] Innervation to the sympathetic muscle of the lower eyelid and to Müller's inferior orbital muscle overlying the inferior orbital fissure travel along branches of the

infraorbital nerve from the pterygopalatine fossa. A dense nerve plexus has been described in the levator aponeurosis,[11] similar to that in the longitudinal ligaments of the vertebral column.[42] These may be afferent in nature, but their function remains unknown. More recently, Kakizaki et al.[58] reported the consistent finding of smooth muscle fibers distributed mainly in the posterior layer of the levator aponeurosis in Caucasians similar to that in the Asian eyelid. They suggested that these may play a role in regulating tension within this structure.

Horner's syndrome results from ipsilateral disruption of sympathetic innervation to the head and neck. It may be caused by a lesion anywhere along the three-neuron oculosympathetic pathway from the brainstem to the eye. The affected pupil is miotic in dim light due to paresis of the dilator muscle. Impaired innervation to sympathetic accessory retractor muscles in both upper and lower eyelids results in mild upper lid ptosis, and mild elevation of the lower lid. In Horner's syndrome resulting from preganglionic sympathetic denervation, there is associated impairment of sweating and vasoconstriction on the ipsilateral face and neck.

Horner's syndrome resulting from injury to the first order neurons is usually seen in the setting of severe central nervous system disease and, as such, presents little diagnostic difficulty. From a practical standpoint, it is more important to be able to determine whether an isolated Horner's syndrome results from involvement of the preganglionic or postganglionic neurons, since the responsible lesions differ considerably. Preganglionic (second-order) Horner's is related to malignancy in up to 50% of cases,[41] and may be the initial sign of occult neoplasm in some cases. Lower cervical trauma is another common cause of damage to preganglionic fibers. Isolated postganglionic (third-order) Horner's, on the other hand, is usually due to causes other than malignant tumor, and thus has a better prognosis. Confirmation and localization of the site of pathology is accomplished with pharmacologic testing. When a postganglionic Horner's results from a lesion in the cavernous sinus, there are usually associated cranial nerve palsies.

Parasympathetic system

As discussed above, parasympathetic nerve fibers serving ocular function originate in the Edinger-Wesphal nucleus and pass with the oculomotor nerve through the superior orbital fissure to the ciliary ganglion where they synapse. Postganglionic fibers then course in the short posterior ciliary nerves to the eye where they innervate the ciliary and sphincter pupillae muscles.

In addition to the control of ocular functions, parasympathetic nerve fibers are also distributed to orbital and paraorbital targets. Preganglionic fibers arising in the superior salivatory nucleus of the facial nerve leave the brain in the nervus intermedius where they join the main facial nerve and pass through the geniculate ganglion. These fibers divide into two pathways, the greater superficial petrosal nerve and the chorda tympani. The latter runs to the submandibular ganglion from which postganglionic fibers innervate the submandibular and sublingual salivary glands. The greater superficial petrosal nerve runs through the middle ear and joins with the deep petrosal nerve carrying sympathetic fibers from the ICA plexus. Together they form the vidian nerve, or nerve of the pterygoid canal (also known as the vidian canal). This nerve enters the canal at the anterolateral edge of the foramen lacerum and runs within it along the line of fusion of the pterygoid process and the body of the sphenoid bone.[91] The canal opens anteriorly into the medial part of the pterygopalatine fossa situated between the margins of the maxillary and sphenoid bones. Here the parasympathetic fibers synapse in the pterygopalatine (sphenpalatine) ganglion. This is a small structure measuring about 5 mm in diameter embedded within fatty tissue of the fossa. Postganglionic fibers leave the ganglion through several routes. The greater and lesser palatine nerves, the nasopalatine nerve, and the pharyngeal nerve pass to secretory glands in the mouth, pharynx, and nose. Another branch joins the maxillary division of the trigeminal nerve (V2). The latter enters the pterygopalatine fossa from the cavernous sinus via the foramen rotundum. It courses laterally and slightly upward to the inferior orbital fissure in company with the infraorbital artery, and divides into the infraorbital and zygomatic nerves. The parasympathetic fibers from the pterygopalatine ganglion are associated with all major branches of the infraorbital nerve. The zygomatic nerve divides into the zygomaticotemporal and zygomaticofacial nerves which pass through foramina in the lateral orbital walls to provide sensory innervation to the temple and upper cheek. A small communicating branch from the zygomaticotemporal branch carries parasympathetic fibers to the lacrimal gland for secretomotor function of tear production.[102,109] Other fibers pass to the meibomian glands in the eyelids, and to the choroidal vasculature.[21]

Small autonomic ganglia have been described within the cavernous sinus along the abducens and lateral autonomic plexuses.[13,113] Based on immunohistochemical staining these appear to be parasympathetic ganglia. Thus, it appears that both sympathetic and parasympathetic fibers may pass into the orbit from the cavernous sinus autonomic plexuses. Bleys et al.[13] found fibers extending from the cavernous sinus to the pterygopalatine parasympathetic ganglion, but could not confirm exact fiber pathways.

The facial nerve

Although the facial nerve is not strictly an orbital nerve, it does supply motor fibers to the eyelid protractors through its temporal and zygomatic branches, and parasympathetic fibers to the lacrimal gland. It, therefore, must be included in any discussion of orbital and eyelid anatomy.

The facial nerve is a mixed nerve with both sensory and motor components. The larger motor root supplies most of the muscles of facial expression, as well as the buccinator, platysma, stapedius, stylohyoideus, and the posterior belly of the digastricus muscles. The smaller sensory root (nervus intermedius) carries special sensory fibers for taste from the anterior tongue and palate, and general sensory fibers from the external auditory meatus, soft palate, and adjacent pharynx. It also carries parasympathetic secretomotor fibers to the submandibular, sublingual, and lacrimal glands. Nerve fibers that will form the facial nerve derive from four general areas in the brain and brainstem; the facial nucleus, the salivatory nucleus, the trigeminal nucleus, and the tractus solitarius.

The cortical motor projection of the facial nerve originates in the inferior portion of the precentral gyrus, in the middle of the motor cortical strip. Fibers extend downward, within the internal capsule, and then pass through the pons within the pyramidal tracts. Most of these fibers cross in the posterior pons to reach the facial nucleus on the opposite side. However, some fibers diverge toward the ipsilateral nucleus. The motor nucleus of the facial nerve is located in the reticular formation of the pons, in the vicinity of the nucleus ambiguus. Within the nucleus, motor cells are arranged in groups representing their muscles of innervation.[115] The nucleus can be divided into an upper segment that supplies the frontalis muscle, the superior portion of the orbicularis muscle, and the corrugator muscle, and a lower segment that supplies the other muscles of facial expression.[53] Cells located in the lower segment receive connections from the pyramidal system that are completely crossed. Those in the upper segment receive both crossed and uncrossed fibers.[20] Other sources of input to the facial nerve subserve non-voluntary movements of the face. Emotional control of musculature is through efferents originating in the extrapyramidal areas of the hypothalmus and globus pallidus projecting in the reticular formation.[72] The facial nucleus also receives afferents from other brain stem nuclei, particularly from sensory centers. Input from the trigeminal nucleus provides the basis for the corneal reflex, and the reflex loop with the acoustic nucleus is responsible for the reflexive eye closure with loud noises. Additional afferent loops from the visual system result in reflex blinking.[78]

Motor axons leave the dorsal surface of the facial nucleus. They run dorsally and medially to the rhomboid fossa where they turn sharply rostrally above the medial longitudinal fasciculus along the medial side of the abducens nucleus. Here, they abruptly arch over the abducens nucleus within the genu of the facial nerve to form an elevation in the rhomboid fossa known as the facial colliculus. Since the motor fibers are not joined by other components of the facial nerve until after they have formed this internal genu around the abducens nucleus, they can be involved by central lesions not affecting other functions of the facial nerve. The motor fibers then course ventrolaterally and caudally, and exit from the brainstem at the cerebellopontine angle, between the olive and the restiform body, at the caudal border of the pons. It leaves the brain adjacent to the acoustic nerve in the cerebellopontine angle, where the facial nerve lies in close contact with the anterior inferior cerebellar artery.[72] This relationship may play a role in the etiology of hemifacial spasm.

Special sensory taste fibers destined for the tongue and palate originate in the gustatory nucleus which is the rostral portion of the nucleus of the tractus solitarius. These join with general sensory fibers from the spinal trigeminal nucleus which will target the ear and postauricular skin, and mucus membranes of the nasopharynx. These then join with parasympathetic fibers from the superior salavatory nucleus which will provide secretory innervation to the lacrimal, submandibular, and sublingual glands. All of these sensory and parasympathetic fibers leave the brain in the nervus intermedius between the motor trunk of the facial nerve and the auditory nerve.

The motor component of the facial nerve and the sensory component (nervus intermediate) enter the internal auditory canal in the petrous portion of the temporal bone and then pass through the facial (fallopian) canal to the geniculate ganglion where the motor branch and the nervus intermedius join into a single trunk. Here sensory fibers synapse, but the motor and parasympathetic fibers pass through. Three branches emerge from the geniculate ganglion. The chorda tympani leaves the geniculate ganglion and passes through the middle ear, across the tympanic membrane between the malleus and incus. It then passes through the petrotympanic fissure into the temporalis fossa where it joins the lingual branch of the mandibular nerve (V3). Special sensory fibers then pass to the tongue for taste. Parasympathetic fibers synapse in the submandibular ganglion and project to the submandibular and sublingual glands.

As discussed earlier, other preganglionic parasympathetic fibers pass through the geniculate ganglion and then continue in the greater superficial petrosal nerve to the pterygopalatine (sphenopalatine) ganglion. From here postganglionic fibers join the maxillary branch of the trigeminal nerve (V2) where they enter the orbit through the inferior orbital fissure within the zygomatic branch. A communicating branch courses up along the lateral orbital wall to provided secretomotor parasympathetic innervation to the lacrimal gland.

The motor branch of the facial nerve passes through the labyrinth section of the facial canal where it runs a serpentine course. As the nerve passes between the cochlea and semicircular canals, it makes an abrupt bend. Here the motor and sensory roots temporarily fuse and the nerve is thickened by the presence of the geniculate ganglion, where the sensory fibers synapse. The motor root passes through the ganglion and then continues downward beside the mastoid air cells, and exits the braincase at the stylomastoid foramen. During facial dissections, the main trunk of the nerve is found anterior to the mid-portion of the earlobe, at a mean depth of about 20 mm from the surface.[101] The nerve ascends from the stylomastoid foramen to the parotid gland at an angle of approximately 45°. Typically, the nerve enters the posterior substance of the gland before it divides into its terminal branches. It continues anteriorly through the parotid gland, crosses the external carotid artery, and divides into two divisions, an upper temporofacial and a lower cervicofacial division. Each trunk further divides, forming a total of 6–9 primary branches just as they emerge from the anterior border of the parotid gland. These further divide into 14–15 distal branches that can be divided into five functional groups based on muscles of innervation.[118] However, numerous intercommunications are seen between some of these major branches. The peripheral facial nerve shows at least six common patterns of branching and intercommunication between these branches.[23,64]

The upper temporofacial division usually subdivides into the temporal, zygomatic, and buccal branches, and forms a plexus deep to the orbicularis muscle. These branches supply the frontalis and orbicularis muscles along their deep surfaces. The temporal branch divides into 2–4 twigs that run in the submuscular plane along a line approximately from just below the tragus of the ear to a point 1.0–1.5 cm above the lateral aspect of the superior orbital rim. The position of the lateral brow is more variable, and is less reliable in determining the position of the nerve.[33] When it leaves the upper pole of the parotid gland, the temporal branch lies deep to the temporoparietal fascia (SMAS) layer. As it crosses the zygomatic arch, it becomes slightly more superficial, as it is invested by layers of the fibrofatty tissue representing the SMAS in this region.[6] The temporal branch courses upward within a cephalad extension of the SMAS along with the superficial temporal artery. This layer is the temporoparietal or superficial temporal fascia, and is continuous with the galea over the cranium to which it fuses along the superficial temporal line. The galea is an aponeurosis joining the frontalis muscle anteriorly, and the occipitalis muscle posteriorly. Between the temporoparietal fascial and the deep temporal fascia over the temporalis muscle is a loose areolar layer, the subaponeurotic plane. This is avascular and does not contain any crossing vessels or nerves.[112] Dissections in the temporal region, as for lateral brow suspension or orbitotomies, should be confined to this plane. However, for extensive myocutaneous rotation procedures where the incision curves upward and around the temporal region, the dissection plane should remain superficial to the temporparietal fascia, within the subcutanous fat, to avoid cutting the temporal and zygomatic nerves. When operating in the temporal region through a coronal incision, the dissection should be within the subaponeurotic plane, between the superficial and deep temporal fascial layers.

The course of the temporal branches of the facial nerve may follow a curved trajectory from the parotid upward, and then forward to the lateral brow. In these individuals the frontal branches lie about 1.0–1.5 cm lateral to the lateral border of the eyebrow. In other cases the frontal nerves run a straighter trajectory, so that the nerve branches lie closer to the lateral canthus.[50] In the latter cases, the anterior and middle rami may be injured during lower eyelid reconstructions using a Tenzel or Mustarde rotational flap. As the temporal branch of the facial nerve approaches the lateral orbit it becomes more superficial, and usually divides into three, or less commonly four, rami. The posterior ramus innervates the anterior auricular and temporoparietal muscles. The anterior and middle rami frequently have anastomotic connections between them, and innervate the frontalis muscle and the upper portion of the orbicularis muscle on their undersurfaces. The nerve runs about 1 cm above the supraorbital rim. In about 60% of individuals a tiny ramus runs medially to innervate the transverse head of the corrugator muscle.[118] Within the eyelid, the fine terminal twigs of the facial nerve run vertically in the postorbicular fascial plane, and penetrate the muscle on its posterior surface. These twigs are routinely cut during surgeries performed through an upper eyelid crease incision.[57] This may explain the occurrence of a weak blink and temporary lagophthalmos following some upper eyelid procedures.

The zygomatic branch of the temporofacial division of the facial nerve may be single or double and crosses the zygomatic arch deep in the subcutaneous fat. In most individuals it divides into 2–6 branches. These pass over the parotid duct and then course over or sometimes through the zygomaticus major and minor muscles.[30] Branches to the eyelid remain at this relatively protected depth to about 5 cm distal to the parotid gland. Here they become more superficial where they innervate the lateral half of the orbicularis muscle. In its course, the zygomatic branch has a variable number of interconnections with the deep buccal branches and sometimes forms a neural plexus. The zygomatic and buccal branches interconnect and frequently co-innervate the orbicularis and upper facial muscles with an unpredictable intermuscular course.[123]

The superficial buccal branches divide from the common trunk of the buccal branch. They pass medially across the malar eminence anterior to the levator labii superioris muscle, and then extend upward along the medial side of the orbicularis muscle in the lower eyelid supplying fibers to these muscles. A small branch continues medially and superiorly, crosses over the medial canthal tendon in company with the angular artery, and supplies the superomedial orbicularis, procerus, and corrugator muscles.[87]

The lower cervicofacial division of the facial nerve gives rise to the marginal mandibular and cervical branches. There is considerable variation in branching pattern, both between individuals and from one side to the other, and in some individuals extensive anastomotic twigs interconnect all the peripheral branches of the facial nerve.[23]

Clinical correlations

Paralysis of the facial nerve is a common neurologic problem with potentially severe ophthalmic consequences. The etiology of seventh nerve dysfunction may be anywhere from the cerebral cortex to the peripheral branches of the facial nerve, and the site of pathology can usually be localized clinically with great accuracy. That portion of the facial nucleus serving the upper face receives crossed and uncrossed impulses from the precentral motor cortex of both hemispheres, while that portion serving the lower face receives mainly crossed fibers from the contralateral hemisphere. Thus, supranuclear lesions affecting the corticopontine pathway to the facial nucleus result in paralysis of the opposite lower facial muscles with sparing of the upper face. This is frequently seen in patients with stroke affecting the cortical, diencephalic, or mesencephalic pathways to the nucleus. Pontine lesions, such as those associated with multiple sclerosis affecting descending fascicular fibers, generally produce complete ipsilateral facial paralysis. Those lesions in the dorsal pons, in the region where the seventh nerve fasciculus arches over the abducens nucleus, may produce sixth nerve palsy, conjugate gaze palsy, and internuclear ophthalmoplegia in addition to facial nerve paralysis. Lesions in the mid pons often associate paralysis of the facial nerve with involvement of the spinal tract of the trigeminal nerve. Ipsilateral taste is usually spared, since these sensory fibers leave the nerve as it enters the pons, and pass to the tractus solitarius.

As the facial nerve leaves the pons in the cerebellopontine angle, it has an intimate relationships with the acoustic nerve (VIII). Expanding lesions in this region, such as meningiomas, neurilemmomas, dermoid cysts, or aneurysms, frequently produce facial paralysis associated with ipsilateral loss of hearing. The roots of the fifth, ninth, and tenth cranial nerves lie nearby and also may become involved. Postinfectious polyneuritis (Guillain-Barré syndrome) is a presumed hypersensitivity or autoimmune response leading to demyelination, edema, and compression of nerve roots within their dural sheaths, resulting in weakness and paresthesias. Cranial nerve involvement is seen in half of all cases, and in some patients the disease may be confined to these nerves. The facial nerve is the most frequently affected, often bilaterally.

Compression of the facial nerve within the circuitous facial canal may occur with neurilemmoma, sarcoidosis, or leukemic infiltrates. Inflammatory processes in adjacent structures, such as mastoiditis or otitis media, also may result in facial nerve weakness. *Herpes zoster* involving the geniculate ganglion (Ramsay Hunt syndrome) causes pain and vesicles within the external auditory meatus and on the tympanic membrane, associated with facial paralysis. The facial nerve is also vulnerable to fractures involving the temporal bone.

Bell's palsy is an idiopathic disorder characterized by acute facial paralysis of the lower motor neuron type that is not associated with other neurologic findings. The etiology may be due to viral infection with edema of the facial nerve within the facial canal. Clinically, the condition may be preceded by pain at the stylomastoid foramen, followed by acute facial paralysis. Orbicularis muscle weakness may result in severe lagophthalmos, corneal exposure, and potential loss of vision. Epiphora from weakness of the lacrimal pump mechanism is a frequent accompanying symptom. Spontaneous recovery of facial nerve function is usual, although in some patients the condition may be permanent.

Hemifacial spasm is characterized by unilateral hyperkinetic tonic spasms of the facial muscles. In about 0.2–0.5% of cases, a posterior fossa tumor may be responsible. In most patients, however, it results from a vascular cross-compression of the facial nerve root in the cerebellopontine angle.[71] Most commonly, the offending vessel is the anterior inferior cerebellar artery, although the posterior inferior cerebellar artery may also cause compression from below. Smaller caliber vessels often show more intimate relationships to the seventh nerve, and may also produce compressive symptoms.[16] It has been suggested that such vascular compression was the result of aging, from arterial elongation and caudal displacement of the brain stem in the posterior fossa.[52] However, vascular loops and elongated arteries may be normal structures present at birth.[16] Hemifacial spasm can be cured surgically in most cases by microvascular decompression, with elevation of the abnormal vessel at the seventh nerve exit root zone.[71] Alternatively, the spasms can be controlled by peripheral chemodenervation with botulinum toxin.[28]

Essential blepharospasm is a variably progressive focal cranial dystonia characterized by bilateral, involuntary, sustained contractions of the orbicularis muscle. It may result in severe visual disability and functional blindness. Not uncommonly it may progress to a segmental distribution with involvement of adjacent focal regions, such as oromandibular dystonia, and torticollis. The etiology is uncertain, but some experimental evidence suggests a neurotransmitter or receptor defect at the level of the basal ganglia. Pharmacologic therapy has proven to be ineffective in most patients, and only partially effective in others. Surgical management consists of radical or limited neurmyectomy.[4] The therapeutic procedure of choice, however, is chemodenervation with botulinum toxin.[29]

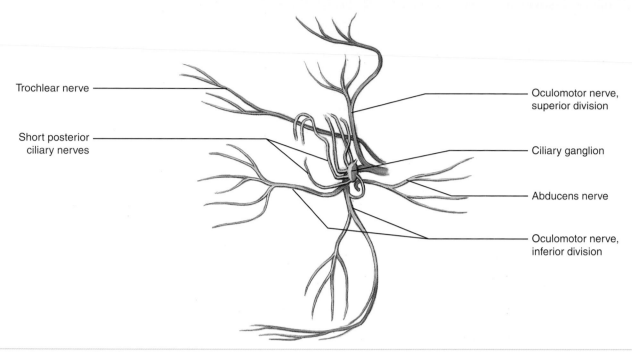

Trochlear nerve

Short posterior
ciliary nerves

Oculomotor nerve,
superior division

Ciliary ganglion

Abducens nerve

Oculomotor nerve,
inferior division

Figure 4-1 Motor nerves, frontal view.

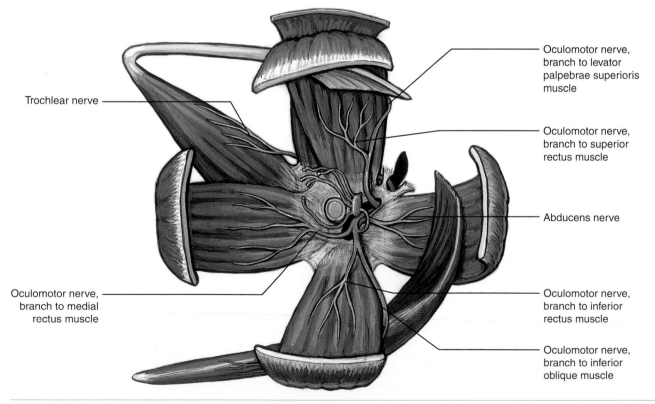

Trochlear nerve

Oculomotor nerve,
branch to levator
palpebrae superioris
muscle

Oculomotor nerve,
branch to superior
rectus muscle

Abducens nerve

Oculomotor nerve,
branch to medial
rectus muscle

Oculomotor nerve,
branch to inferior
rectus muscle

Oculomotor nerve,
branch to inferior
oblique muscle

Figure 4-2 Motor nerves, frontal view with extraocular muscles.

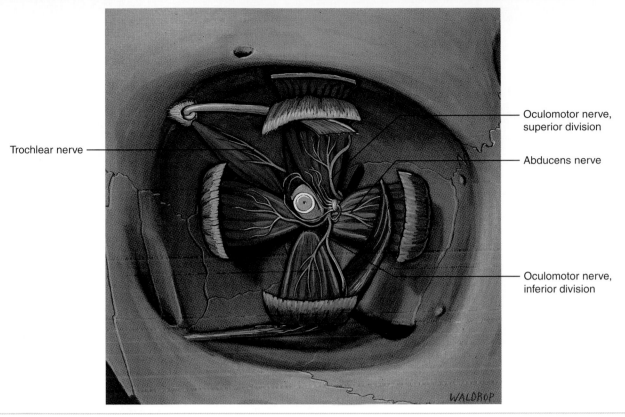

Trochlear nerve

Oculomotor nerve, superior division

Abducens nerve

Oculomotor nerve, inferior division

WALDROP

Figure 4-3 Motor nerves, frontal view, composite with extraocular muscles and orbital bones.

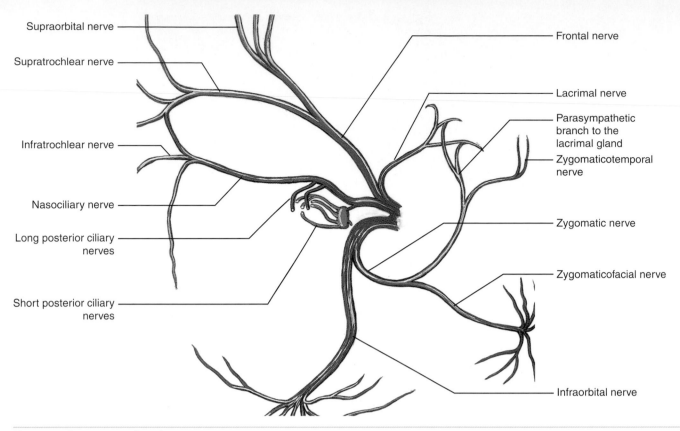

Supraorbital nerve

Supratrochlear nerve

Infratrochlear nerve

Nasociliary nerve

Long posterior ciliary nerves

Short posterior ciliary nerves

Frontal nerve

Lacrimal nerve

Parasympathetic branch to the lacrimal gland

Zygomaticotemporal nerve

Zygomatic nerve

Zygomaticofacial nerve

Infraorbital nerve

Figure 4-4 Sensory nerves, frontal view.

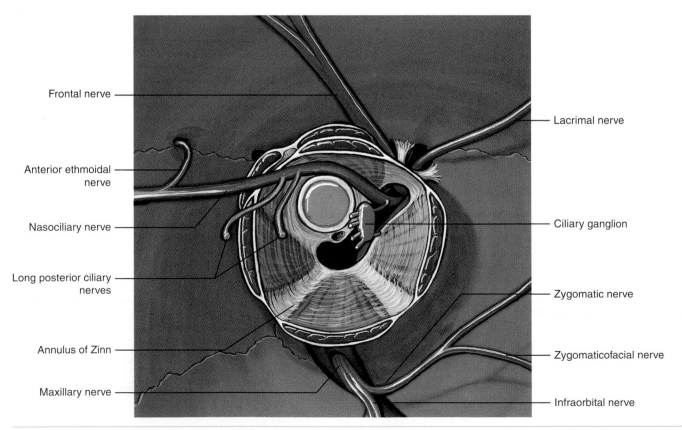

Frontal nerve

Anterior ethmoidal nerve

Nasociliary nerve

Long posterior ciliary nerves

Annulus of Zinn

Maxillary nerve

Lacrimal nerve

Ciliary ganglion

Zygomatic nerve

Zygomaticofacial nerve

Infraorbital nerve

Figure 4-5 Sensory nerves, frontal view, orbital apex.

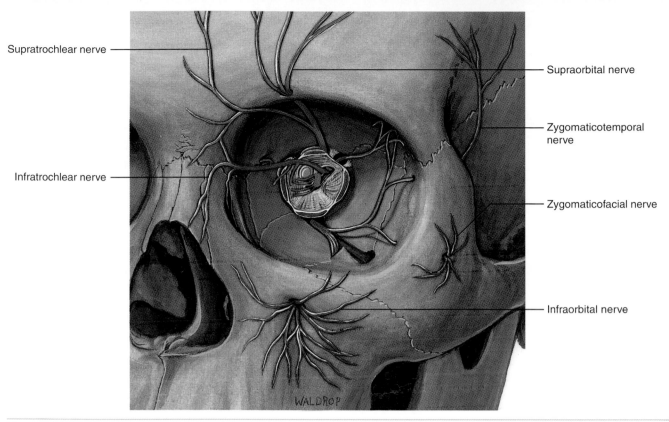

Supratrochlear nerve

Infratrochlear nerve

Supraorbital nerve

Zygomaticotemporal nerve

Zygomaticofacial nerve

Infraorbital nerve

Figure 4-6 Sensory nerves, frontal periorbital view with orbital bones.

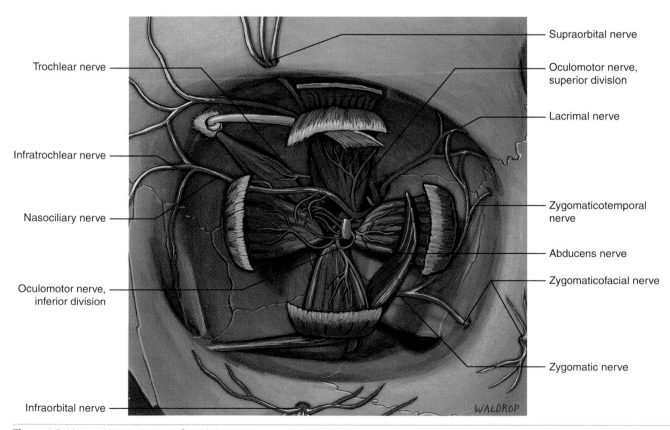

Trochlear nerve

Infratrochlear nerve

Nasociliary nerve

Oculomotor nerve, inferior division

Infraorbital nerve

Supraorbital nerve

Oculomotor nerve, superior division

Lacrimal nerve

Zygomaticotemporal nerve

Abducens nerve

Zygomaticofacial nerve

Zygomatic nerve

Figure 4-7 Motor and sensory nerves, frontal view.

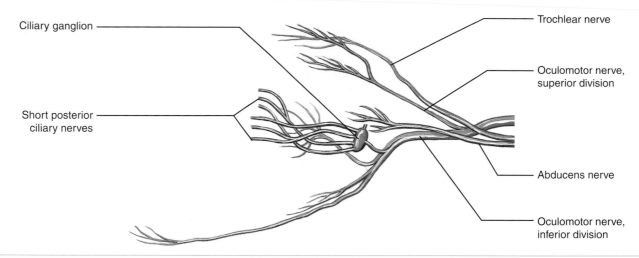

Ciliary ganglion

Short posterior
ciliary nerves

Trochlear nerve

Oculomotor nerve,
superior division

Abducens nerve

Oculomotor nerve,
inferior division

Figure 4-8 Motor nerves, lateral view.

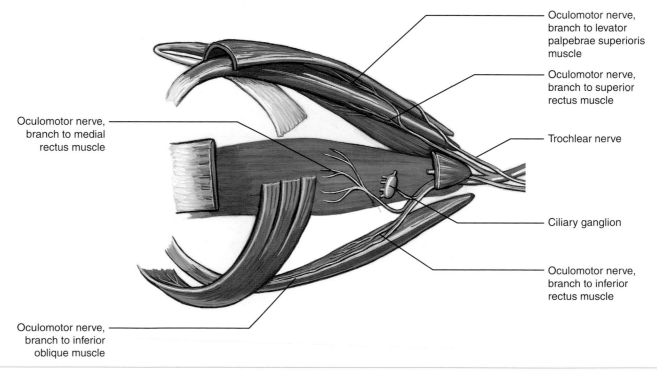

Oculomotor nerve,
branch to medial
rectus muscle

Oculomotor nerve,
branch to inferior
oblique muscle

Oculomotor nerve,
branch to levator
palpebrae superioris
muscle

Oculomotor nerve,
branch to superior
rectus muscle

Trochlear nerve

Ciliary ganglion

Oculomotor nerve,
branch to inferior
rectus muscle

Figure 4-9 Motor nerves, lateral view with extraocular muscles.

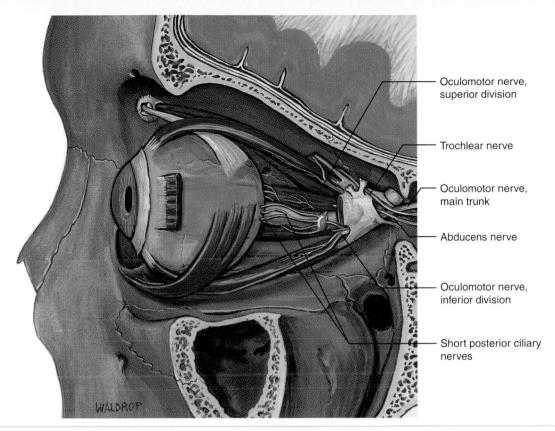

Oculomotor nerve,
superior division

Trochlear nerve

Oculomotor nerve,
main trunk

Abducens nerve

Oculomotor nerve,
inferior division

Short posterior ciliary
nerves

Figure 4-10 Motor nerves, lateral composite view with extraocular muscles, globe and orbital bones.

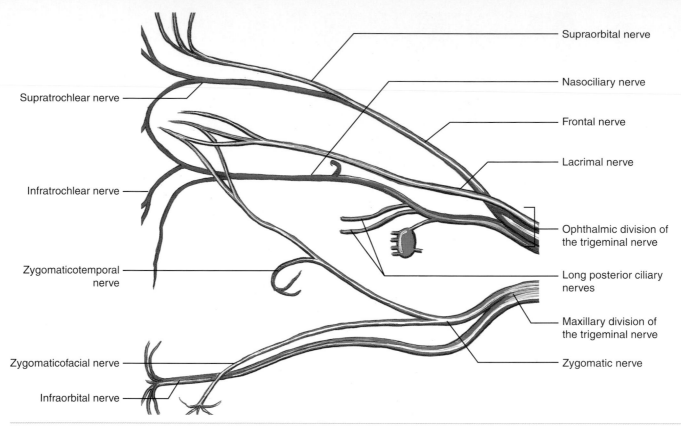

Supraorbital nerve

Nasociliary nerve

Frontal nerve

Lacrimal nerve

Supratrochlear nerve

Ophthalmic division of the trigeminal nerve

Infratrochlear nerve

Long posterior ciliary nerves

Zygomaticotemporal nerve

Maxillary division of the trigeminal nerve

Zygomaticofacial nerve

Zygomatic nerve

Infraorbital nerve

Figure 4-11 Sensory nerves, lateral view.

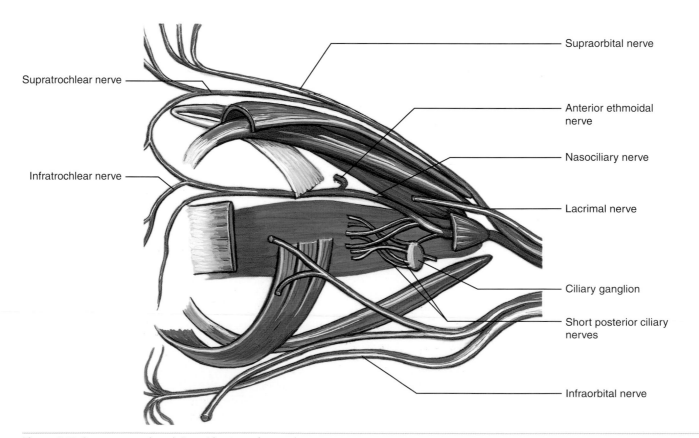

Supraorbital nerve

Supratrochlear nerve

Anterior ethmoidal nerve

Nasociliary nerve

Infratrochlear nerve

Lacrimal nerve

Ciliary ganglion

Short posterior ciliary nerves

Infraorbital nerve

Figure 4-12 Sensory nerves, lateral view with extraocular muscles.

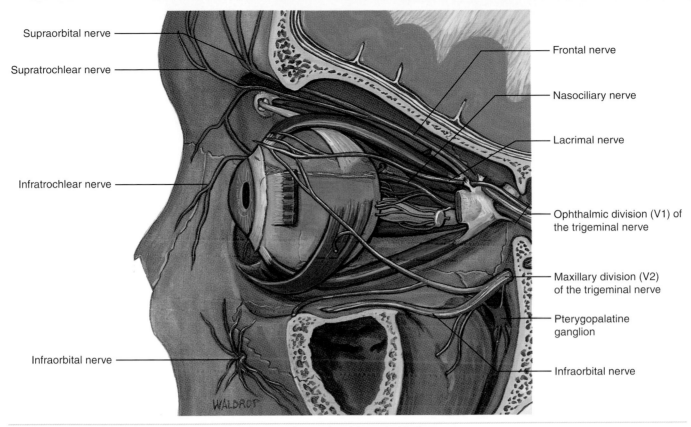

Supraorbital nerve

Supratrochlear nerve

Infratrochlear nerve

Infraorbital nerve

Frontal nerve

Nasociliary nerve

Lacrimal nerve

Ophthalmic division (V1) of the trigeminal nerve

Maxillary division (V2) of the trigeminal nerve

Pterygopalatine ganglion

Infraorbital nerve

WALDROP

Figure 4-13 Sensory nerves, lateral composite view with extraocular muscles, globe and orbital bones.

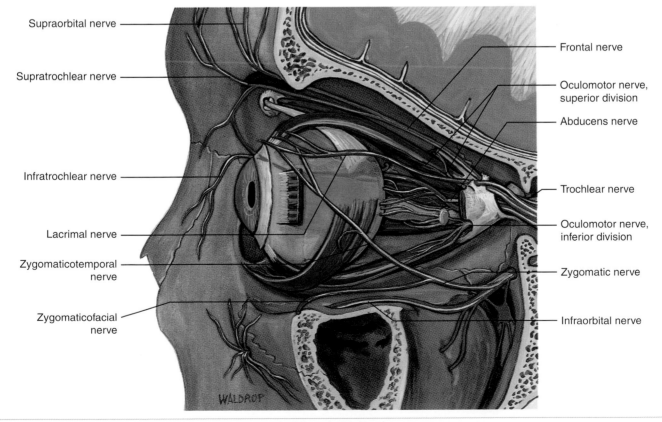

Supraorbital nerve

Supratrochlear nerve

Infratrochlear nerve

Lacrimal nerve

Zygomaticotemporal nerve

Zygomaticofacial nerve

Frontal nerve

Oculomotor nerve, superior division

Abducens nerve

Trochlear nerve

Oculomotor nerve, inferior division

Zygomatic nerve

Infraorbital nerve

WALDROP

Figure 4-14 Motor and sensory nerves, lateral composite view with globe and orbital bones.

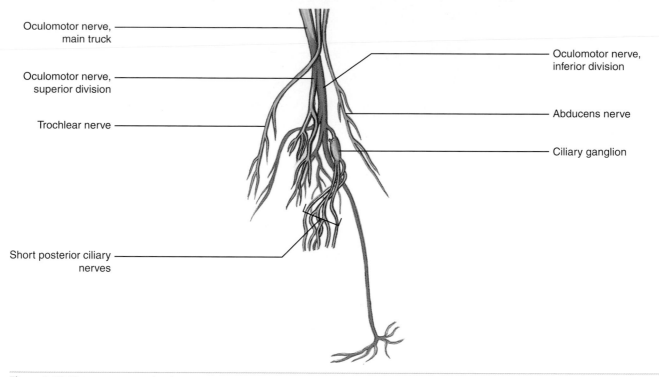

Oculomotor nerve,
main truck

Oculomotor nerve,
superior division

Trochlear nerve

Short posterior ciliary
nerves

Oculomotor nerve,
inferior division

Abducens nerve

Ciliary ganglion

Figure 4-15 Motor nerves, superior view.

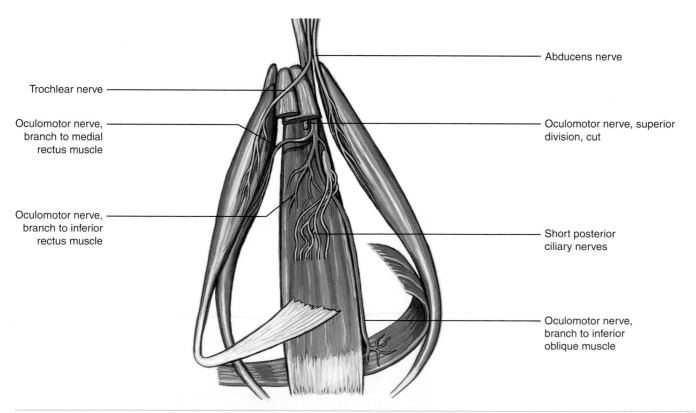

Trochlear nerve

Oculomotor nerve,
branch to medial
rectus muscle

Oculomotor nerve,
branch to inferior
rectus muscle

Abducens nerve

Oculomotor nerve, superior
division, cut

Short posterior
ciliary nerves

Oculomotor nerve,
branch to inferior
oblique muscle

Figure 4-16 Motor nerves, superior view with extraocular muscles.

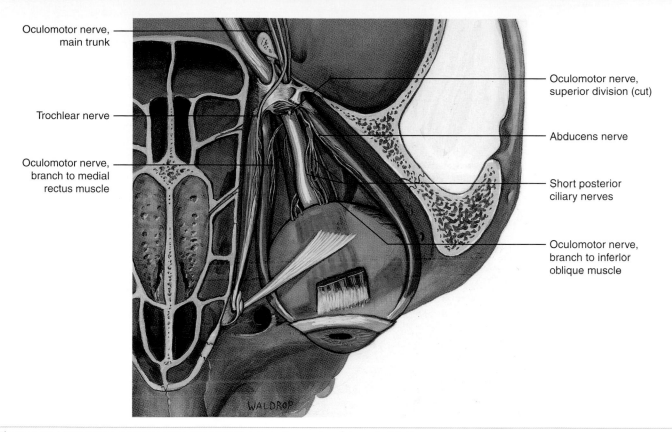

Oculomotor nerve,
main trunk

Trochlear nerve

Oculomotor nerve,
branch to medial
rectus muscle

Oculomotor nerve,
superior division (cut)

Abducens nerve

Short posterior
ciliary nerves

Oculomotor nerve,
branch to inferlor
oblique muscle

WALDROP

Figure 4-17 Motor nerves, superior composite view with extraocular muscles, globe and orbital bones.

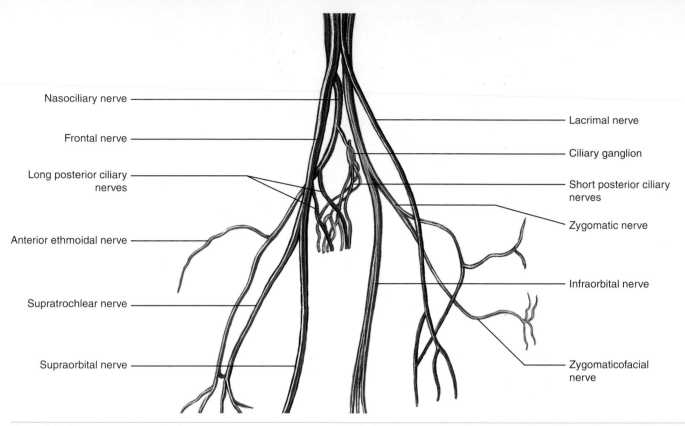

Figure 4-18 Sensory nerves, superior view.

Nasociliary nerve

Frontal nerve

Long posterior ciliary nerves

Anterior ethmoidal nerve

Supratrochlear nerve

Supraorbital nerve

Lacrimal nerve

Ciliary ganglion

Short posterior ciliary nerves

Zygomatic nerve

Infraorbital nerve

Zygomaticofacial nerve

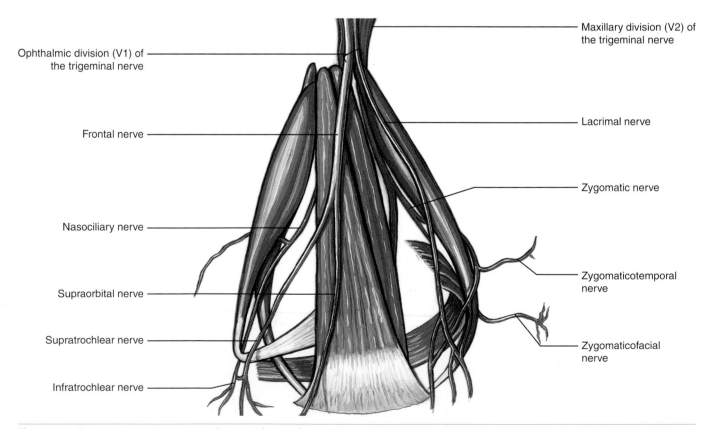

Figure 4-19 Sensory nerves, superior view with extraocular muscles.

Ophthalmic division (V1) of the trigeminal nerve

Frontal nerve

Nasociliary nerve

Supraorbital nerve

Supratrochlear nerve

Infratrochlear nerve

Maxillary division (V2) of the trigeminal nerve

Lacrimal nerve

Zygomatic nerve

Zygomaticotemporal nerve

Zygomaticofacial nerve

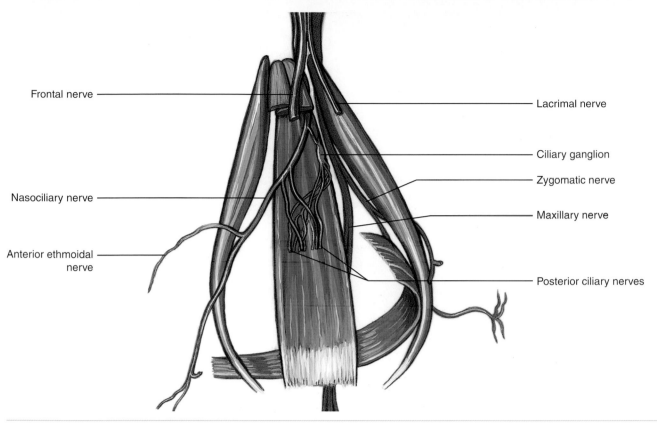

Frontal nerve

Lacrimal nerve

Ciliary ganglion

Zygomatic nerve

Nasociliary nerve

Maxillary nerve

Anterior ethmoidal
nerve

Posterior ciliary nerves

Figure 4-20 Sensory nerves, superior view with extraocular muscles, central dissection.

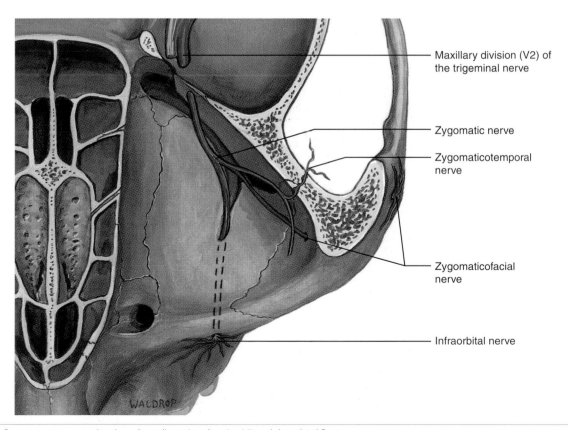

Maxillary division (V2) of
the trigeminal nerve

Zygomatic nerve

Zygomaticotemporal
nerve

Zygomaticofacial
nerve

Infraorbital nerve

WALDROP

Figure 4-21 Sensory nerves, superior view, deep dissection showing V3 and the orbital floor.

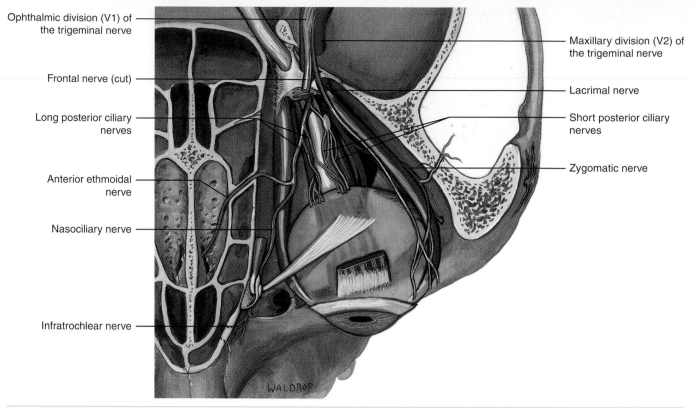

Ophthalmic division (V1) of
the trigeminal nerve

Frontal nerve (cut)

Long posterior ciliary
nerves

Anterior ethmoidal
nerve

Nasociliary nerve

Infratrochlear nerve

Maxillary division (V2) of
the trigeminal nerve

Lacrimal nerve

Short posterior ciliary
nerves

Zygomatic nerve

WALDROP

Figure 4-22 Sensory nerves, superior composite view, with extraocular muscles, globe and orbital bones.

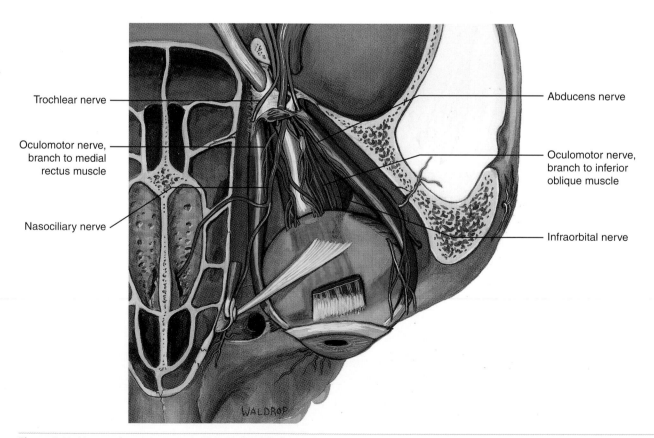

Trochlear nerve

Oculomotor nerve,
branch to medial
rectus muscle

Nasociliary nerve

Abducens nerve

Oculomotor nerve,
branch to inferior
oblique muscle

Infraorbital nerve

WALDROP

Figure 4-23 Motor and sensory nerves, superior composite view, with extraocular muscles, globe and orbital bones.

References

1. Abad JM, Alvarez F, Blazquez MG: An unrecognized neurological syndrome: sixth nerve palsy and Horner's syndrome due to traumatic intracavernous carotid aneurysm. *Surg Neurol* 16:141, 1981.

2. Adams ME, Linn J, Yousry I: Pathology of the ocular motor nerves III, IV, and VI. *Neuroimag Clin N Am* 18:261, 2008.

3. Anderson DR, Hendrickson A: Effect of intraocular pressure on rapid axoplasmic transport in monkey optic nerve. *Invest Ophthalmol Vis Sci* 13:771, 1974.

4. Anderson RL, Parinely JR: Surgical management of blepharospasm. *Surv Ophthalmol* 49:501, 1988.

5. Anderson RL: The blepharocardiac reflex. *Arch Ophthalmol* 96:1418, 1978.

6. Appiani E, Delfino MC: Observations on orbitofrontal rhytidectomy. *Ann Plast Surg* 18:398, 1987.

7. Apt L, Isenberg SJ, Gaffney WL: The oculocardiac reflex in strabismus surgery. *Am J Ophthalmol* 76:533, 1973.

8. Arey LB: *Developmental Anatomy*. 7th ed. Philadelphia, WB Saunders, 1966, pp 532–534.

9. Aschner B: Über einen bisher noch nicht beschreibenen reflex vom Auge auf Kreislauf und Atmung: Vershwinden des Radial impulses bei Druck auf das Auge. *Wien Klin Wochenschr* 21:1529, 1908.

10. Axenfeld T: Zweite Demonstrations-Situng. *Berl Dtsch Ophthal Ges* 34:300, 1907.

11. Baljet B, van der Werf F, Otto AJ: Autonomic pathways in the orbit of the human fetus and the rhesus monkey. *Doc Ophthalmol* 72:247, 1989.

12. Blanc VF, Hardy JF, Milot J, Jacob JL: The oculo-cardiac reflex: A graphic and statistical analysis in infants and children. *Can Anesth Soc J* 30:360, 1983.

13. Bleys RLA, Janssen LM, Groen JG: The lateral sellar nerve plexus and its connections in humans. *J Neurosurg* 95:102, 2001.

14. Bomberg BB: Autonomic control of lacrimal protein secretion. *Invest Ophthalmol Vis Sci* 20:110, 1981.

15. Bosomworth PP, Ziegler CH, Jacoby J: The oculocardiac reflex in eye muscle surgery. *Anesthesiology* 19:7, 1958.

16. Brunsteins DB, Ferreri AJM: Microsurgical anatomy of the VI and VII cranial nerves and related arteries in the cerebellopontine angle. *Surg Radiol Anat* 12:259, 1990.

17. Chung MS, Kim HJ: Locational relationship of the supraorbital notch or foramen, intraorbital and mental foramina in Koreans. *Acta Anat Basel* 154:162, 1995.

18. Collin JRO, Beard C, Wood I: Terminal course of nerve supply to Muller's muscle in the rhesus monkey and its clinical significance. *Am J Ophthalmol* 87:234, 1979.

19. Cooper ERA: The development of the nuclei of the oculomotor and trochlear nerves (somatic efferent column). *Brain* 69:50, 1946.

20. Crosby EC, deJonge BR: Experimental and clinical studies of the central connections and central relationships of the facial nerve. *Ann Otolaryngol* 72:735, 1963.

21. Cuthbertson S, LeDoux MS, Jones J, et al: Localization of preganglionic neurons that innervate neurons of the pterygopalatine ganglion. *Invest Ophthalmol Vis Sci* 44:3713, 2003.

22. Daroff RB: Ocular motor manifestations of brainstem and cerebellar dysfunction. In: Smith, JL (ed): *Neuro-Ophthalmology: Symposium of the University of Miami and the Bascom Palmer Eye Institute*, Vol. 5. Hallendale, FL, Huffman, 1971, p 104.

23. Davis RA, Anson BJ, Budinger JM, Kuith LE: Surgical anatomy of the facial nerve and parotid gland based upon a study of 350 cervicofacial halves. *Surg Gynecol Obstet* 102:385, 1956.

24. Demer JL, Miller JM, Poukens V, et al: Evidence for fibromuscular pulleys of the recti extraocular muscles. *Invest Ophthalmol* 36:1125, 1995.

25. DiDio LJA, Baptista CAC, Teofilovski-Parapid G: Anatomical variations of the abducent nerve in humans. *Arch Ital Anat Embryol* 95:167, 1990.

26. Dolman PJ, Glazer LC, Harris GJ, et al: Mechanisms of visual loss in severe proptosis. *Ophthalm Plast Reconstr Surg* 7:256, 1991.

27. Ducasse A, Delattre JF, Segal A, et al: Anatomical basis of the surgical approaches to the medial wall of the orbit. *Anat Clin* 7:15, 1985.

28. Dutton JJ: Treatment of hemifacial spasm and essential blepharospasm with botulinum toxin. In: Wilkins RH, Rengachary SS (eds): *Neurosurgery Update I*. New York, McGraw-Hill, 1990, pp 138–141.

29. Dutton JJ, Buckley EG: Long-term results and complications of botulinum A toxin in the treatment of blepharospasm. *Ophthalmology* 95:1529, 1988.

30. Erbli KM, Hayran M, Mas N, et al: The relationship of the parotid duct to the buccal and zygomatic branches of the facial nerve; an anatomical study with parameters of clinical interest. *Folia Morphol (Warsz)* 66:109, 2007.

31. Erdogmus S, Govsa F: Anatomy of the supraorbital region and the evaluation of it for the reconstruction of facial defects. *J Craniofac Surg* 18:104, 2007.

32. Erdogmus S, Govsa F, Celik S: Innervation features of the extraocular muscles. *J Craniofac Surg* 18:1439, 2007.

33. Fatah MF: Innervation and functional reconstruction of the forehead. *Br J Plast Surg* 44:351, 1991.

34. Foerster O, Gagel O, Mahoney W: Über die Anatomie, Physiologie und Pathologie der Pupillarinnervation. *Verh Dtsch Ges Inn Med* 48:386, 1936.

35. Gacek RR: Localization of neurons supplying the extraocular muscles in the kitten using horseradish peroxidase. *Exp Neurol* 44:381, 1974.

36. Gay AJ, Newman NM, Keltner JL, Stroud MH: *Eye Movement Disorders*. St. Louis, CV Mosby, 1974.

37. Goldstein JE, Cogan DG: Diabetic ophthalmoplegia with special reference to the pupil. *Arch Ophthalmol* 64:592, 1960.

38. Gönül E, Timurkaynak E: Inferolateral microsurgical approach to the orbit: An anatomical study. *Minim Invasive Neurosurg* 42:137, 1999.

39. Govsa F, Kayalioglu G, Ertuk M, Ozgur T: The superior orbital fissure and its contents. *Surg Radiol Anat* 21:181, 1999.

40. Grimes P, vonSallmann L: Comparative anatomy of the ciliary nerves. *Arch Ophthalmol* 64:81, 1960.

41. Grimson BS, Thompson HS: Raeder's syndrome: A clinical review. *Surv Ophthalmol* 24:199, 1980.

42. Groen GJ, Baljet B, Boekelaar AB, Drukker J: Branches of the thoracic sympathetic trunk in the human fetus. *Anat Embryol (Berl)* 176:401, 1987.

43. Harris FS, Rhoton AL, Jr: Anatomy of the cavernous sinus: A microsurgical study. *J Neurosurg* 45:169, 1976.

44. Hartmann B, Kremer I, Gutman I, et al: Cavernous sinus infection manifested by Horner's syndrome and isolated sixth nerve palsy. *J Clin Neuro Ophthalmol* 7:223, 1987.

45. Hervouet F: Development normal de l'oeil et de ses annexes. II. Embryologie du nerf optique. In: Dejean C, Hervouet F, Leplat G (eds): *L'Embryologie de L'Oeil et sa Teratologie.* Paris, Masson, 1958, pp 171–219.

46. Hogan MJ, Alvarrado JA, Weddell JE: *Histology of the Human Eye—An Atlas and Textbook.* Philadelphia, WB Saunders, 1971.

47. Hogg ID: Observations of the development of the nucleus of Edinger-Westphal in man and the albino rat. *J Comp Neurol* 126:567, 1966.

48. Hu K, Kwak H, Song W, et al: Branching patterns of the infraorbital nerve and topography within the infraorbital space. *J Craniofac Surg* 17:1111, 2006.

49. Iaconetta G, Fusco M, Cavallo LM, et al: The abducens nerve: Microanatomic and endoscopic study. *Oper Neurosurg* 61:ONS7, 2007.

50. Ishikawa Y: An anatomical study on the distribution of the temporal branch of the facial nerve. *J Cranio Max Surg* 18:287, 1990.

51. Izci Y, Gonul E: The microsurgical anatomy of the ciliary ganglion and its clinical importance in orbital traumas: An anatomic study. *Minim Invasive Neurosurg* 49:156, 2006.

52. Jannetta PJ, Moller M, Moller AR: Disabling positional vertigo. *The New Engl J Med* 310:1700, 1984.

53. Jannetta PJ: Cranial nerve compression in hemifacial spasm. In: Youmans JR (ed): *Neurological Surgery: A Comprehensive Reference Guide to the Diagnosis and Management of Neurosurgical Problems.* 2nd ed., Vol 6. Philadelphia, WB Saunders Co, 1982, pp 3773–3775.

54. Joffe WS, Gay AJ: The oculorespiratory cardiac reflex in dogs. *Invest Ophthalmol* 5:550, 1966.

55. Jonas JB, Mardin CY, Schlötzer-Schrechardt U, et al: Morphometry of the human lamina cribrosa surface. *Invest Ophthalmol Vis Sci* 32:401, 1991.

56. Jonas JB: *Biomorphometrie des Nervus opticus.* Stuttgart, Enke-Verlage, 1989.

57. Jordan DR, Anderson RL: The facial nerve in eyelid surgery (letter). *Arch Ophthalmol* 107:1114, 1989.

58. Kakizaki H, Madge SN, Malhotra R, Selva D: The levator aponeurosis contains smooth muscle fibers: New findings in Caucasians. *Ophthal Plast Reconstr Surg* 25:267, 2009.

59. Katsev DA, Drews RC, Rose BT: An anatomical study of retrobulbar needle path length. *Ophthalmology* 96:1221, 1989.

60. Kazkayasi M, Ergin A, Ersoy M, et al: Microscopic anatomy of the infraorbital canal, nerve, and foramen. *Otolaryngol Head Neck Surg* 129:692, 2003.

61. Kerr FW, Hollowell OW: Location of pupillomotor and accommodation fibers in the oculomotor nerve: Experimental observations on paralytic mydriasis. *J Neurosurg Psychiatr* 27:473, 1968.

62. Kerr FW: The pupil-functional anatomy and clinical correlation. In: Smith JL (ed): *Neuro-Ophthalmology.* 4th ed. St. Louis, CV Mosby, 1968, pp 44–80.

63. Khurana AK, Khurana I, Yadav RN, et al: An experimental model of oculorespiratory reflex. *Br J Ophthalmol* 76:76, 1992.

64. Kim YS, Suh YS, Kim W, Chun CS: Branching pattern of the facial nerve in the parotid gland. *J Korean Surg Soc* 62:453, 2002.

65. Kimura K: Foramina and notches on the supraorbital margin in some racial groups. *Acta Anat* 52:203, 1977.

66. Klooster J, Beckers HJ, Ten Tusscher MP, et al: Sympathetic innervation of the rat choroids: An autoradiographic tracing and immunohistochemical study. *Ophthalmic Res* 28:36, 1996.

67. Kobet K: Cerebral spinal fluid recovery of lidocaine and bupivacaine following respiratory arrest subsequent to retrobulbar block. *Ophthalm Surg* 18:11, 1987.

68. Kuchiiwa S, Kuchiiwa T, Suzuki T: Comparative anatomy of the accessory ciliary ganglia in mammals. *Anat Embryol* 180:199, 1989.

69. Leston JM: Functional anatomy of the trigeminal nerve. *Nurochirugie* 55:99, 2009 (in French).

70. Lilequist B: The subarachnoid cisterns: An anatomic and roentgenographic study. *Acta Radiol (Suppl)* 185:1, 1959.

71. Loesser JD, Chen J: Hemifacial spasm: Treatment by microsurgical facial nerve decompression. *Neurosurgery* 13:141, 1983.

72. Malone B, Maisel RH: Anatomy of the facial nerve. *Am J Otolaryngol* 9:494, 1988.

73. Mann I: *The Development of the Human Eye.* 3rd ed. New York, Grune and Stratton, 1964, pp 189–255.

74. Manson PN, Lazarus RB, Morgan R, Iliff N: Pathways of sympathetic innervation to the superior and inferior (Müller's) tarsal muscles. *Plast Reconstr Surg* 78:33, 1986.

75. Matarasso A: The oculocardiac reflex in blepharoplasty surgery. *Plast Reconstr Surg* 83:243, 1989.

76. Matsumoto Y, Tanabe T, Ueda S, Kawata M: Immunohistochemical and enzymehistochemical studies of pepidergic, aminergic and cholinergic innervation of the lacrimal gland of the monkey (Macaca fuscata). *J Auton Nerv Syst* 37:207, 1992.

77. Mendelblatt FI, Kirsch RE, Lemberg L: A study comparing methods of preventing the oculocardiac reflex. *Am J Ophthalmol* 53:506, 1962.

78. Miehlke A: *Surgery of the Facial Nerve.* 2nd ed. Philadelphia, WB Saunders, 1973, pp 7-21, 147–174.

79. Mikelberg FS, Drance SM, Schulzer M, et al: The normal human optic nerve. Axon count and axon diameter distribution. *Ophthalmology* 96:1325, 1989.

80. Mikelberg FS, Yidegiligne HM, White VA, Schuler M: Relationships between optic nerve axon number and axon diameter to scleral canal area. *Ophthalmology* 98:60, 1991.

81. Miyazaki S: Bilateral innervation of the superior oblique muscle by the trochlear nucleus. *Brain Res* 348:52, 1985.

82. Miyazaki S: Location of motoneurons in the oculomotor nucleus and the course of their axons in the oculomotor nerve. *Brain Res* 348:57, 1985.

83. Moonie GT, Rees DL, Elton D: The oculocardiac reflex during strabismus surgery. *Can Anesth Soc J* 11:621, 1964.

84. Munden PM, Carter KD, Nerad JA: The oculocardiac reflex during enucleation. (Letter). *Am J Ophthalmol* 111:378, 1991.

85. Nadeau SE, Trobe JD: Pupil-sparing oculomotor palsy. A brief review. *Ann Neurol* 13:143, 1983.

86. Nathan H, Ouaknine G, Kosary IZ: The abducens nerve: Anatomical variations in its course. *J Neurosurg* 41:561, 1979.

87. Nemoto Y, Sekino Y, Kaneko H: Facial nerve anatomy in eyelid and periorbit. *Jpn J Ophthalmol* 45:445, 2001.

88. Nicoll JVM, Acharya A, Ahlen K, et al: Central nervous system complications after 6000 retrobulbar blocks. *Anesth Analg* 66:1298, 1987.

89. Nordin M: Sympathetic discharges in the human supraorbital nerve and the relation to sudo- and vasomotor responses. *J Physiol* 423:241, 1990.

90. Oikawa S, Kawagishi K, Yokouchi K, et al: Immunohistochemical determination of the sympathetic pathway in the orbit via the cranial nerves in humans. *J Neurosurg* 101:1037, 2004.

91. Osawa S, Photon AL Jr, Seker A, et al: Microsurgical and endoscopic anatomy of the vidian canal. *Neurosurgery* 64(Suppl. 2):385, 2009.

92. Ozanics V, Jakobiec FA: Prenatal development of the eye and its adnexa. In: Duane, TD, Jaeger EM (eds): *Biomechanical Foundations of Ophthalmology*. Philadelphia, Lippincott, 1988, pp 1–86.

93. Ozveren MF, Sam B, Akdemir I, et al: Duplication of the abducens nerve at the petroclinoid region: An anatomic study. *Nruosurg* 52:645, 2003.

94. Parkinson D: Bernard Mitchell, Horner syndrome and others? *Surg Neurol* 11:221, 1979.

95. Petzetakis M: Reflexe oculo-respiratoire et reflex oculovasomoteur a l'etat normal. *Bull Mem Soc Med Hosp Paris* 37:816, 1914.

96. Porter JD, Guthrie BL, Sparks DL: Innervation of monkey extraocular muscles: Localization of sensory and motor neurons by retrograde transport of horseradish peroxidase. *J Comp Neurol* 218:208, 1983.

97. Reese BE, Guillery RW, Marzi CA, Tassinari G: Position of axons in the cat's optic tract in relation to their retinal origin and chiasmatic pathway. *J Comp Neurol* 306:539, 1991.

98. Rhodes RH: Development of the optic nerve. In: Jakobiec FA (ed): *Ocular Anatomy, Embryology, and Teratology*. Philadelphia, Harper & Row, pp 601–638.

99. Rhoton AL, Hardy DG, Chambers SM: Microsurgical anatomy and dissection of the sphenoid bone, cavernous sinus, and sellar region. *Surg Neurol* 1:63, 1978.

100. Roberti F, Boari N, Mortini P, Caputy AJ: The pterygopalatine fossa: An anatomic report. *J Craniofac Surg* 18:586, 2007.

101. Rudolph R: Depth of the facial nerve in face lift dissections. *Plast Reconstr Surg* 85:537, 1990.

102. Ruskell GL: The orbital branches of the pterygopalatine ganglion and their relationship with internal carotid nerve branches in primates. *J Anat* 106:323, 1970.

103. Ruskell GL: The distribution of autonomic post-ganglionic nerve fibers to the lacrimal gland in monkeys. *J Anat* 109:229, 1971.

104. Ruskell GL: Access of autonomic nerves through the optic canal, and their orbital distribution in man. *Anat Rec* 275:973, 2003.

105. Rusu MC, Pop F: The anatomy of the sympathetic pathway through the pterygopalatine fossa in humans. *Ann Anat* 192:17, 2010.

106. Sacks JG: Peripheral innervation of extraocular muscles. *Am J Ophthalmol* 95:520, 1983.

107. Sakamoto M: Embryology of the 3rd, 4th and 6th cranial nerves. *Acta Soc Ophthalmol Jap* 57:146, 1953.

108. Schott GD: Neurogenic facial pain. *Trans Ophthalmol Soc UK* 100:252, 1980.

109. Segade LAG, Quintanilla JS: Distribution of postganglionic parasympathetic fibers originating in the pterygopalatine ganglion in the maxillary and ophthalmic nerve branches of the trigeminal nerve; HRP & WGA-HRP study in the guinea pig. *Brain Res* 522:327, 1990.

110. Sevel D: Development of the nerves of the extraocular muscles. In: Reinecke RD (ed): *Strabismus II*. Orlando, Grune and Stratton, 1986.

111. Sinnreich Z, Nathan H: The ciliary ganglion in man (anatomical observations). *Anat Anz* 150:287, 1981.

112. Stuzin JM, Wagstrom L, Kawamoto HK, Wolfe SA: Anatomy of the frontalis branch of the facial nerve: The significance of the temporal fat pad. *Plast Reconstr Surg* 83:265, 1989.

113. Suzuki N, Hardeba JE: Anatomical basis for a parasympathetic and sensory innervation of the intracranial segment of the internal carotid artery in man. Possible implications for vascular headache. *J Neurol Sci* 104:19, 1991.

114. Swanson MW: Neuroanatomy of the cavernous sinus and clinical correlations. *Optom Vis Sci* 67:891, 1990.

115. Szentagothai J: The representation of the facial and scalp muscles in the facial nucleus. *J Comp Neurol* 88:207, 1948.

116. Thakker MM, Huang J, Possin DE, et al: Human orbital sympathetic nerve pathways. *Ophthal Plast Reconstr Surg* 24:360, 2008.

117. Thompson HS: Adie's syndrome: Some new observations. *Trans Am Ophthalmol Soc* 75:587, 1977.

118. Tzafetta K, Terzis JK: Essays on the facial nerve: Part I. Microanatomy. *Plast Reconstr Surg* 125:879, 2010.

119. Umansky F, Nathan H: The lateral wall of the cavernous sinus. *J Neurosurg* 56:228, 1982.

120. Umansky F, Eldin J, Valarezo A: Dorello's canal: A microanatomical study. *J Neurosurg* 75:294, 1991.

121. Umansky F, Valarezo A, Elidan J: The microsurgical anatomy of the abducens nerve in its intracranial course. *Laryngoscope* 102:1285, 1992.

122. Unsold R, Stanley JA, Degroot J: The CT-topography of retrobulbar anesthesia. Anatomic clinical correlation of complications and suggestions of modified technique. *Graefes Arch Clin Exp Ophthalmol* 217:125, 1981.

123. Vasilic D, Barker JH, Blagg R, et al: Facial transplantation; an anatomic and surgical analysis of the periorbital functional unit. *Plast Reconstr Surg* 125:125, 2010.

124. Villain M, Segnarbieux F, Bonnel F, et al: The trochlear nerve: Anatomy by microdissection. *Surg Radiol Anat* 15:169, 1993.

125. Wang BC, Bogart B, Hillman DE, Turndorf H: Subarachnoid injection—A potential complication of retrobulbar block. *Anesthesiology* 71:845, 1989.

126. Warwick J: Representation of the extra-ocular muscles in the oculomotor nucleus of the monkey. *J Comp Neurol* 98:449, 1953.

127. Warwick R: The ocular parasympathetic nerve supply and its mesencephalic sources. *J Anat* 70:71, 1936.

128. Webster RC, Gaunt JM, Hamdan US, et al: Supraorbital and supratrochlear notches and foramina: Anatomical variations and surgical relevance. *Laryngoscope* 96:311, 1986.

129. Weninger WJ, Muller GB: The sympathetic nerves of the parasellar region: Pathways to the orbit and brain. *Acta Anat* 160:254, 1997.

130. Yu HG, Chung H, Yoon TG, et al: Stellate ganglion block increases blood flow into the optic nerve head and the peripapillary retina in humans. *Auton Neurosci* 109:53, 2003.

131. Zhang Y, Liu H, Liu E, et al: Microsurgical anatomy of the ocular motor nerves. *Surg Radiol Anat* 32:623, 2010.

CHAPTER 5

Arterial Supply to the Orbit

Embryology

Establishment of the ophthalmic arterial system is complex and the ocular and orbital branches derive from different sources. Undifferentiated orbital vessels containing nucleated red blood cells can be recognized in the mesenchyme surrounding the optic vesicle before the 3 mm embryonic stage.[38] By the 4 mm (28-day) stage, the internal carotid artery is already present at the sides of the developing brain, and a branch from this forms a primitive dorsal opththalmic artery. The hyaloid artery arises from this branch and extends along the inferior side of the optic stalk. A fine anastomotic vascular net develops around the optic stalk from this hyaloid system and supplies arterial blood to the developing optic nerve and eye. One branch of this net will later become the central retinal artery. A more distal branch of the dorsal ophthalmic artery gives rise to the temporal posterior ciliary artery.[40] The primitive dorsal ophthalmic artery will eventually become the first portion of the definitive adult ophthalmic artery.

At about the 9 mm (36-day) stage a second branch arises from a more distal segment of the internal carotid artery, from the region of the future anterior cerebral vessels. This is the primitive ventral ophthalmic artery. It enters the region of the orbit and gives rise to the nasal ciliary arteries that supply the developing choroid. In the 16–19 mm (46-day) embryonic stage, the temporociliary branch of the dorsal ophthalmic artery and the nasociliary branch of the ventral ophthalmic artery fuse around the optic stalk to form a ring. Eventually the dorsal ophthalmic artery becomes dominant as most of the ventral artery regresses, so that the blood supply to the eye derives only from the primitive dorsal ophthalmic artery (now the definitive ophthalmic artery) via its central retinal branch to the retina, and the ciliary branches to the choroid. At this stage, the ophthalmic artery supplies blood only to the optic nerve, the retina, and the choroid, but not to any other orbital structures.

During the 12–14 mm (38–41-day) embryonic stage a new vessel, the stapedial artery, arises from the first part of the internal carotid siphon. It branches into a superior and an inferior ramus.[29,40] The superior ramus gives rise to the middle meningeal artery that supplies the dura of the middle cranial fossa, and another branch that passes into the developing orbit through the region of the future, but as yet unossified, greater sphenoid wing. In the orbit, this branch of the stapedial artery becomes the supraorbital ramus (not to be confused with the supraorbital artery of adult human anatomy). It then gives rise to three branches: the lacrimal artery, the frontal artery, and the ethmoidal artery.[5] During the

20–24 mm (48–51-day) stages, the internal carotid origin of the stapedial artery begins to regress. The superior ramus becomes annexed by the maxillary branch of external carotid artery system to form the definitive middle meningeal artery.[18]

At the 24 mm (51-day) stage the optic nerve is surrounded by anastomotic twigs forming an arterial ring that arises from the origin of the central retinal artery and the two posterior ciliary arteries.[26] Connections are also established between the lacrimal branch of the supraorbital ramus of the stapedial system and these ophthalmic arterial twigs. At this stage, the supraorbital ramus, bringing blood to extra-global orbital structures, receives most of its blood from the external carotid system via the maxillary artery, with a small contribution from the internal carotid system via the ophthalmic artery perioptic network. As the ophthalmic artery continues to mature in the orbit, it completely annexes the branches of the supraorbital ramus by dilation of one of its anastomotic twigs connected to the lacrimal artery. This anastomotic twig becomes the second portion of the ophthalmic artery. The stapedial artery, and the connection between the supraorbital ramus in the orbit and the middle meningeal artery begin to regress, leaving the orbital branches of the supraorbital ramus supplied primarily by the ophthalmic artery. Thus, through this series of annexations and regressions, the dual blood supply to the eye and orbit, via both internal and external carotid systems, become the single ophthalmic artery from the internal carotid artery alone.

The upper twigs of the perioptic arterial ring are larger and better developed than those of the lower portion. The definitive course of the adult ophthalmic artery, whether over or under the optic nerve, is established at this time as most of the small anastomotic branches degenerate leaving one predominant channel as the major arterial trunk, usually in the upper half of the ring. The annexed part of the supraorbital ramus of the old stapedial system becomes part of the adult ophthalmic artery, and it's frontal, lacrimal, and ethmoidal branches become branches of the ophthalmic arterial system. Simultaneously, the root of the supraorbital ramus connecting these orbital vessels to the stapedial system completely atrophies,[39] thus leaving the ophthalmic artery as the only source of blood into the orbit, supplying the globe as well as other orbital structures. This is a uniquely primate condition. However, in 30–45% of human adults this former connection between the ancient stapedial (now middle meningeal) artery and the new ophthalmic artery may persist as the meningolacrimal artery[5,34] which passes through the meningolacrimal (also known as Hyrtl's or the lacrimal) foramen in the greater wing of the sphenoid bone.

In 55–70% of normal individuals, the meningolacrimal artery regresses completely, so that there is no connection to the middle meningeal artery, which now arises from the maxillary artery. A new vessel sometimes develops as an anastomotic connection between the root of the middle meningeal artery in the middle cranial fossa and the lacrimal artery in the orbit, passing through the superior orbital fissure. This vessel has been referred to as the sphenoidal artery or the recurrent meningeal artery, although blood flow through this vessel appears to be predominantly into the orbit, not out of it. Gillian[19] proposed the term "accessory ophthalmic artery" to more accurately reflect its function. This vessel, present only in humans and orangutans, had long been considered to be the real homologue of the primitive stapedial system. However, anatomic evidence suggests that this represents a true neomorphic vessel, with the regressed meningolacrimal artery representing the original superior ramus of the stapedial system.[5] As noted above, in humans the meningolacrimal artery usually atrophies, possibly due to hemodynamic alterations related to closure of the bony lateral orbital wall. However, occasionally part of the arterial segment between the ophthalmic and the lacrimal arteries also regresses, leaving the middle meningeal artery via the recurrent branch as the only source of blood for the lacrimal artery watershed.[26] In 1–2% of normal individuals the anastomotic branch from the ophthalmic artery to the superior ramus of the stapedial system may also regress, leaving the middle meningeal artery, via the recurrent orbital branch, as the major arterial source to all non-ocular orbital structures through the lacrimal, frontal and ethmoidal vessels. In such cases, the ophthalmic artery continues to supply the globe through the central retinal and ciliary arteries.[32] Finally, in rare instances, the ophthalmic artery may arise from the middle meningeal artery with no connection at all to the internal carotid system.[36]

In early embryonic development, the initial branch of the ophthalmic trunk, the hyaloid artery, lies in close association with the ventral surface of the optic stalk, and becomes enclosed within the depths of the developing optic fissure. This fissure develops as a partial longitudinal invagination that extends along the optic stalk from the forebrain to the rim of the optic cup. It finally closes over during the 12–20 mm (6–9-week) embryonic stages, leaving the hyaloid artery running to the optic vesicle within a central canal inside the optic stalk. Upon emerging from the distal end of the stalk, the hyaloid vessel traverses the optic vesicle to reach the lens placode and rim of the optic cup where it forms an extensive vascular net. Simultaneously, small vessels develop within the mesenchyme to form a fine network around the outer surface of the optic cup. These are the choriocapillary vessels.

The ciliary vessels arise from the primitive dorsal and ventral ophthalmic arteries, which fuse around the optic stalk to form the hyaloid network. After the emergence of the hyaloid vessel (central retinal artery), the ciliary branches proceed forward to the optic cup as the long posterior ciliary arteries. Near the posterior portion of the optic cup a series of small branches emerge from these vessels to form the short posterior ciliary arteries. These latter vessels establish communication with the posterior choriocapillary net in the region of the developing optic nerve head. The long posterior ciliary vessels continue forward to the rim of the optic cup, where they communicate with the circular net supplied by the terminal hyaloid vessels. This choriocapillary network also communicates via four branches (the future vortex veins) with the developing venous system. By the 20–24 mm (7-week) stage, the optic cup has established a dual blood supply; from the internal carotid artery via the central retinal and ciliary vessels; and from the external carotid artery via the maxillary, middle meningeal, and meningolacrimal vessels.

During the 60 mm (12-week) fetal stage the hyaloid artery, its vast anastomotic system around the developing lens, and its anterior circular communications with the choriocapillary network, begin to regress. By the end of this process, the ciliary vessels lose all communications anteriorly with the central retinal arterial system, and remain as the principal arterial supply to the choroid. At the 100 mm (15-week) stage, two small buds appear at the base of the hyaloid artery within a small mound, Burgmeister's papilla, at the site of the future optic disc. These later become the superior and inferior main retinal arterioles of the central retinal artery. They further branch and ramify within Burgmeister's papilla and grow peripherally in the nerve fiber layer to reach the ora serrata by the 8th month of gestation. By this time the intravitreal portion of the hyaloid system has largely atrophied, and Burgmeister's papilla has collapsed to leave the optic disc and its central physiologic cup.

Adult arterial system

In the adult, the vascular supply to the orbit derives primarily from the internal carotid artery, and consists of a complex system of vessels branching from the orbital apex forward. The internal carotid artery passes through the petrous portion of the temporal bone in the carotid canal, and enters the middle cranial fossa through the upper portion of the foramen lacerum. It proceeds upward in the cavernous sinus along the posterior clinoid process and then turns sharply horizontally. The artery runs forward in the sinus in a groove along the body of the sphenoid bone called the carotid sulcus. The abducens nerve is along its lateral side, and the artery is surrounded by sympathetic filaments of the carotid plexus derived from the superior cervical ganglion. At the level of the anterior clinoid process the carotid artery makes an upward turn to form the carotid siphon, passing just medial to the oculomotor, trochlear, and ophthalmic nerves. Here it gives off several small, but important cavernous branches. The most important of these is the meningohypophyseal artery.[21,44] This usually gives off three additional branches: the tentorial artery that supplies the lateral tentorium and the intracavernous oculomotor and trochlear nerves, the inferior hypophyseal artery that supplies the pituitary gland, and the dorsal meningeal artery that supplies the clival region and the abducens nerve. An inferior cavernous sinus branch has occasionally been described, supplying the ophthalmic division of the trigeminal nerve and the gasserian ganglion.[27] These cavernous branches are important, principally for their involvement in carotid-cavernous fistulas, and in aneurysm formation. Fistulas may develop spontaneously or due to trauma, and may be of the high-flow or low-flow type.[35] Low-flow fistulas usually form in the small branch vessels of the posterior cavernous sinus, and commonly shunt relatively low volumes of blood to the inferior petrosal sinus.[20] High-flow fistulas are typically found in the anterior cavernous sinus directly affecting the carotid artery.[42] These cause increased pressure in the cavernous sinus and reversed flow in the ophthalmic veins, thus resulting in the symptoms of retinal ischemia, orbital congestion, and an audible bruit.

After turning upward in the anterior cavernous sinus, the carotid artery perforates the dura at the medial aspect of the anterior clinoid process, and turns backward inferior to the optic nerve. As it does so, it gives off its first major branch, the ophthalmic artery. In about 5% of individuals, the ophthalmic artery (OA) may arise extradurally within the cavernous sinus, from the carotid artery before the latter penetrates the dura of the sinus roof to become intradural.[13,44]

The intracranial portion of the ophthalmic artery is approximately 2.5–5 mm in length, and measures about 2 mm in diameter. It emerges from the medial side of the carotid trunk below the optic nerve, usually within the intradual space just after the carotid artery pierces the dura to emerge from the cavernous sinus on the medial side of the anterior clinoid process. In about 5% of cases, the ophthalmic artery may arise from the extradual portion of the carotid artery between the inferior and superior dural rings[14] (see Chapter 1). The ophthalmic artery enters the optic canal inferomedially, perforates the inner layers of dura surrounding the optic nerve, usually within the canal, and runs within a split in the dural sheath where the latter is fused to periorbita. As the artery passes through the optic canal it usually moves laterally to emerge at the inferolateral portion of the orbital optic foramen. Within the optic canal the artery is separated from the optic nerve by a layer of dura, and is somewhat compressed against the inferior canal wall. Here it may be further compressed by increased CSF pressure in the subarachnoid space. Clinical observations using Doppler echography have demonstrated increased blood flow in the ophthalmic artery following anterior optic nerve sheath fenestration (Dr. Patrick Flaherty, personal communication).

Inoue et al.[28] reported that in 8% of their anatomic sample the ophthalmic artery arose within the cavernous sinus below the anterior clinoid process. In these cases it passed through the SOF and annulus of Zinn instead of the optic canal. In some of their cases a second hypoplastic ophthalmic artery arose in the normal supraclinoid area and followed the normal pathway. Heyreh[22] reported a rare third variation where the optic nerve enters the orbit through a duplicate optic canal.

On the orbital side of the optic canal the ophthalmic artery gradually pierces the outer layers of dura to emerge extradurally within the intraconal orbital compartment. It passes into the oculomotor foramen of the annulus of Zinn lateral, superolateral, or inferior to the optic nerve.[43] A small recurrent branch emerges from the ophthalmic artery, and turns backward through the annulus of Zinn and the central superior orbital fissure. This anastomoses with the inferolateral trunk of the cavernous branch of the carotid artery to help supply the lateral neural wall of the cavernous sinus. In some cases this is the main arterial supply to this region.[32]

The ophthalmic artery carries the major blood supply to the orbit in 96% of individuals. In about 3%, the middle meningeal artery shares equally in providing blood through an enlarged recurrent meningeal branch. In 1% of individuals the ophthalmic artery does not arise from the carotid artery, but rather its orbital connection to the middle meningeal artery provides the only source of arterial blood to the orbit.[22] In rare instances the maxillary artery fails to annex the embryonic stapedial system, so that the ophthalmic artery becomes the sole source of blood to the middle meningeal artery by retrograde flow. In addition to the middle meningeal connection, the external carotid system contributes collateral blood flow to the orbit through four other anastomotic channels. These are between, (1) the anterior deep temporal artery and the lacrimal artery through the zygomaticotemporal branch; (2) the superficial temporal artery and the supraorbital branch of the frontal artery; (3) the infraorbital artery and the ophthalmic inferior muscular artery; and (4) the angular artery and the dorsal nasal terminal branch of the ophthalmic artery. Of these, only the first two may carry significant arterial flow into the orbit.

The intraorbital ophthalmic artery

The ophthalmic artery can be divided into three anatomic portions within the orbit.[23] The first portion runs anteriorly from the optic canal, usually inferolateral to the optic nerve. In about 30% of individuals, the artery may enter the orbit inferiorly or even inferonasal to the optic nerve. The ophthalmic artery continues forward to a bend where the vessel begins to turn over or under the nerve. The anatomy of the short second portion depends upon whether the artery runs a course over the optic nerve (seen in about 81% of individuals, range 72–95%), or under it (seen in 19% of individuals, range 5–28%).[4,26] In the over the nerve pattern, the second portion runs upward along the lateral side of the nerve and crosses over it to where the artery again turns in an anterior direction. In the under the nerve pattern the artery turns medially and crosses beneath the nerve. The third and longest portion begins as the artery turns anteriorly and extends along the superomedial orbital wall to its terminal branches.[17] For much of this portion, the artery lies between the superior oblique muscle and the optic nerve and measures about 0.5–1.0 mm in diameter. Just posterior to the junction of the optic nerve and sclera, 10–15 mm behind the trochlea, the ophthalmic artery passes out of the rectus muscle cone into the superomedial extraconal space. In 75–80% of individuals it passes between the medial rectus and the superior oblique muscles and continues forward along the medial orbital wall.[7] In most cases (80%) the artery forms a major loop, either horizontally or vertically, as it passes through the intermuscular septum of the medial rectus fascial system. This loop forms a convoluted arterial channel immediately below the superior oblique muscle. It probably allows for movement of the extraocular muscles without stress on the vessel. In about 7% of individuals the artery reenters the muscle cone in the anterior orbit, and then exits again near the trochlea. In 20–25% of normal individuals the ophthalmic artery does not exit the muscle cone until it approaches the trochlea. In such cases the artery does not usually form a prominent loop. Regardless of its exact orbital course, the ophthalmic artery exits the orbit inferior to the trochlea to emerge at the superomedial orbital rim.

Within the orbit, the ophthalmic artery gives off branches to ocular, orbital, extraorbital, and intracranial structures. The order of branching along the arterial tree varies considerably, especially between the over-optic-nerve and under–optic-nerve patterns. There is no single branching sequence that can be considered "normal." Instead, it is better to refer to certain patterns as more "usual" than others.[1,24] Because of the variability in branching sequence of the ophthalmic artery, it is pointless to attempt a description of these in order of origin. In Table 5-1 the "usual" sequence is given for the over-optic-nerve and under-optic-nerve patterns. In the descriptions that follow, these branches are considered within topographic groups,[41] without reference to specific branching order. Branches in the ocular group include the central retinal artery, the posterior ciliary arteries, and small collateral vessels to the optic nerve. Branches in the orbital group include the lacrimal artery, branches to the extraocular muscles, vessels to the periosteum, and orbital fat. Branches in the extraorbital group are the ethmoidal, palpebral, supraorbital, supratrochlear, and dorsal nasal arteries. Finally, branches in the dural group consists of the two recurrent meningeal branches.

Table 5-1 The most common branching orders of the ophthalmic artery

Order of origin	
Over the optic nerve	
1	Central retinal artery
2	Lateral posterior ciliary artery
3	Lacrimal artery
4	Muscular branch to the superior rectus and levator palpebrae superioris muscles
5	Posterior ethmoidal and supraorbital arteries
6	Medial posterior ciliary artery
7	Medial muscular branch
8	Muscular branch to the superior oblique and medial rectus muscles
9	Branch to areolar tissue
10	Anterior ethmoidal artery
11	Inferior medial palpebral artery
12	Superior medial palpebral artery
13	Dorsal nasal artery
Under the optic nerve	
1	Lateral posterior ciliary artery
2	Central retinal artery
3	Medial muscular branch
4	Medial posterior ciliary artery
5	Lacrimal artery
6	Muscular branch to the superior rectus and levator palpebrae superioris muscles
7	Posterior ethmoidal and supraorbital arteries
8	Muscular branch to the superior oblique and medial rectus muscles
9	Anterior ethmoidal artery
10	Branch to areolar tissue
11	Inferior medial palpebral artery
12	Superior medial palpebral artery
13	Dorsal nasal artery

Ocular branches of the ophthalmic artery

The central retinal artery (CRA) arises as the first or second branch of the ophthalmic artery, usually from the inferolateral side of the first or second segments. It measures 0.1–0.4 mm in diameter.[41] The CRA usually arises directly from the OA, but may sometimes arise from a common trunk shared with the lateral posterior ciliary artery, and less commonly from the lacrimal artery. It runs a redundant course along the lateral side of the optic nerve and pierces the dura and substance of the nerve 7–15 mm behind the globe. The central retinal artery usually enters the nerve inferolaterally, but in 30% of cases may enter inferiorly or inferonasally. The artery travels within the subarachnoid space for 1 mm or more and then penetrates the substance of the optic nerve via a small channel lined with pia mater. On reaching the center of the nerve the CRA turns anteriorly and runs forward within a narrow canal to the optic disc in company with the central retinal vein. At the disc it branches into several arterioles that supply blood to the retina and to the superficial anterior optic nerve.[37] In some individuals, on entering the optic nerve the CRA gives rise to a small branch directed retrograde toward the optic canal. This branch narrows and may divide further before finally disappearing within the substance of the nerve. Although its function has not been established, this branch appears to supply blood to the proximal portions of the orbital optic nerve.

The posterior ciliary arteries arise from the first and second portions of the ophthalmic artery.[17] They vary from 1–5 in number, with 30–50% of individuals having three (medial, lateral, and superior). However, at least two, one medial and one lateral, are present in 95% of individuals. These divide into a variable number of short posterior ciliary arteries, ranging from 10–20.[25] These vessels are about 0.4–0.7 mm in diameter.[31] The short ciliary arteries are highly convoluted and run along the optic nerve in two groups, the paraoptic and distal groups. The paraoptic group is immediately adjacent to the nerve and supplies blood to the orbital optic nerve. These vessels pierce the sclera on either side of the optic nerve head. The distal group runs a short distance away from the nerve and penetrates the sclera medially and laterally on either side of the optic disc. Within the eye the short posterior ciliary arteries supply blood to the prelaminar and laminar portions of the optic nerve head. They also supply the choroid, RPE, and the outer 130 μm of the retina. The long posterior ciliary arteries emerge from the OA and course on either side of the optic nerve to enter the sclera medially and laterally more peripherally than the short arteries. They course in the suprachoroidal space to the ciliary body and iris. Anteriorly, the posterior ciliary arteries anastomose with branches of the anterior ciliary arteries entering the globe from within the rectus muscles from the muscular arteries.

A number of tiny branches from the ophthalmic and posterior ciliary arteries pierce the dura of the optic nerve to form a fine arborizing plexus on the pia mater. These provide the chief arterial supply to the optic nerve. These vessels are potentially susceptible to compression from increased intraorbital and subarachnoid pressure.

Orbital branches of the ophthalmic artery

The orbital branches of the ophthalmic artery supply intraorbital structures other than the optic nerve and globe. The arterial branches to the extraocular muscles are numerous and variable, but generally they arise from the inferior surface of the ophthalmic artery, and occasionally from the lacrimal artery as two main arterial trunks.[8] These trunks are conceptual only, and the vessels associated with them may arise from a true common trunk, independently, or in various combinations from the same approximate zone. The lateral or superior muscular trunk arises from the second portion of the ophthalmic artery as it crosses over the optic nerve or from the junction of the second and third portions when it crosses under the optic nerve. It may also originate from the base of the lacrimal branch, either alone or in common with other major branches, such as additional lateral ciliary vessels. The lateral muscular artery arises from the ophthalmic artery in 60% of cases and from the lacrimal artery in 40%.[16] It supplies the lateral rectus muscle and may also send branches to the superior rectus and levator muscles. The branch to the levator muscle occasionally arises from the supraorbital artery. Less commonly, the lateral muscular trunk may also send branches to others of the extraocular muscles, such as the inferior oblique. In general, the muscular arteries measure about 0.3–0.4 mm in diameter.[31]

The medial or inferior muscular trunk usually arises near the beginning of the third portion of the ophthalmic artery. It usually sends branches to the medial and inferior rectus muscles, and may also supply the inferior oblique muscle. A small muscular branch directly from the third portion of the ophthalmic artery supplies the superior oblique. An accessory, or in some cases the only branch to the levator muscle sometimes originates here as well.

As the muscular arterioles approach the muscle bellies on their conal surfaces they run within longitudinal grooves between the fascicular bundles and arborize into fine vessels that penetrate the conal surface. Within the substance of each rectus muscle several larger branches continue forward as the anterior ciliary arteries. There are two such vessels associated with each of the rectus muscles, except for the lateral rectus which usually has only one. As the anterior ciliary arteries run forward they move to the orbital surface immediately beneath the muscle sheath. At the tendinous insertions these vessels penetrate the sclera to anastomose with the anterior uveal circulation. Small branches from these vessels also supply the bulbar conjunctiva and superior fornix.

The lacrimal artery usually arises as a separate branch from the second portion of the ophthalmic artery, close to the origin of the central retinal artery, but this branch may be absent in as many as 30% of cases. The artery courses laterally and superiorly between the superior and lateral rectus muscles into the superolateral extraconal space. Here it measures 0.3–1.0 mm in diameter.[41] Just before it turns anteriorly along the superolateral orbital wall it is joined by the accessory ophthalmic (recurrent meningeal) artery in up to 70% of individuals. In 10% of individuals the meningolacrimal (sphenoidal) artery branches off from the lacrimal artery and passes through a separate bony foramen (Hyrtl's canal) in the greater wing of the sphenoid bone. Both the accessory ophthalmic and the meningolacrimal branches anastomose intracranially with a branch of the middle meningeal artery.[30]

The lacrimal artery then continues forward in company with the lacrimal nerve along the upper border of the lateral rectus muscle. It gives rise to muscular, zygomatic and glandular branches.[13,41] Sometimes some of the short posterior

ciliary arteries can arise from the lacrimal artery as well. Muscular arteries supply the lateral and superior rectus/levator muscle complex. Just posterior to the lacrimal gland a branch descends along the lateral orbital wall and divides into two vessels, the zygomaticotemporal and zygomaticofacial arteries. These penetrate the lateral orbital wall through foramina with the same names where they anastomose with branches of the transverse facial and superficial temporal arteries forming a rich subdermal vascular net in the lateral temporal and cheek region.[2] The lacrimal artery divides into numerous branches that supply the lacrimal gland. One terminal branch continues through the gland or passes inferiorly around it, penetrates the orbital septum, and divides to form the superior and inferior lateral palpebral arteries. These run along the upper and lower eyelids as the arterial arcades and anastomose with the medial palpebral vessels. The inferior lateral palpebral artery also anastomoses with branches of the facial artery.

As noted earlier in the discussion of embryology, in some cases the lacrimal arterial supply derives exclusively from the external carotid system via the meningolacrimal artery passing through the lacrimal (Hyrtl's) formaen.[9] This opening is situated in the greater sphenoid wing 5-10 mm lateral to the SOF.[41] In some cases the lacrimal artery may have a dual blood supply from both the ophthalmic artery and the meningolacrimal artery.[6] Occasionally, multiple small branches are present that pass through several small foramina in the same area. Rarely, the lacrimal artery may originate from the deep temporal branch of the external carotid system through a vessel that penetrates the greater sphenoid wing to anastomose with the zygomaticotemporal artery.[31]

In addition to the major branches of the ophthalmic artery, tiny vessels enter the posterior orbit through the optic canal, the superior orbital fissure, and through perforating foramina in the sphenoid bone. These vessels are derived from the cavernous branches of the carotid artery and supply periorbita, the annulus of Zinn, the posterior extraocular muscles, and fat in the orbital apex. Some of them anastomose with orbital branches of the ophthalmic artery. Small vessels arising from the first portion of the ophthalmic artery, the posterior ciliary arteries, the central retinal artery, and the muscular arteries supply blood to the ciliary ganglion and motor nerves to the extraocular muscles.[12] These vessels measure only 40–60 μm in diameter and vary considerably in number and configuration.

Extraorbital branches of the ophthalmic artery

The extraorbital branches of the ophthalmic artery supply structures outside the orbit proper. The small posterior ethmoidal artery measures only about 0.3–0.5 mm in diameter. It arises near the junction of the second and third portions of the ophthalmic artery in 75% of cases where it is present.[10] In 25% of individuals who have this vessel it arises from the supraorbital artery or, less frequently, from the anterior ethmoidal artery. It may be absent in up to 50% of individuals,[45] or may be multiple. This vessel extends across the orbit medially, usually passes over, but sometimes under the superior oblique muscle, and exits through the posterior ethmoidal foramen 5–10 mm anterior to the optic canal, and 10–15 mm behind the anterior ethmoidal foramen. Before entering the posterior ethmoidal foramen it often gives off one or more accessory muscular branches to the superior oblique, superior rectus, or levator muscles. The artery primarily supplies the mucosa of the posterior ethmoid air cells, and then passes intracranially through a small foramen to supply the dura of the posterior half of the anterior cranial fossa.

The larger and more constant anterior ethmoidal artery measures about 0.6–0.7 mm in diameter. It arises from the middle of the third portion of the ophthalmic artery, near where the latter crosses beneath the superior oblique muscle. Occasionally it may originate from the supraorbital artery or other branches. The vessel may be absent in less than 2% of cases,[10] and rarely may be multiple. In 98% of individuals the anterior ethmoidal artery passes under the superior oblique muscle *en route* to the medial wall. It travels with the anterior ethmoidal nerve through the anterior ethmoidal foramen. This vessel supplies the mucosa of the anterior ethmoid air cells, the frontal sinus, and the lateral wall of the nose and nasal septum. A small meningeal branch from this vessel penetrates the roof of the ethmoid sinus near the cribriform plate, and runs within the falx cerebri as the anterior meningeal (anterior falcine) artery with branches to the dura of the anterior cranial fossa.

The main trunk of the ophthalmic artery continues forward in the superomedial extraconal orbital space as the nasofrontal artery. Just before reaching the trochlea it divides into two branches. The supratrochlear artery continues forward above the trochlea, and the dorsal nasal artery passes between the trochlea and the medial canthal tendon. Just before leaving the orbit the dorsal nasal artery gives rise to the medial palpebral artery. The latter further divides into the medial superior and medial inferior palpebral arteries that enter the eyelids above and below the medial canthal tendon.

The supraorbital artery arises from the second or third portion of the ophthalmic artery. It may be absent in 10–20% of normal individuals. The artery passes into the extraconal space on the medial side of the midportion of the superior rectus and levator muscles. Here it measures about 0.8–1.0 mm in diameter. Although the supraorbital artery primarily supplies extraorbital structures, it does give off small muscular branches to the superior oblique, superior rectus, and levator muscles. The artery runs anteriorly with the supraorbital nerve to exit the orbit at the supraorbital foramen or notch. The main trunk enters the corrugator muscle and divides into superficial and deep branches. The superficial branch continues through the orbicularis and frontalis muscles, and pierces the frontalis and the superficial galea about 40–60 mm above the orbital rim to enter the subcutaneous fat plane.[15] It divides into 2–3 branches that supply muscles of the brow and forehead, and the scalp to the vertex of the skull. The supraorbital artery anastomoses with branches of the superficial temporal artery laterally, and with the supratrochlear and angular arteries medially. The deep branch of the supraorbital artery turns laterally from the supraorbital foramen, and runs within the deep subgaleal fascia just above periosteum to supply the pericranium along the supraorbital rim.

The supratrochlear and dorsal nasal arteries are the terminal twigs of the OA.[26] The supratrochlear artery is about 0.8 mm in diameter and runs in the superomedial orbit to the orbital rim. Here it pierces the orbital septum just above the level of the trochlea. The nerve then passes deep to the frontalis and orbicularis muscles, and just above the corrugator muscle. It turns superiorly to supply the medial forehead and scalp. In 13% of individuals the supratrochlear and supraorbital arteries exit the orbit as a single vessel and separate immediately after exiting from the supraorbital foramen or notch.[15]

The dorsal nasal artery penetrates the orbital septum just below the supratrochlear artery about 10–12 mm above the medial canthal ligament. It supplies the nasal bridge, the central forehead and scalp near the midline, and anastomoses with the contralateral dorsal nasal artery. The supratrochlear and dorsal nasal arteries have rich anastomotic connections across the nasal bridge, with the angular artery of the facial system,[11,41] and with the frontal branch of the superficial temporal artery.

The eyelid arterial arcades

The arterial supply to the eyelids form part of a vast anastomotic periorbital network supplied by both the internal and external carotid systems. Medially the terminal ophthalmic artery gives rise to the medial superior and inferior palpebral arteries, and laterally the lacrimal artery gives rise to the lateral palpebral arteries (see Chapter 8). These medial and lateral palpebral vessels join to form the arterial arcades in the upper and lower eyelids. In the upper eyelid a marginal arcade runs within or just anterior to the tarsal plate about 2–3 mm from the lid margin. A peripheral arcade, generally appearing as one or more fine serpentine vessels, is located along the anterior surface of Müller's accessory retractor muscle at the superior border of the tarsus. The peripheral arcade lies immediately beneath the levator aponeurosis. During eyelid surgery if these vessels are seen it indicates a disinsertion and retraction of the aponeurosis, or a thin transparent distal aponeurosis. The two upper eyelid arcades are interconnected by vertical arterial branches that supply the tarsal plates, orbicularis muscle, conjunctiva, and skin. In the lower eyelid usually only the marginal arcade is present and it is located about 2 mm from the lid margin. A peripheral arcade is occasionally seen as a variant in some individuals. An anastomotic network of fine vessels interconnects the arterial arcades with the anterior ciliary vessels through the palpebral conjunctiva around the superior and inferior fornices. Tiny branches may join the arcades from the maxillary artery via the infraorbital artery, and from the superficial temporal artery via the frontal, zygomatico-orbital, and transverse facial branches.

Dural branches of the ophthalmic artery

Several recurrent branches from the initial portion of the OA turn backward and course through the annulus of Zinn. One supplies dura of the cavernous sinus, intracranial optic nerve, and tentorium, and another forms an anastomotic connection with the inferolateral trunk of the intracavernous carotid artery. A small branch supplies the intracanalicular portion of the optic nerve.

Anastomotic connections of the orbital arterial system

Around the orbital rim extensive anastomotic connections between the internal and external carotid systems bring collateral blood supply to the orbit. The facial artery arises from the external carotid artery in the carotid triangle below the angle of the jaw. It courses forward and upward over the mandible, across the cheek to the angle of the mouth, and then ascends along the side of the nose, where it becomes the angular artery along the medial canthus. Here it anastomoses with branches of the infraorbital, dorsal nasal, and supratrochlear arteries.

As the external carotid artery continues to ascend it divides behind the neck of the mandible into its two main terminal trunks, the internal maxillary and superficial temporal arteries. The internal maxillary artery gives rise to numerous branches that supply deep structures of the face.[33] Of particular importance for the orbit is the infraorbital branch which arises in the pterygopalatine fossa at the posterior inferior orbital fissure. The infraorbital artery enters the orbit and the infraorbital groove, and passes forward in the infraorbital canal in company with the infraorbital nerve. It emerges on the face at the infraorbital foramen about 4 mm below the central inferior orbital rim. *En route* to its terminal branches, the infraorbital artery gives rise to one or more small vessels within the orbit. These penetrate periorbita about 13–17 mm posterior to the infraorbital rim, and may result in brisk bleeding during inferior orbital wall dissection if not recognized and cauterized.[3] In 86% of individuals they supply the inferior oblique and inferior rectus muscles, where they anastomose with the inferior muscular branch of the ophthalmic artery. Occasionally this may be the sole source of blood to the inferior oblique muscle.[10] Additional branches may supply the lacrimal sac, and others may pass downward to supply the mucosa of the maxillary sinus. On the face, the infraorbital artery supplies the lower eyelid and upper cheek, and anastomoses with branches from the angular and palpebral arteries.

The superficial temporal and maxillary arteries represent the terminal branches of the external carotid system. The superficial temporal artery gives rise to several vessels, the parietal, frontal, zygomaticoorbital, and transverse facial arteries. The last four vessels branch off at various levels in front of the ear and anastomose with the zygomaticofacial, zygomaticotemporal, and infraorbital vessels from the orbit and the internal carotid system. They form superficial subdermal and deep suborbicularis muscle vascular nets over the lateral orbit and cheek. The superficial temporal artery is a major trunk measuring 2 mm in diameter. It originates 1 cm in front of the bony external auditory canal, and approximately 6–7 cm posterior to the lateral orbital rim.[41] As it crosses the zygomatic process, it is covered by the auricularis muscle, and is accompanied by the auriculotemoral nerve, which lies immediately behind it. Just above the zygomatic process and in front of the ear, the artery becomes more superficial, lying below the skin and within the superfical temporal fascia. It continues to ascend in the temple about 1 cm anterior to the ear. Here it can be palpated easily, and may be biopsied in suspected cases of temporal arteritis.

The frontal branch of the superficial temporal artery crosses the forehead just above the lateral brow. It supplies the frontalis muscle, skin, and pericranium, and anastomoses with twigs of the supraorbital artery. The zygomaticoorbital branch runs along the upper border of the zygomatic arch and between the deep and superficial temporal fascial layers to supply the orbicularis muscle at the lateral canthus. Here it anastomoses with the zygomaticofacial artery, and the

lateral palpebral branches of the lacrimal artery. The transverse facial artery arises from the superficial temporal artery just inferior to the zygomatic arch. It courses transversely across the side of the face between the zygomatic arch and the parotid duct to supply the parotid gland and masseter muscle, and anastomoses with branches of the zygomaticofacial and infraorbital artery, and with the inferior palpebral arcade.

Clinical correlations

The anastomotic connections between the internal and external carotid systems are of clinical significance. During orbital surgery periosteal elevation along the lateral orbital wall will sometimes encounter brisk arterial bleeding from disruption of the meningolacrimal or the zygomaticotemporal arteries passing through the sphenoid bone. These usually stop with gentle pressure. During surgery on the orbital floor for blow out fracture repair or with decompression surgery, bleeding may occur from tearing of the anastomotic branches between the infraorbital artery and inferior muscular arteries.

Giant-cell or temporal arteritis is the most common vasculitis. It is characterized by focal occlusive granulomatous inflammations of medium and small arteries that primarily affect cranial vessels of elderly patients. Although the superficial temporal artery is frequently involved, the ophthalmic, posterior ciliary, and central retinal artery, and more rarely, cerebral, aortic and coronary arteries may also be affected. The diagnosis is made by clinical history in an elderly patient with an elevated erythrocyte sedimentation rate, and on a temporal artery biopsy, although the latter may be negative in many individuals. Because of possible involvement of the internal carotid and ophthalmic artery trunk, the only alternate arterial flow to orbital structures may be via anastomotic branches through the involved, but still patent, superficial temporal artery. Compression of the temporal artery for several minutes prior to biopsy may help to ascertain the patency of blood supply to the retina from the ophthalmic artery. If the patient develops amaurosis with compression of the superficial temporal artery, it is likely that the ophthalmic artery is non-patent. In such cases, the biopsy should not be undertaken on that side.

Orbital vessels may be involved in the formation of arteriovenous shunts. Their effect on orbital structures depends largely upon the site of the shunt and the volume-rate of blood flow. Slow-flow shunts increase venous pressure leading to venous dilatation and orbital edema, and may result in thrombosis. High-flow shunts may cause orbital swelling, pulsatile proptosis, chemosis, dilated epibulbar veins, increased intraocular pressure, and ocular ischemia. A-V shunts may be congenital, but more commonly are acquired either spontaneously or following head trauma. The shunt is usually located outside the orbit near the cavernous sinus, with arterial blood passing directly to the orbital veins by retrograde filling. Distention and increased pressure in the cavernous sinus may result in diplopia from cranial nerve palsies, usually the third and sixth. Less frequently the shunt is located within the orbit, associated with congenital A-V malformations.

Capillary hemangiomas are congenital hamartomas of vascular channels. They are common vascular tumors in childhood where they may involve skin, eyelid structures, or occur in the deep orbit. Clinical symptoms vary from just a cosmetic blemish to large disfiguring masses. Ptosis, proptosis, strabismus, and visual impairment may be associated findings. These tumors usually undergo a proliferative phase followed by slow involution. Cavernous hemangiomas are benign vascular neoplasms of large endothelial-lined vascular channels presenting most commonly as orbital lesions in young to middle aged adults. They are characterized by slowly progressive painless proptosis, sometimes associated with diplopia and decreased vision.

Orbital mucormycosis is an aggressive opportunistic fungal infection of the paranasal sinuses that frequently extends to involve the orbit. Debilitated and immunosuppressed patients, especially those with uncontrolled diabetes and ketoacidosis, are particularly susceptible. The organism invades vascular lumina leading to inflammatory occlusion, infarction, and ischemic necrosis. Proptosis, motility restriction, and visual loss from central retinal artery occlusion confirm massive orbital infection. The disease may spread intracranially through the superior orbital fissure to the cavernous sinuses, and in untreated cases is frequently fatal.

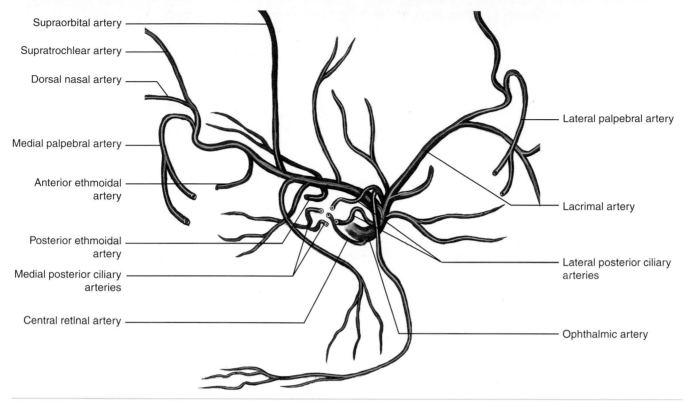

Supraorbital artery

Supratrochlear artery

Dorsal nasal artery

Medial palpebral artery

Anterior ethmoidal artery

Posterior ethmoidal artery

Medial posterior ciliary arteries

Central retinal artery

Lateral palpebral artery

Lacrimal artery

Lateral posterior ciliary arteries

Ophthalmic artery

Figure 5-1 Orbital arteries, frontal view.

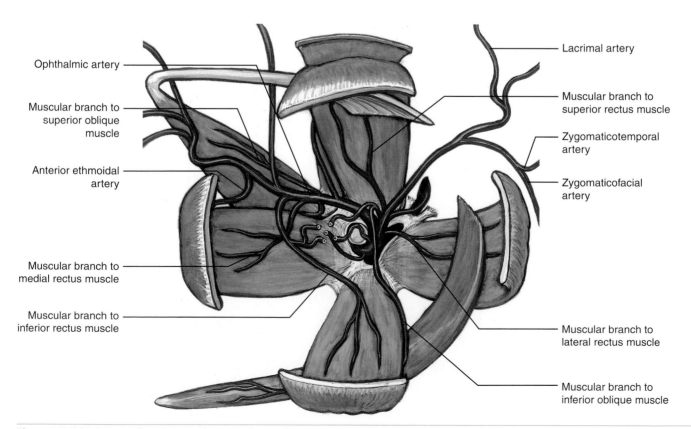

Ophthalmic artery

Muscular branch to superior oblique muscle

Anterior ethmoidal artery

Muscular branch to medial rectus muscle

Muscular branch to inferior rectus muscle

Lacrimal artery

Muscular branch to superior rectus muscle

Zygomaticotemporal artery

Zygomaticofacial artery

Muscular branch to lateral rectus muscle

Muscular branch to inferior oblique muscle

Figure 5-2 Orbital arteries, frontal view with extraocular muscles.

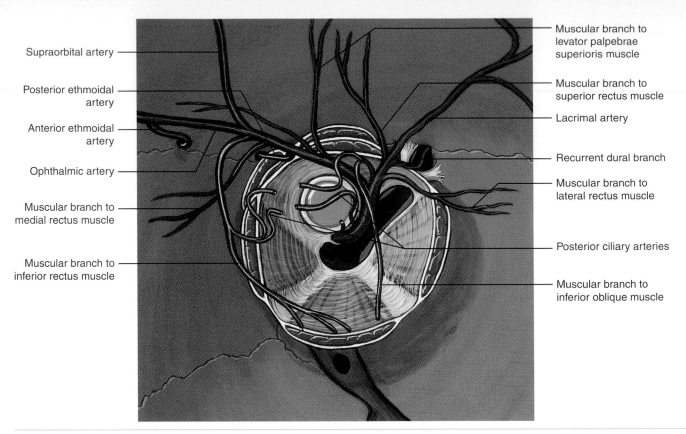

Supraorbital artery

Posterior ethmoidal artery

Anterior ethmoidal artery

Ophthalmic artery

Muscular branch to medial rectus muscle

Muscular branch to inferior rectus muscle

Muscular branch to levator palpebrae superioris muscle

Muscular branch to superior rectus muscle

Lacrimal artery

Recurrent dural branch

Muscular branch to lateral rectus muscle

Posterior ciliary arteries

Muscular branch to inferior oblique muscle

Figure 5-3 Orbital arteries, frontal view, orbital apex.

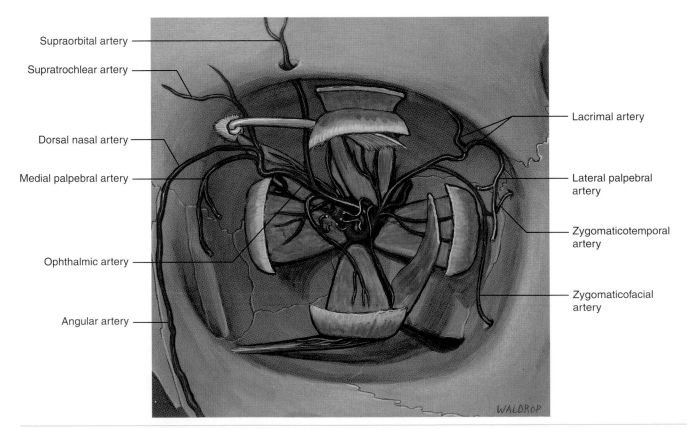

Supraorbital artery

Supratrochlear artery

Dorsal nasal artery

Medial palpebral artery

Ophthalmic artery

Angular artery

Lacrimal artery

Lateral palpebral artery

Zygomaticotemporal artery

Zygomaticofacial artery

WALDROP

Figure 5-4 Orbital arteries, frontal composite view with extraocular muscles and orbital bones.

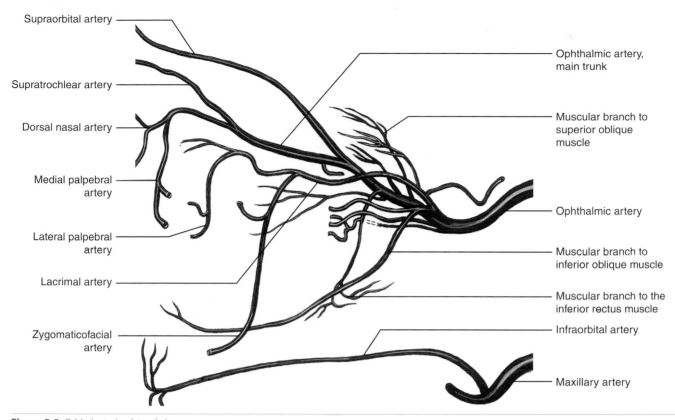

Supraorbital artery

Supratrochlear artery

Dorsal nasal artery

Medial palpebral artery

Lateral palpebral artery

Lacrimal artery

Zygomaticofacial artery

Ophthalmic artery, main trunk

Muscular branch to superior oblique muscle

Ophthalmic artery

Muscular branch to inferior oblique muscle

Muscular branch to the inferior rectus muscle

Infraorbital artery

Maxillary artery

Figure 5-5 Orbital arteries, lateral view.

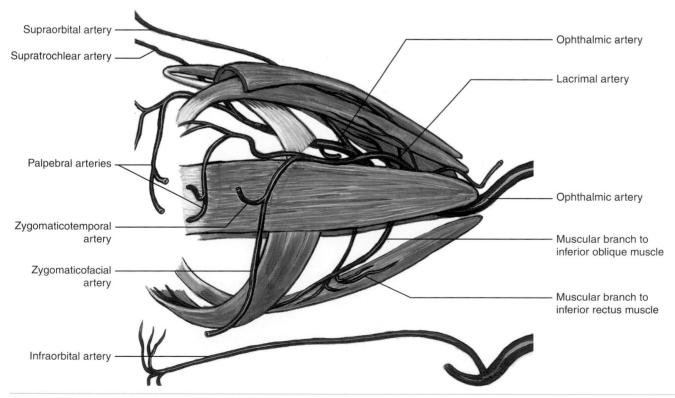

Supraorbital artery

Supratrochlear artery

Palpebral arteries

Zygomaticotemporal artery

Zygomaticofacial artery

Infraorbital artery

Ophthalmic artery

Lacrimal artery

Ophthalmic artery

Muscular branch to inferior oblique muscle

Muscular branch to inferior rectus muscle

Figure 5-6 Orbital arteries, lateral view with extraocular muscles.

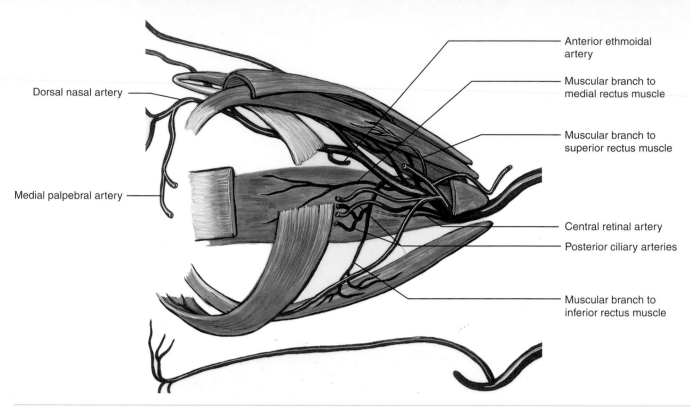

Dorsal nasal artery

Medial palpebral artery

Anterior ethmoidal artery

Muscular branch to medial rectus muscle

Muscular branch to superior rectus muscle

Central retinal artery

Posterior ciliary arteries

Muscular branch to inferior rectus muscle

Figure 5-7 Orbital arteries, lateral view, lateral rectus muscle removed.

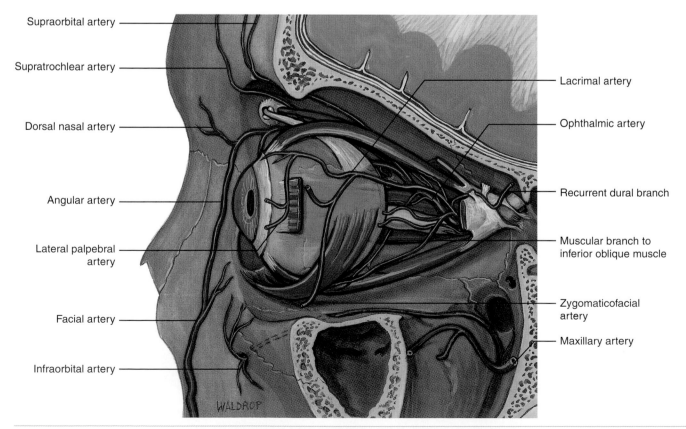

Supraorbital artery

Supratrochlear artery

Dorsal nasal artery

Angular artery

Lateral palpebral artery

Facial artery

Infraorbital artery

Lacrimal artery

Ophthalmic artery

Recurrent dural branch

Muscular branch to inferior oblique muscle

Zygomaticofacial artery

Maxillary artery

WALDROP

Figure 5-8 Orbital arteries, lateral composite view, with extraocular muscle, globe and orbital bones.

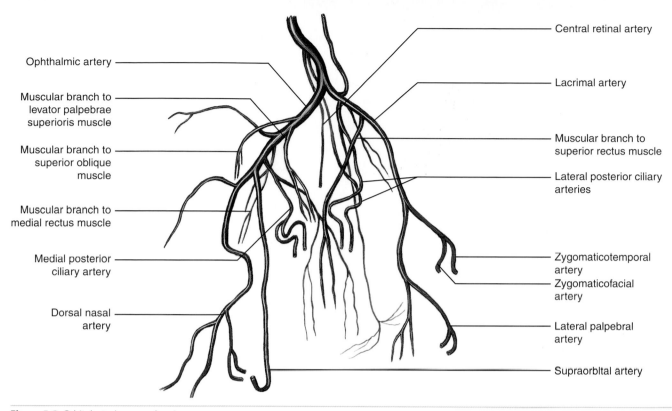

Central retinal artery

Ophthalmic artery

Lacrimal artery

Muscular branch to
levator palpebrae
superioris muscle

Muscular branch to
superior rectus muscle

Muscular branch to
superior oblique
muscle

Lateral posterior ciliary
arteries

Muscular branch to
medial rectus muscle

Medial posterior
ciliary artery

Zygomaticotemporal
artery

Zygomaticofacial
artery

Dorsal nasal
artery

Lateral palpebral
artery

Supraorbltal artery

Figure 5-9 Orbital arteries, superior view.

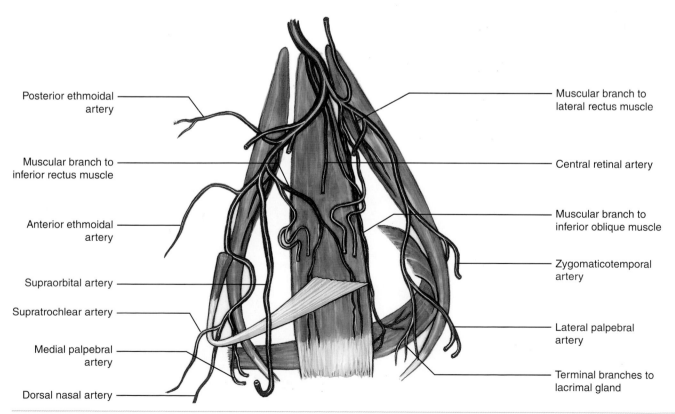

Posterior ethmoidal
artery

Muscular branch to
lateral rectus muscle

Muscular branch to
inferior rectus muscle

Central retinal artery

Anterior ethmoidal
artery

Muscular branch to
inferior oblique muscle

Supraorbital artery

Zygomaticotemporal
artery

Supratrochlear artery

Medial palpebral
artery

Lateral palpebral
artery

Dorsal nasal artery

Terminal branches to
lacrimal gland

Figure 5-10 Orbital arteries, superior view, with extraocular muscles.

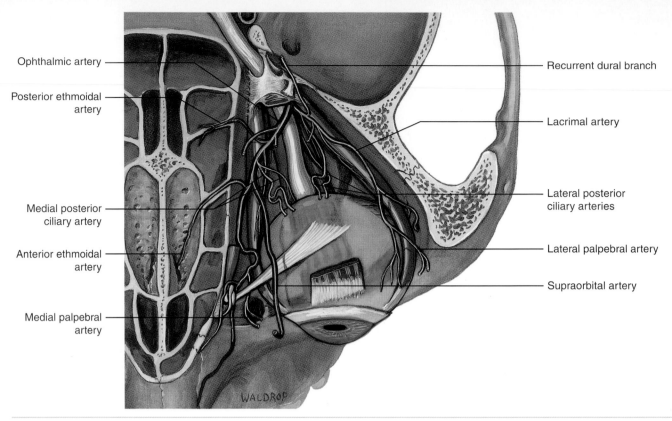

Figure 5-11 Orbital arteries, superior composite view with extraocular muscles, globe and orbital bones.

Ophthalmic artery

Posterior ethmoidal artery

Medial posterior ciliary artery

Anterior ethmoidal artery

Medial palpebral artery

Recurrent dural branch

Lacrimal artery

Lateral posterior ciliary arteries

Lateral palpebral artery

Supraorbital artery

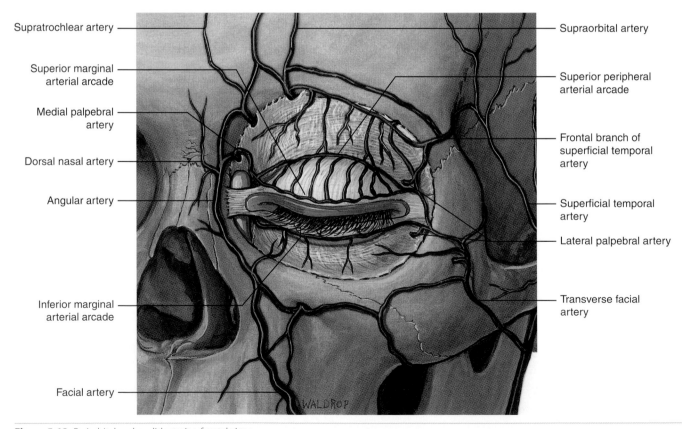

Figure 5-12 Periorbital and eyelid arteries, frontal view.

Supratrochlear artery

Superior marginal arterial arcade

Medial palpebral artery

Dorsal nasal artery

Angular artery

Inferior marginal arterial arcade

Facial artery

Supraorbital artery

Superior peripheral arterial arcade

Frontal branch of superficial temporal artery

Superficial temporal artery

Lateral palpebral artery

Transverse facial artery

References

1. Bergin MP: A spatial reconstruction of the orbital vascular pattern in relation with the connective tissue system. *Acta Morphol Neerl Scand* 20:117, 1982.

2. Bozikov K, Show-Dunn J, Soutar DS, Arnez ZM: Arterial anatomy of the lateral orbital and cheek region and arterial supply to the "peri-zygomatic perforator arteries" flap. *Surg Radiol Anat* 30:17, 2008.

3. Coulter VL, Holds JB, Anderson RL: Avoiding complications of orbital surgery: The orbital branches of the infraorbital artery. *Ophthalm Surg* 21:141, 1990.

4. DeSantis M, Anderson KJ, King DW, Nielsen J: Variability in relationships of arteries and nerves in the human orbit. *Anat Anz* 157:227, 1984.

5. Diamond MK: Homologies of the meningeal-orbital arteries of humans: A reappraisal. *J Anat* 178:223, 1991.

6. Ducasse A, Delattre JF, Flament JB, Hureau J: The arteries of the lacrimal gland. *Surg Radiol Anat* 6:287, 1984.

7. Ducasse A, Delattre JF, Segal A, et al: Anatomical basis of the surgical approaches to the medial wall of the orbit. *Anat Clin* 7:15, 1985.

8. Ducasse A, Flament JB, Delattre JF, Avisse C: Arterial blood supply and innervation of the rectus muscles of the eyeball. *J Fr Ophtalmol* 24:382, 2001.

9. Duccasse A, Segal A, Delattre JF, Flament JB: La participation de l'art,re carotide externe ... la vascularisation orbitaire. *J Fr Ophtalmol* 8:333, 1985.

10. Ducasse A, Segal A, El Ladki S, Flament JB: Vascularisation arterielle et innervation de la glande lacrymale. *Ophthalmologie* 4:129, 1990.

11. Edizer M, Beden U, Icten N: Morphological parameters of the periorbital arterial arcades and potential clinical significance based on anatomical identification. *J Craniofac Surg* 20:209, 2009.

12. Eliskova M: Blood vessels of the ciliary ganglion in man. *Br J Ophthalmol* 57:766, 1973.

13. Erdogmus S, Govsa F: Importance of the anatomic features of the lacrimal artery for orbital approaches. *J Craniofac Surg* 16:957, 2005.

14. Erdogmus S, Govsa F: Anatomic features of the intracranial and intracanalicular portions of the ophthalmic artery: For the surgical procedures. *Neurosurg Rev* 29:21, 2006.

15. Erdogmus S, Govsa F: Anatomy of the supraorbital region and the evaluation of it for the reconstruction of facial defects. *J Craniofac Surg* 18:104, 2007.

16. Erdogmus S, Govsa F: Arterial vascularization of the extraocular muscles on its importance of orbital approaches. *J Craniofac Surg* 18:1125, 2007.

17. Erdogmus S, Govsa F: Anatomic characteristics of the ophthalmic and posterior ciliary arteries. *J Neuroophthalmol* 28:320, 2008.

18. Gailloud P, Gregg L, Ruiz DSM: Developmental anatomy, angiography, and clinical implications of orbital arterial variations involving the stapedial artery. *Neuroimag Clin N Am* 19:169, 2009.

19. Gillilan LA: The collateral circulation of the human orbit. *Arch Ophthalmol* 65:684, 1961.

20. Halbach VV, Hieshima GB, Higashida RT, Reicker M: Carotid cavernous fistulae: Indications for urgent treatment. *AJR* 149:587, 1987.

21. Harris FS, Rhoton AL: Anatomy of the cavernous sinus. *J Neurosurg* 45:169, 1976.

22. Hayreh SS, Dass R: The ophthalmic artery. I. Origin and intracanalicular course. *Br J Ophthalmol* 46:65, 1962.

23. Hayreh SS, Dass R: The ophthalmic artery. II. Intra-orbital course. *Br J Ophthalmol* 46:165, 1962.

24. Hayreh SS: The ophthalmic artery. III. Branches. *Br J Ophthalmol* 46:212, 1962.

25. Hayreh SS: Posterior ciliary artery circulation in health and disease. The Weisenfeld Lecture. *Invest Ophthalmol Vis Sci* 45:749, 2004.

26. Hayreh SS: Orbital vascular anatomy. *Eye* 20:1130, 2006.

27. Hollingshead WWH: *Anatomy for Surgeons: The Head and Neck.* 3rd ed. Philadelphia, Harper and Row, 1982, p 52.

28. Inoue T, Rhoton AL Jr, Theele D, Barry ME: Surgical approaches to the cavernous sinus: A microsurgical study. *Neurosurg* 26:903, 1990.

29. Krause W: Zur Entwicklungsgeschichte der Arteria ophthalmica beim Menschen. *Z Anat Entwicklungsgesch, Berlin* 119:311, 1956.

30. Kuru Y: Meningeal branches of the ophthalmic artery. *Acta Radiol Diag* 6:241, 1967.

31. Lang J, Kageyama I: The ophthalmic artery and its branches, measurements and clinical importance. *Surg Radiol Anat* 12:83, 1990.

32. Lasjaunias P, Brismar J, Moret J, Theron J: Recurrent cavernous branches of the ophthalmic artery. *Acta Radiol Diag* 19:553, 1978.

33. Lasjaunias P, Vignaud J, Hasso AN: Maxillary artery blood supply to the orbit: Normal and pathologic aspects. *Neuroradiol* 9:87, 1975.

34. Lee HY, Chung IH: Foramen meningo-orbitale and its relationships with the middle meningeal artery. *Korean J Anat* 33:99, 2000.

35. Leonard TJK, Moseley IF, Sanders MD: Ophthalmoplegia in carotid cavernous sinus fistulas. *Br J Ophthalmol* 68:128, 1984.

36. Liu Q, Rhoton AL Jr: Middle meningeal origin of the ophthalmic artery. *Neurosurg* 49:401, 2001.

37. Mackenzie PJ, Cioffi GA: Vascular anatomy of the optic nerve head. *Can J Ophthalmol* 43:308, 2008.

38. Mann I: *The Development of the Human Eye.* New York, Grune and Stratton, 1964.

39. Moret J, Lasjaunias P, Theron J, Merland JJ: The middle menigeal artery. Its contribution to the vascularization of the orbit. *J Neuroradiol* 4:225, 1977.

40. Padget DH: The development of the cranial arteries in the human embryo. *Contr Embryol Carnegie Instn, Washington* 32:205, 1948.

41. Perrini P, Cardia A, Raser K, Lanzini G: A microsurgical study of the anatomy and course of the ophthalmic artery and its possible dangerous anastomoses. *J Nueurosurg* 106:142, 2007.

42. Phelps CD, Thompson HS, Ossoinig KC: The diagnosis and prognosis of atypical carotid-cavernous fistula (red-eyed shunt syndrome). *Am J Ophthalmol* 93:423, 1982.

43. Reymond J, Kwiatkowski J, Wysocki J: Clinical anatomy of the superior orbital fissure and the orbital apex. *J Cranio-Maxillofac Surg* 36:346, 2008.

44. Rhoton AL, Hardy DG, Chambers SM: Microsurgical anatomy and dissection of the sphenoid bone, cavernous sinus, and sellar region. *Surg Neurol* 1:63, 1978.

45. Stock AL, Collins HP, Davideson TM: Anatomy of the superficial temporal artery. *Head Neck Surg* 2:466, 1980.

CHAPTER 6

Venous and Lymphatic Systems

Embryology

Beginning in the 5 mm (4-week) embryonic stage, small blood spaces appear within the orbital mesenchyme simultaneous with development of the arterial hyaloid system. These coalesce to form venous channels. They drain posteriorly into a plexus of blood spaces that form along the outer part of the cerebral vesicle, and communicate with a large space lying medial to the gasserian ganglion, the future cavernous sinus.

As the optic fissure closes during the 12–20 mm (5–7- week) stages, the choriocapillary network forms and establishes communication posteriorly with the developing orbital arterial system, and anteriorly with the circular net around the rim of the optic cup. This choriocapillary network also develops four orbital branches at the equator of the optic vesicle. These are the future vortex veins. They communicate with two main venous blood spaces in the orbit, the supraorbital and infraorbital plexuses. The latter both drain posteriorly into the cavernous sinus. By the 18 mm (6-week) embryonic stage, these orbital plexuses coalesce as the superior and inferior ophthalmic veins.

During the 100 mm (15-week) fetal stage the intravitreal portion of the arterial hyaloid system atrophies, and Burgmeister's papilla collapses to leave the optic disc and its central physiologic cup. Small arterial buds from the hyaloid vessel form at the base of Burgmeister's papilla and ramify to establish the retinal arterial circulation. The retinal veins form simultaneously as small vascular channels that finally open into two main trunks on the optic disc. These run into the optic nerve, coalesce as a single central retinal vein, and emerge, usually near the central retinal artery, to join the developing ophthalmic venous system.

The venous drainage system in the adult

In the adult, the orbital venous drainage bed is very complex with a high degree of individual variation.[22] Veins from the eye and orbit drain into a diffuse network of interconnected branches. In contrast to the more or less orderly topographic arrangement of the arterial system, orbital veins are less well defined and considerably more variable, except for the major trunks. An extensive microvascular network interconnecting the arterial and venous systems, and in close association with the connective tissue system of the orbit, has been described.[3] It's exact physiologic role remains conjectural.

Unlike the arterial system in the orbit, the veins maintain an intimate relationship with the complex orbital fascial systems.[4,5] Throughout their courses the veins travel within these septal layers, and the larger vessels are further supported by fascial slings. This arrangement appears to prevent excessive stretching, and helps prevent collapse of the delicate venous walls by ocular motility and variations in intraorbital pressure.[8] However, this may also make the veins more vulnerable to orbital fibrosis and enlarging muscles or masses, resulting in changes in venous flow and possible vascular congestion, as, for example, in Graves' orbital disease.

Although the major drainage of orbital blood is backward to the cavernous sinus, secondary flow occurs into the pterygoid venous plexus through the inferior orbital fissure, and in some cases may even drain forward to the facial venous system. In achondroplastic dwarfs, orbital venous flow is consistently anterior,[30] possibly due to vascular outflow compression from stenosis of cranial foramina.

The orbital veins do not generally follow a course parallel to arteries as in other parts of the body, but form a separate morphologic system.[9] The major exceptions are the central retinal, lacrimal, and ethmoidal veins, and the anterior portion of the superior ophthalmic vein, which do follow their respective arterial channels. As with the arterial system, drainage is derived from three sources—extraorbital, orbital, and ocular sites. In the posterior third of the orbit the veins are situated peripherally, and for the most part are surrounded and supported by fibrous connective tissue septa.[4–6] Only a few small caliber veins traverse the central intraconal space near the orbital apex. This contrasts with the arterial system in the apex where major vessels are primarily situated centrally.

The superior ophthalmic vein

The orbital venous system is composed of two major vessels, the superior and inferior ophthalmic veins. The superior ophthalmic vein (SOV) is the largest vein in the orbit and provides the major channel for venous drainage. It originates from a series of tributaries in the superomedial part of the orbit as two roots.[15] The superior root begins at the supraorbital and supratrochlear veins draining the forehead and scalp. The inferior root joins the orbital system with the angular branch of the facial vein that drains to the external jugular system.[23] The superior and inferior medial palpebral veins carry blood from the eyelids and join the inferior root near its junction with the angular vein. These anterior tributaries join to form the superior ophthalmic vein posterior to the trochlea and medial to the tendinous insertion of the superior rectus muscle.[15]

It is frequently stated that the orbital veins do not contain valves, and that blood flow within them depends largely upon local pressure gradients. However, Zhang and Stringer[46] noted the presence of multiple valves along the superior ophthalmic vein, and additional valves in its two main tributaries, the angular and supraorbital veins. Orientation of the valve cusps was compatible with blood flow from the angular vein and superior ophthalmic vein backward toward the cavernous sinus. Valves have not been identified in the inferior ophthalmic vein.

The superior ophthalmic vein runs posteriorly just medial and inferior to the superior oblique muscle, and along its route, it receives a number of tributaries.[10] These include the medial ophthalmic vein, the superior vortex vein, the anterior ethmoidal vein, the central retinal vein, the lacrimal vein, some muscular veins, and sometimes the inferior ophthalmic vein. As the superior ophthalmic vein continues posteriorly it is supported by a prominent hammock-like sling formed by connective tissue septa of the medial, superior, and lateral rectus suspensory systems.[27] This sling is suspended from periorbita along the superolateral wall, and joins the orbital roof between the levator and superior oblique muscles (see Chapter 7). It has extensive connections with the fascial system around the superior oblique muscle along the superomedial wall, and with the lateral rectus system. It also has interconnections directly to the sheath of the superior rectus muscle. The superior ophthalmic vein is, therefore, layered between the superior rectus muscle and this fascial hammock. Thickening of the superior rectus muscle, as in Graves' orbitopathy or with inflammatory myositis, may compress the vein against this sling, resulting in orbital venous congestion.[24]

At the mid-orbit just behind the globe, the superior ophthalmic vein moves laterally between the optic nerve and superior rectus muscle. In this segment it is joined by the superior medial and superior lateral vortex veins, a vein from the superior rectus muscle, and by the anterior ethmoidal vein. The exit sites of the vortex veins generally lie 14–17 mm behind the insertions of the rectus muscles. The number of vortex veins varies from four to as many as ten.[29,38] However, there is always at least one in each of the four quadrants of the eye between the rectus muscles, and there are more than four in 65% of normal individuals.[28] Multiple vortex veins are present in the nasal quadrants more commonly than in the temporal quadrants. Experimental studies in monkeys have shown that normal choroidal circulation is reduced to 73% of normal after destruction of two vortex veins and to 49% after destruction of three veins.[21] Another study showed that following destruction of three or more vortex veins intraocular pressure rose to 60 mm Hg.[18] The presence of multiple vortex veins in each quadrant may reduce potential complications from traumatic or surgical vortex vein damage.

The superior ophthalmic vein is 2–3 mm in diameter but may be dilated to 5–10 mm in the central orbit. It narrows again toward the orbital apex. Murakami et al.[31] suggested that this portion of the vessel may function as a reservoir for venous blood in the orbit, and it may play a role in regulating orbital hemodynamics. As the superior ophthalmic vein proceeds backward along the lateral edge of the superior rectus muscle, it is joined by a lateral collateral vessel from the inferior ophthalmic vein, and by the lacrimal vein which runs along the upper border of the lateral rectus muscle

from the lacrimal gland. The central retinal vein exits from the substance of the optic nerve inferomedially or medially. It frequently branches within the optic nerve sheath into numerous small vessels that initially run in the subdural space,[7] then coalesce into one or more vessels that penetrate the dura and drain into the superior ophthalmic vein near the orbital apex. Occasionally, the central retinal vein may continue directly to the cavernous sinus,[42] but it always has at least some anastomotic connections with the ophthalmic veins or posterior collateral vein.[2]

The superior ophthalmic vein continues posteriorly along the lateral edge of the superior rectus muscle, exits the muscle cone, and passes above the heads of the lateral rectus muscle. The exact pathway of the SOV through the SOF seems to be somewhat controversial in the literature. The vein usually leaves the orbit through the superior orbital fissure above the annulus of Zinn, where it is anchored to the lateral surface of the annulus by several fibrous bands. Reymond et al.[35] noted that the SOV coursed lower in 6% of their study sample, passing through the annular tendon adjacent to the abducens nerve, and Cheung and McNab[15] stated that in their anatomic series the vein passed through the annulus of Zinn. In an earlier study, Natori and Rhoton[32] reported that the SOV passes through the SOF below the annular tendon. Clearly the pathway is variable.

The superior ophthalmic vein enters the anterior cavernous sinus venous plexus. The sinus venous spaces are an endothelial-lined plexus of venous channels within a split in the dura along the body of the sphenoid bone. It is composed of a diffusely anastomotic system of variously-sized venules lacking smooth muscle surrounding the intracavernous portion of the carotid artery,[11] and is not the trabecular structure previously believed.[26] Any increased venous pressure within the cavernous sinus, as with a carotid-cavernous or dural-cavernous fistula, results in dilatation of the superior ophthalmic vein and its tributaries, clearly evident on computed tomography or magnetic resonance images.

The inferior ophthalmic vein

The inferior ophthalmic vein (IOV) originates in the anterior medial orbit as a diffuse venous plexus along the orbital floor, between the globe and the inferior rectus muscle. The plexus receives small branches from the medial and inferior rectus muscles, and the inferior oblique muscle. It is also joined at this point to the superior ophthalmic vein by the medial collateral vessel. As the vein proceeds posterolaterally crossing over the inferior rectus muscle, it is joined by the inferior medial and inferior lateral vortex veins, and muscular branches from the lateral rectus muscle. The net of small vessels located outside the muscle cone along the orbital floor collects veins from the lower eyelid and the lacrimal sac, and communicates with the inferior ophthalmic system via a branch passing around the lateral side of the inferior rectus muscle.

The inferior ophthalmic vein continues to run backward along the lateral border of the inferior rectus muscle, and here it is often joined to the superior ophthalmic vein through the lateral collateral branch. In the posterior orbit the inferior ophthalmic vein gives off small branches inferiorly which divide into smaller vessels. These pass through the substance of Müller's orbital muscle within the inferior orbital fissure, and join the pterygoid venous plexus. Here they anastomose with branches from the infraorbital vein through which blood once again communicates with the facial system. Müller's orbital muscle is an atavistic remnant from earlier mammalian and early primate evolution where the posterior orbit was still open to the temporalis fossa, but bridged by a fibrous and smooth muscle membrane. While the function of Müller's orbital muscle in humans remains unknown, it may help mediate autonomic regulation of orbital blood flow dynamics through compression of these draining vessels. Although hypertrophy of Müller's orbital muscle in Graves' orbitopathy has not been demonstrated as it has for the sympathetic tarsal muscles, nevertheless, this might represent a partial mechanism for the orbital congestion seen in that disease.

The main trunk of the inferior ophthalmic vein passes backward and dilates into several broad venous sinuses immediately inferior to the annulus of Zinn. These channels maintain intimate contact with the annulus above and with Müller's orbital muscle which forms a sling just below them. As these sinuses continue backward toward the cavernous sinus they coalesce into a large dilated channel. At this level Müller's smooth muscle fibers no longer contact the adjacent orbital bones. Rather, they pass from the inferior annulus of Zinn medially, to the floor and lateral wall of the cavernous sinus laterally, partially enclosing the inferior venous sinus. It is tempting to speculate a role for Müller's muscle in modulating venous outflow here. In some individuals, the inferior ophthalmic vein may pass upward around the lateral rectus muscle to join the superior ophthalmic vein as the latter empties into the cavernous sinus.

The medial ophthalmic vein

A medial ophthalmic vein has been described in 30–40% of normal individuals.[10,15] When present, it arises in the superomedial orbit from branches of the superior ophthalmic and angular veins, and runs along the superomedial orbital wall in the extraconal space. It receives tributaries from the medial and superior rectus muscles. In the posterior orbit it rejoins the superior ophthalmic vein as the latter passes through the superior orbital fissure to the cavernous sinus, or it may drain directly into the cavernous sinus. On venograms this vessel may be mistaken for a displaced superior ophthalmic vein.[9] A superior medial ophthalmic vein is sometimes also present anteriorly, arising from the angular vein and draining into the superior ophthalmic vein in the mid-orbit.

The middle ophthalmic vein

The middle ophthalmic vein (veine ophthalmique moyenne) described by Henry[23] arises as a muscular branch from the medial rectus muscle, receives tributaries from the collateral veins, and drains the inferior orbital net. It extends backward just above the level of the inferior ophthalmic vein. It passes lateral to the muscle cone at the apex and drains into the inferior ophthalmic vein or directly into the cavernous sinus. Its presence is quite variable, and may be absent in 80% or more of individuals.[9]

The collateral veins

A system of collateral veins interconnects the superior and inferior ophthalmic venous systems. Henry[23] described four such collateral veins. The most important and consistent are the medial and lateral.[15] The medial collateral vein is situated in the medial intraconal space and interconnects the inferior and superior ophthalmic veins. The lateral collateral vein lies in the lateral intraconal space and interconnects the inferior ophthalmic vein with the superior ophthalmic or the lacrimal vein.

The cavernous sinus

The cavernous sinuses lie within the middle cranial fossa, on either side of the body of the sphenoid bone (see Chapter 1). They extend from the superior orbital fissure to the apex of the petrous portion of the temporal bone. The cavernous sinuses represent extradural parasellar spaces between the endosteum of the sphenoid bone and the dura propria continuous with the tentorium cerebelli.[39,40] They contain the internal carotid artery, the three extraocular motor nerves, the first two of the trigeminal nerve branches, and an extensive venous system.[41] The cavernous sinus is a plexus of various-sized interconnected venules that receive blood from the ophthalmic veins, the sphenopalatine sinus, cerebral veins, tributaries of the middle meningeal veins, and the superior petrosal sinus.[37] From the cavernous sinuses blood drains into the transverse sinus by way of the superior petrosal sinus, into the internal jugular vein through the inferior petrosal sinus, and it may flow retrograde into the angular vein through the ophthalmic venous system. They also communicate with the pterygoid venous plexus via tributaries passing through the foramen Vesalins, foramen ovale, and foramen lacerum. The two sinuses are interconnected by the anterior and posterior intercavernous sinuses which cross the midline in front of and behind the hypophysis to form the circular sinus.[25] They are further connected by the basal plexus joining the inferior petrosal sinuses.[14]

Clinical correlation of the venous system

Orbital varices are dilated venous channels. They are considered to represent one end of a spectrum of developmental venous anomalies that also includes lymphangiomas. These lesions usually present with proptosis that often is exacerbated with changes in head position or valsalva. When large or when they undergo thrombosis, they may cause motility restriction or optic nerve compression. Orbital veins may also be involved in the formation of arteriovenous malformations and arterioveous shuts, discussed in Chapter 5.

The lymphatic system

Embryology

The embryology of lymphatic vessels is still a matter of debate. Some researchers have argued that they arise from mesenchymal spaces where primary lymph sacs and vessels develop. Centripetal extensions make connections with the venous system. Others have argued that primary lymph sacs bud off from primitive veins and that lymphatic vessels grow out by endothelial budding to form a lymphatic vascular plexus.[44] More recent studies have suggested that both models may apply to various portions of the lymphatic system.[45] Whatever the exact mechanism, the lymphatic vasculature initially forms in association with the anterior cardinal vein, at the junction of the jugular and primitive subclavian veins.[33] These initial lymphatic sacs are first seen in the 14–20 mm (6–7-week) embryonic stages. Lymphatic endothelial cells migrate from the cardinal vein to form the primitive lacrimal sacs along the anteroposterior embryonic axis.[45] The system becomes separated from the blood vasculature, and lymphatic endothelial cells sprout from the sacs to give rise to the lymphatic vessel network.

The adult lymphatic system

In the adult, lymphatic vessels are located in almost all tissues that have blood vessels. The major exceptions are the central nervous system, bone marrow, and the retina, all of which lack lymphatics. They are also lacking in avascular tissues such as the epidermis, cartilage, and the cornea. The lymphatic system consists of a network of delicate vessels lined by a single layer of extensively overlapping endothelial cells with endothelial cell leaflets linked by discontinuous cell-cell junctions that open in response to increased interstitial fluid pressure.[1,12] Lymphatic capillaries lack a basement membrane and supporting smooth muscle pericytes, making them extremely permeable. They drain into larger precollecting and collecting trunks that do contain these structures. Collecting trunks also have internal valves that prevent backflow.

The lymphatic system transports fluids, plasma macromolecules, and cells extravasated from blood vessels, returning them via collecting vessels into larger trunks that eventually empty into the blood circulatory system. Lymphatics are also an important component of the immune system where they transport antigens and white blood cells from tissues to lymph nodes located along their pathway through which they pass, and to the tonsils, Peyer's patches, the spleen, and the thymus. They also serve as a major pathway for the spread of metastatic cells from cancers.

The lymphatic vessels in the eyelids form a deep system that drains the tarsus and conjunctiva, and a superficial system that receives lymph from the orbicularis muscle and skin. According to classic interpretation drainage from the lateral two-thirds of the upper eyelid, lateral one-third of the lower eyelid, and lateral one-half of the conjunctiva is into the preauricular nodes. The medial one-third of the upper eyelid, medial two-thirds of the lower eyelid, and medial one-half of the conjunctiva drain into the submandibular nodes, and ultimately to the anterior and deep cervical nodes.

In a recent study by Nijhawan et al.[32A] using TC99m sulfur colloid lymphoscintigraphy, 72% of patients demonstrated first order drainage into the preauricular lymph nodes regardless of where around the eyelids the injection was given. 90% of their study population did not show the classic drainage pattern.

The orbitomalar retaining ligament along the inferior orbital rim is the principal suspensory structure for the infraorbital soft tissues, but it also separates the lymphatic drainage fields of the lid from that of the cheek.[34] This explains why significant lower eyelid edema is often seen to stop at the orbital rim.

The human orbit has long been thought to be devoid of lymphatic vessels and nodes. Recent experimental studies have confirmed the absence of such structures in the monkey orbit.[20] Nevertheless, orbital edema in humans does resolve, probably via several routes. Excess fluid and proteins in the intraconal space may pass to the extraconal space. From here they can diffuse along connective tissue septal planes to the conjunctival lymphatic system, and thereby drain to the anterior and deep cervical nodes. From the posterior orbit, fluid and protein may also drain along the vascular and neural structures to the cavernous sinus, and even to the contralateral orbit across the intercavernous sinus system. This posterior pathway may provide the route for spread of orbital cellulitis, resulting in meningitis and cavernous sinus thrombosis, and may explain the rare occurrence of contralateral orbital akinesia and decreased vision following retrobulbar anesthesia.[20]

Sherman et al.[36] identified orbital lymphatic vessels in the monkey using microscopy and enzyme histochemistry. These were located in the conjunctiva, lacrimal glands, and in the dura and arachnoid of the optic nerve. Positive staining suggestive of lymphatic vessels was also identified in the orbital apex. However, no lymphatics were found in the extraocular muscles or in the retrobulbar fat. Similar findings were reported in the human orbit using specific lymphatic endothelium staining.[19] It is now abundantly clear that lymphatics do occur in at least some portions of the human orbit, and this in part helps to explain drainage of orbital edema fluid, and may also explain the occurrence of orbital lymphangiomas.[17] Using specific immunohistochemical markers, Cursiefen et al.[16] demonstrated the presence of lymphatic endothelium in an orbital lymphangioma.

In a recent report, Camelo et al.[13] demonstrated that rhodamine-conjugated liposomes injected into the vitreous cavity of Lewis rats drained into conjunctival lymphatics and into the cervical lymph nodes. This suggests a more complicated lymphatic drainage pattern from the eye in some mammals, and possibly the orbit as well, than has previously been appreciated.

Clinical correlations of the lymphatic system

Lymphangiomas are benign malformations of the lymphatic system. They are composed of thin-walled dilated endothelial-lined lymphatic vascular channels filled with proteinaceous lymph fluid. Endothelial differentiation is confirmed by immunohistochemistry. Acute increase in size can be triggered by infections and by bleeding into the vascular spaces. About 60% of lymphangiomas are located in the head and neck, where they are found most commonly in areas where the primitive lymph sacs originally formed during embryogenesis. The mechanism of their formation is unclear. Possible mechanisms may be related to a failure to connect with or separate from the venous system, or abnormal budding of lymphatic endothelial cells, or sequestration of lymphatic anlage during embryonic development in regions without regular connection to the normal lymphatic system. Sequestered anlage are assumed to possess the potential for further growth, but loss of connection to the primary lymphatic buds prevents development of draining lymphatic vessels. Hyperplasia of transformed lymphatic endothelial cells, or dysregulation of growth factors, may allow growth of the lymphangioma.[43]

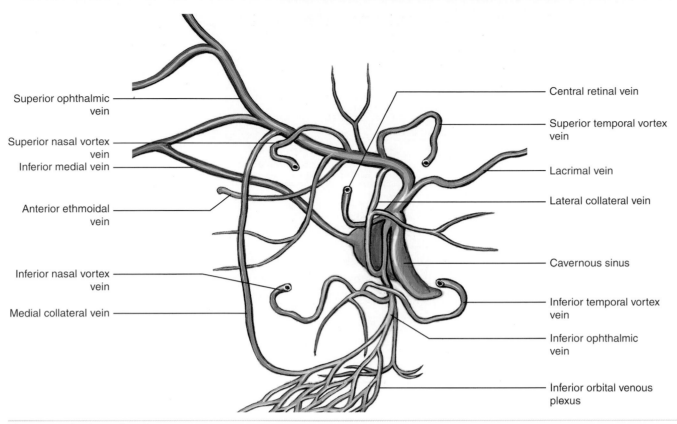

Superior ophthalmic vein

Superior nasal vortex vein

Inferior medial vein

Anterior ethmoidal vein

Inferior nasal vortex vein

Medial collateral vein

Central retinal vein

Superior temporal vortex vein

Lacrimal vein

Lateral collateral vein

Cavernous sinus

Inferior temporal vortex vein

Inferior ophthalmic vein

Inferior orbital venous plexus

Figure 6-1 Orbital veins, frontal view.

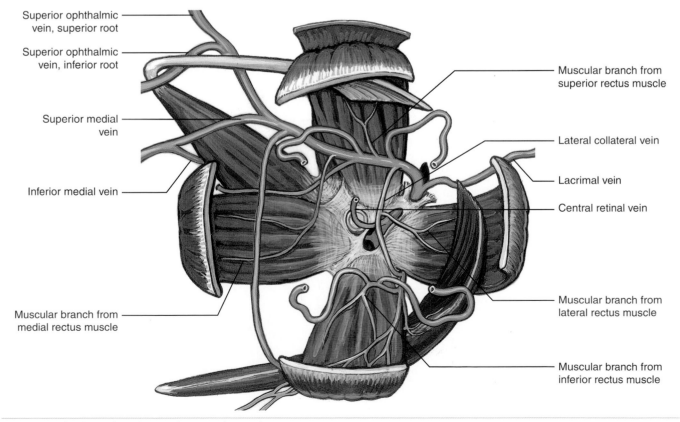

Superior ophthalmic vein, superior root

Superior ophthalmic vein, inferior root

Superior medial vein

Inferior medial vein

Muscular branch from medial rectus muscle

Muscular branch from superior rectus muscle

Lateral collateral vein

Lacrimal vein

Central retinal vein

Muscular branch from lateral rectus muscle

Muscular branch from inferior rectus muscle

Figure 6-2 Orbital veins, frontal view with extraocular muscles.

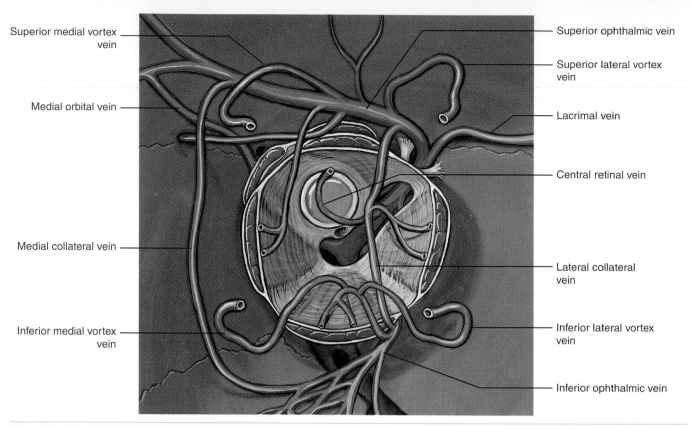

Superior medial vortex vein

Medial orbital vein

Medial collateral vein

Inferior medial vortex vein

Superior ophthalmic vein

Superior lateral vortex vein

Lacrimal vein

Central retinal vein

Lateral collateral vein

Inferior lateral vortex vein

Inferior ophthalmic vein

Figure 6-3 Orbital veins, frontal view, orbital apex.

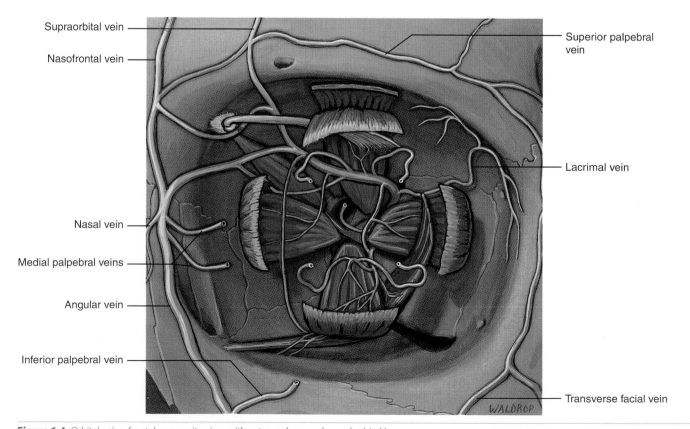

Supraorbital vein

Nasofrontal vein

Nasal vein

Medial palpebral veins

Angular vein

Inferior palpebral vein

Superior palpebral vein

Lacrimal vein

Transverse facial vein

WALDROP

Figure 6-4 Orbital veins, frontal composite view with extraocular muscles and orbital bones.

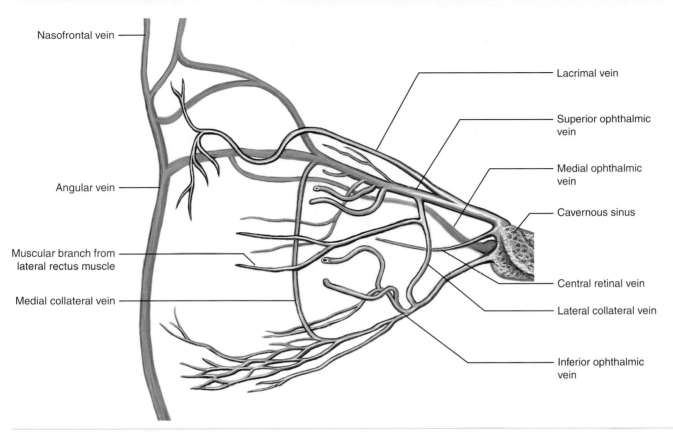

Nasofrontal vein

Angular vein

Muscular branch from lateral rectus muscle

Medial collateral vein

Lacrimal vein

Superior ophthalmic vein

Medial ophthalmic vein

Cavernous sinus

Central retinal vein

Lateral collateral vein

Inferior ophthalmic vein

Figure 6-5 Orbital veins, lateral view.

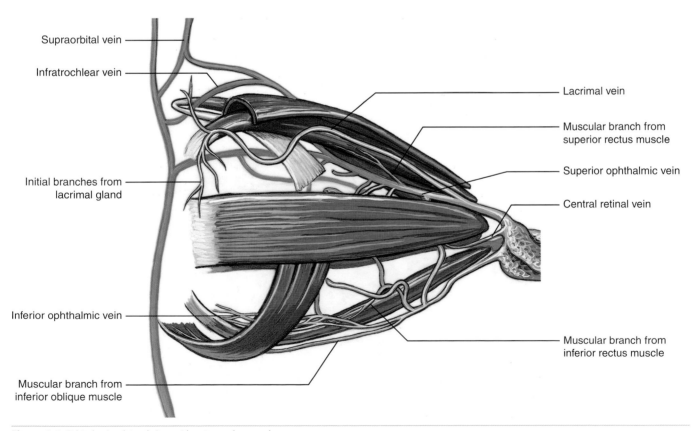

Supraorbital vein

Infratrochlear vein

Initial branches from lacrimal gland

Inferior ophthalmic vein

Muscular branch from inferior oblique muscle

Lacrimal vein

Muscular branch from superior rectus muscle

Superior ophthalmic vein

Central retinal vein

Muscular branch from inferior rectus muscle

Figure 6-6 Orbital veins, lateral view with extraocular muscles.

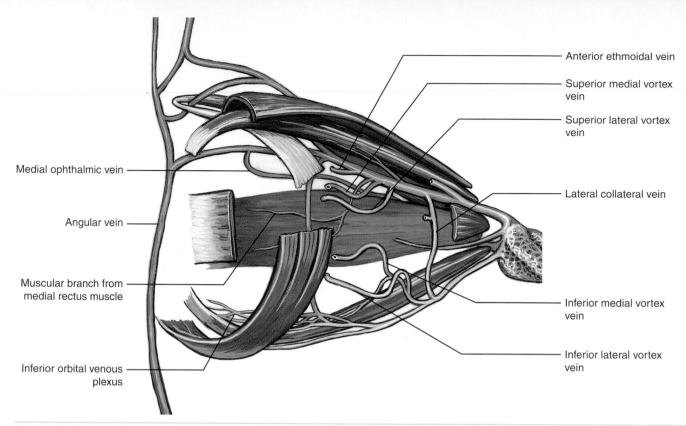

Anterior ethmoidal vein

Superior medial vortex vein

Superior lateral vortex vein

Medial ophthalmic vein

Lateral collateral vein

Angular vein

Muscular branch from medial rectus muscle

Inferior medial vortex vein

Inferior lateral vortex vein

Inferior orbital venous plexus

Figure 6-7 Orbital veins, lateral view, lateral rectus muscle removed.

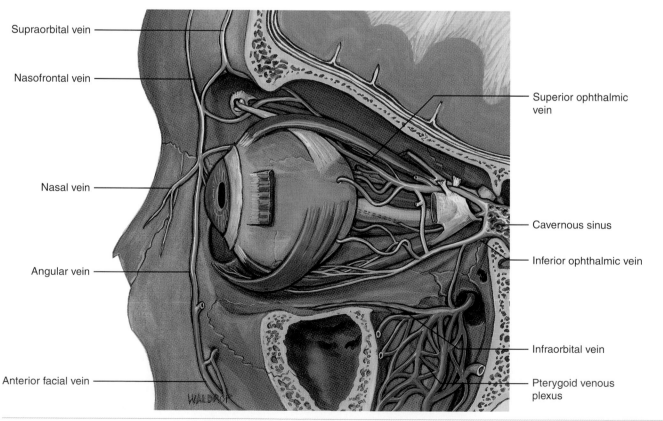

Supraorbital vein

Nasofrontal vein

Superior ophthalmic vein

Nasal vein

Angular vein

Cavernous sinus

Inferior ophthalmic vein

Infraorbital vein

Anterior facial vein

Pterygoid venous plexus

Figure 6-8 Orbital veins, lateral composite view, with extraocular muscles, globe and orbital bones.

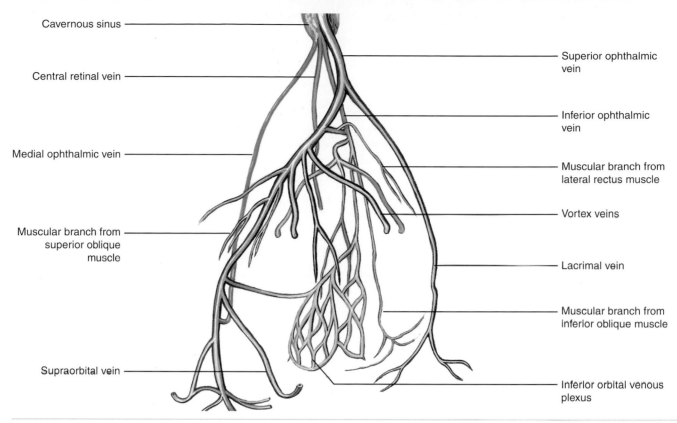

Cavernous sinus

Central retinal vein

Medial ophthalmic vein

Muscular branch from
superior oblique
muscle

Supraorbital vein

Superior ophthalmic
vein

Inferior ophthalmic
vein

Muscular branch from
lateral rectus muscle

Vortex veins

Lacrimal vein

Muscular branch from
inferior oblique muscle

Inferior orbital venous
plexus

Figure 6-9 Orbital veins, superior view.

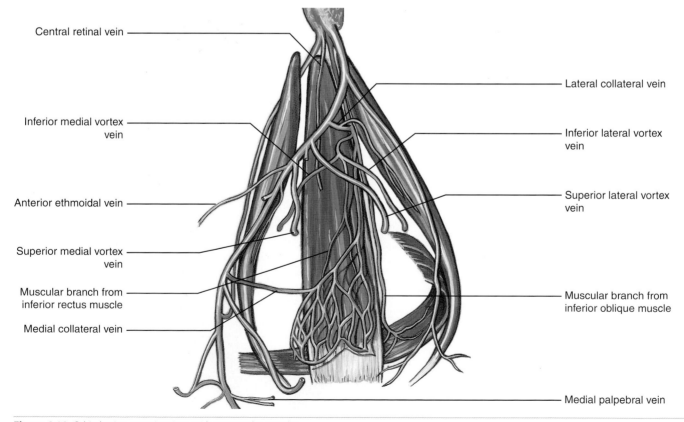

Central retinal vein

Inferior medial vortex
vein

Anterior ethmoidal vein

Superior medial vortex
vein

Muscular branch from
inferior rectus muscle

Medial collateral vein

Lateral collateral vein

Inferior lateral vortex
vein

Superior lateral vortex
vein

Muscular branch from
inferior oblique muscle

Medial palpebral vein

Figure 6-10 Orbital veins, superior view, with extraocular muscles.

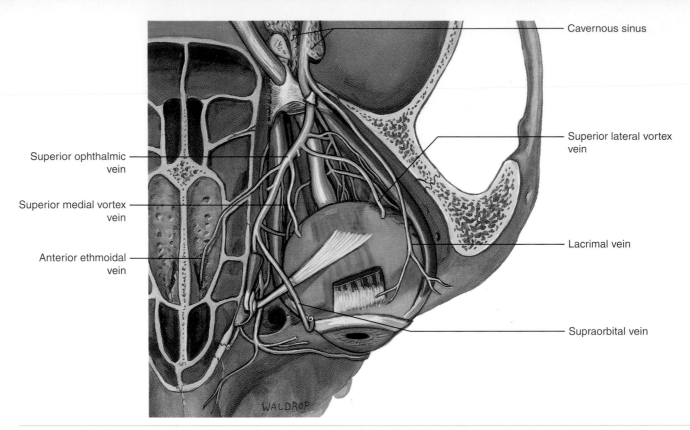

Cavernous sinus

Superior lateral vortex vein

Superior ophthalmic vein

Superior medial vortex vein

Anterior ethmoidal vein

Lacrimal vein

Supraorbital vein

WALDROP

Figure 6-11 Orbital veins, superior composite view with extraocular muscles, globe and orbital bones.

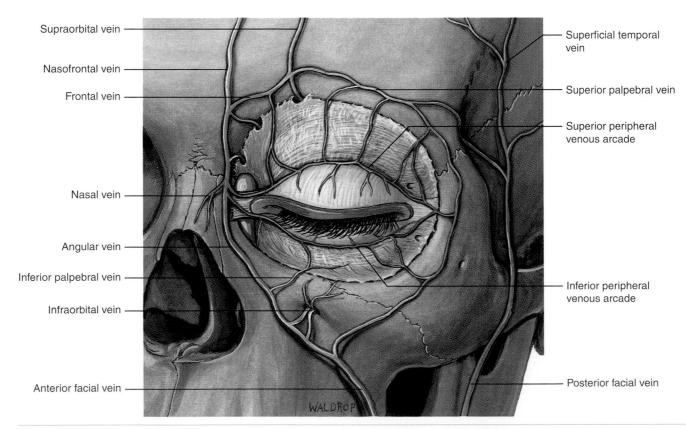

Supraorbital vein

Nasofrontal vein

Frontal vein

Nasal vein

Angular vein

Inferior palpebral vein

Infraorbital vein

Anterior facial vein

Superficial temporal vein

Superior palpebral vein

Superior peripheral venous arcade

Inferior peripheral venous arcade

Posterior facial vein

WALDROP

Figure 6-12 Periorbital and eyelid veins, frontal view.

References

1. Baluk P, Fuxe J, Hashizume H, et al: Functionally specialized junctions between endothelial cells of lymphatic vessels. *J Exp Med* 204:2349, 2007.

2. Bergin MP: A literature review of the vascular system in the human orbit. *Acta Morphol Neerl Scand* 19:273, 1981.

3. Bergin MP: Microvessels in the human orbit in relation to the connective tissue system. *Acta Morphol Neerl Scand* 20:139, 1982.

4. Bergin MP: Relationships between the arteries and veins and the connective tissue system in the human orbit. I. The retrobulbar part of the orbit: apical region. *Acta Morphol Neerl Scand* 20:1, 1982.

5. Bergin MP: Relationships between the arteries and veins and the connective tissue system in the human orbit. II. The retrobulbar part of the orbit: Septal complex region. *Acta Morphol Neerl Scand* 20:17, 1982.

6. Bergin MP: Some histologic aspects of the structure of the connective tissue system and its relationships with the blood vessels in the human orbit. *Acta Morphol Neerl Scand* 20:293, 1982.

7. Bergin MP: A spatial reconstruction of the orbital vascular pattern in relation with the connective tissue system. *Acta Morphol Neerl Scand* 20:117, 1982.

8. Bleeker GM: Changes in the orbital tissues and muscles dysthyroid ophthalmopathy. *Eye* 2:193, 1988.

9. Brismar J: Orbital phlebography. III. Topography of the orbital veins. *Acta Radiol (Diangn) Stockh)* 15:577, 1974.

10. Brismar J: Orbital phlebography. II. Anatomy of the superior ophthalmic vein and its tributaries. *Acta Radiol (Diagn) (Stockh)* 15:481, 1974.

11. Browder J., Kaplan HA: *Cerebral Dural Sinuses and Their Tributaries.* Springfield, IL, CC Thomas, 1976.

12. Butler MG, Isogai S, Weinstein BM. Lymphatic development. *Birth Defects Res* 87:222, 2009.

13. Camelo S, Lajavardi L, Bochot A, et al: Drainage of fluorescent liposomes from the vitreous to cervical lymph nodes via conjunctival lymphatics. *Ophthalmic Res* 40:145, 2008.

14. Carpenter MB: *Core Text of Neuroanatomy*, 2nd ed. Baltimore, Williams and Wilkins, 1978, p 335.

15. Cheung N, McNab AA: Venus anatomy of the orbit. *Invest Ophthalmol Vis Sci* 44:988, 2003.

16. Cursiefen C, Schlötzer-Schrehardt U, Breitender-Geleff S, Holbach LM: Orbital lymphangioma with positive immunohistochemistry of lymphatic endothelial markers (vascular endothelial growth factor receptor 3 and podoplanin). *Graefes Arch Clin Exp Ophthalmol* 239:628, 2001.

17. Dickinson AJ, Gausas RE: Orbital lymphatics: Do they exist? *Eye* 20:1145, 2006.

18. Doi N, Uemura A, Nakao K: Complications associated with vortex vein damage in scleral buckling surgery for rhegmatogenous retinal detachment. *Jpn J Ophthalmol* 43:232, 1999.

19. Gausas RE, Gonnering RS, Lemke BN, et al: Identification of human orbital lymphatics. *Ophthal Plast Reconstr Surg* 15:252, 1999.

20. Getrick JJ, Wilson DG, Dortzbach RK, et al: A search for lymphatic drainage of the monkey orbit. *Arch Ophthalmol* 107:255, 1989.

21. Hayreh SS, Baines JAB: Occlusion of the vortex veins. An experimental study. *Br J Ophthalmol* 57:217, 1973.

22. Hayrey SS: Orbital vascular anatomy. *Eye* 20:1130, 2006.

23. Henry JGM: Contribution a l'etude de l'anatomie des vaisseaux de l'orbite et de la loge caverneuse-pas injection de matieres plastiques du tendon de Zinn et de la capsule de Tenon. These de Paris, 1959. Cited by Bergin MP. *Vascular architecture in the human orbit.* Lisse, Netherlands, Swets and Zeitlinger, BV, 1982.

24. Hudson HL, Levin L, Feldon SE: Graves exophthalmos unrelated to extraocular muscle enlargement. *Ophthalmology* 98:1495, 1991.

25. Kaplan JR, Browder J, Krieger AJ: Intercavernous connections of the cavernous sinus. The superior and inferior circular sinuses. *J Neurosurg* 45:166, 1976.

26. Kline LB, Acker JD, Post MJD: Computed tomographic evaluation of the cavernous sinus. *Ophthalmology* 89:374, 1982.

27. Koornneef L: The architecture of the musculo-fibrous apparatus in the human orbit. *Acta Morphol Neerl Scand* 15:35, 1977.

28. Kutoglu T, Valcin B, Rocabiyik N, Ozan H: Vortex veins: anatomic investigations on human eyes. *Clin Anat* 18:269, 2005.

29. Lim MC, Bateman JB, Glasgow BJ: Vortex vein exit sites. Scleral coordinates. *Ophthalmology* 102:942, 1995.

30. Mueller SM, Reinertson JE: Reversal of emissary vein blood flow in achondroplastic dwarfs. *Neurology* 30:769, 1980.

31. Murakami K, Murakami G, Komatsu A, et al: Gross anatomical study of veins in the orbit. *Acta Soc Ophthalmol Jpn* 95:31, 1991.

32. Natori Y, Rhoton AL Jr: Microsurgical anatomy of the superior orbital fissure. *Neurosurg* 36:762, 1995.

32A. Nijhawan N, Marriott C, Harvey JT: Lymphatic drainage patterns of the human eyelid assessed by lymphoscintigraphy. *Ophthal Plast Reconstr Surg* 26:281, 2010.

33. Oliver G, Srinivasan RS: Lymphatic vasculature development. *Ann NY Acad Sci* 1131:75, 2008.

34. Pesa JE, Garza J: The malar septum: the anatomic basis of malar mounds and malar edema. *Aesthet Plast Surg* 17:11, 1997.

35. Reymond J, Kwiatowski J, Wysocki J: Clinical anatomy of the superior orbital fissure and the orbital apex. *J Craniomaxillofac Surg* 36:346, 2008.

36. Sherman DD, Gonnering RS, Wallow IHL, et al: Identification of orbital lymphatics: enzyme histochemical light microscopy and electron microscopic studies. *Ophthal Plast Reconstr Surg* 9:153, 1993.

37. Swanson MW: Neuroanatomy of the cavernous sinus and clinical correlations. *Optom Vis Sci* 67:891, 1990.

38. Takahashi K, Muraoka K, Sutoh N, et al: Posterior routes of choroidal venous drainage. *Rinsho Ganka (Jpn J Clin Ophthalmol)* 50:161, 1996.

39. Taptas JN: The so-called cavernous sinus: a review of the controversy and its implications for neurosurgeons. *Neurosurgery* 11:712, 1982.

40. Taptas JN: La loge ostéo-durale parasellaire et les éléments vasculaires et nerveux qui la traversent. *Neurochirurgie* 36:201, 1990.

41. Umansky F, Nathan H: The lateral wall of the cavernous sinus: With special reference to the nerves related to it. *J Neurosurg* 56:228, 1982.

42. Whitnall SE: *Anatomy of the Human Orbit and Accessory Organs of Vision.* 2nd ed. London, Oxford Medical Publishers, 1932.

43. Wiegand S, Eivazi B, Barth PJ, et al: Pathogenesis of lymphangiomas. *Virchows Arch* 453:1, 2008.

44. Wigle JT, Oliver G: Prox1 function is required for the development of the murine lymphatic system. *Cell* 98:769, 1999.

45. Wilting J, Aref Y, Huang R, et al: Dual origin of avian lymphatics. *Dev Biol* 292:165, 2006.

46. Zhang J, Stringer MD: Ophthalmic and facial veins are not valveless. *Clin Exp Ophthalmol* 38:502, 2010.

CHAPTER 7

Orbital Fat and Connective Tissue Systems

An extensive system of connective tissue forms a framework for compartmentalization and support of orbital structures. It is essential for maintaining appropriate anatomic relationships between structural components, and for allowing precise and coordinated ocular movements.[2,18,20–24,32,34] Some connective tissue septa are aligned with directions of force that resist displacement of extraocular muscles during contraction. These allow only a small amount of sideslip of the rectus muscle points of tangency over the globe during extremes of gaze, while maintaining relative stability of muscle planes with respect to the orbital walls.[35] Other fascial elements suspend and support delicate orbital vascular and neural elements. In general, the orbital veins follow an intimate course within orbital septal compartments. However, no such relationship exists for most of the arteries.

All orbital structures, including periorbita, globe, optic nerve, and extraocular muscles, are involved in the organization and suspension of these extensive connective tissue septal systems. Disruption in any one portion of the orbit may have widespread effects in other regions of the orbit. Thus, long-term deformities may be associated with trauma or certain operative procedures, such as enucleation surgery. In particular, late enophthalmos and superior sulcus deformity may result primarily from volumetric displacement of major orbital structures due to loss or alteration in suspensory septa formerly associated with the globe, posterior Tenon's capsule, or the distal optic nerve. It has been suggested that vascular hemodynamics remains unchanged in the anophthalmic orbit, and that atrophy of orbital fat plays a minimal role in the development of such deformities in most patients.[27,28] It is clear, however, that progressive fat atrophy may contribute significantly to such deformities in some individuals.

Although intimately linked throughout the orbit, for discussion here the connective tissue structures may be visualized as forming several distinct anatomic systems. These include the orbital fat, the bulbar fascia or Tenon's capsule, the anterior orbital suspensory system, and the posterior orbital septal system.

Embryology

Development of the connective tissue system begins with differentiation of the extraocular muscles.[25] Between the 35 mm (9-week) embryonic and 75 mm (13-week) fetal stages the muscles are surrounded by collagenous fibers formed by condensations of the orbital mesenchyme.[32] These are the rudimentary muscle capsules.[22,23] Additional condensations are seen surrounding blood vessels and nerves. By the 80 mm stage the anterior portion of Tenon's capsule is well developed, but the posterior portion is not fully formed until the 5th month of gestation.[33] Primordia of the connective tissue septa appear at the 112 mm stage (4th month), independent of the muscular, vascular, and neuronal fascial layers. Between the 112 mm and the 200 mm stages (4th to 6th month), the septa rapidly organize and establish extensive relationships with the developing periorbita. Adipose cells arise around capillary beds between septal condensations, and fine connective tissue capsules form around adipose islands. By 6 months of gestation the basic adult plan of orbital connective tissue septa can be recognized, but further differentiation continues between the 6th and 9th months. During this period, the intermuscular septum develops anteriorly, and extensive septal connections form between the extraocular muscles, adjacent orbital walls, and the rectus muscle pulley systems become organized. The levator–superior rectus septal complex to the orbital roof forms, and connective tissue associated with the superior ophthalmic vein hammock and the superior oblique muscle sling become fully developed.

Orbital fat

Orbital fat fills the space surrounding the eye, extraocular muscles, nerves, blood vessels, and the lacrimal gland. The adipose lobules fall into several vaguely defined anatomic compartments: a central intraconal compartment between the four rectus muscles, a peripheral extraconal compartment between the rectus muscles and the bony orbital walls, and an anterior peribulbar compartment.[28,47] Connective tissue septa surround individual fat lobules, and blood vessels and nerve fibers run within these septal membranes. The entire system provides support for intraorbital structures, while also allowing free movement of these structures along these sliding fat lobules.[13] Unlike white adipose tissue in other parts of the body, in the orbit the fat does not appear to play a role in providing energy reserve, and does not undergo reduction in mass during periods of illness and fasting.[3]

In the intraconal compartment near the orbital apex these lobules are larger and surrounded by thin weakly developed fibrous membranes with little collagen and no elastin.[41] The lobules are of various shapes, but are frequently elongated mainly in the longitudinal direction, but also in the radial direction to a lesser extent. More peripherally, between the muscles, around the globe, and in the extraconal space, the fat lobules become smaller with thicker and denser well developed fibrous septa between them.[3,20,47] Although there is no distinct well-defined and continuous intermuscular septum separating the intraconal and extraconal fat compartments, nevertheless, there may be a functional or physiological distinction between the two regions based on anatomic microstructure of the collagenous membranes.

In the anterior orbit the interlobular septa blend with the fascial membranes of the anterior suspensory systems of the rectus muscles that form the so-called pulleys described by Demer,[6,7,10] and proposed to contribute to the function of muscle insertions. These connections allow a more unified and coordinated movement of anterior orbital structures with ocular rotation.

Anterior to the muscle insertions, a thin ring of peribulbar fat lobules separates Tenon's capsule from the orbital walls. An extension of fat from the intraconal compartment projects into the inferior lateral extraconal space between the lateral and inferior rectus muscles, beneath the inferior oblique muscle.[41] This may contribute to the lateral lower eyelid steatoblepharon seen in some older patients. An anterior extension of superior extraconal fat passes down into the upper eyelid between the levator aponeurosis and the orbital septum forming the preaponeurotic fat pocket. In the area of Whitnall's ligament there is a significant increase in collagen and elastin within the fat septa.[41]

Wolfram-Gabel and Kahn[47] noted that the thin extraconal fat continued without separation into the upper and lower eyelids as the retroseptal fat pockets. However, Rohrich et al.,[38] using a methylene blue diffusion technique, reported that when injected into the lower eyelid fat pockets dye did not diffuse posteriorly beyond the mid globe. They described a "circumferential intraorbirtal retaining ligament" (CIRL) that separated the upper and lower fat pads from the orbital extraconal fat compartment. This structure appears to be closely related to the fascial connective tissue suspensory system of the extraocular muscles. The exact function of the CIRL is not clear, but the authors suggested that it might play a role in anterior orbital globe and other tissue support.

It has been noted that preaponeurotic fat in the eyelids appears more yellow than the white fat that fills the rest of the orbit and the nasal eyelid pocket. Sires et al.[42] showed a 4-fold higher amount of β-carotene and leuten in preaponeurotic fat compared to nasal orbital fat. However, the anatomic or physiologic basis for this difference is not clear.

Tenon's capsule

Tenon's capsule is a dense, elastic, fibrovascular connective tissue layer that surrounds the globe, except over the cornea. It also invests the anterior portions of the extraocular muscle insertions. This structure begins near the perilimbal sclera anteriorly and extends around the globe to the optic nerve where it blends with fibers of the dural sheath and sclera. Anterior to the insertion of the rectus muscles, about 2 mm behind the corneal limbus, Tenon's capsule originates and is firmly adherent to episclera. Over the surface of the globe, Tenon's capsule is separated from episclera by a loose potential space that provides a smooth surface for ocular motility. It was the discovery of this capsule by Tenon,[44] and its popularization by O'Farrall and Bonnet (cited in Snyder)[43] that

led to development of modern enucleation techniques, and abandonment of more barbaric and anatomically mutilating surgery.

In the posterior and mid-orbit the extraocular muscles lie outside Tenon's capsule. *En route* from the orbital apex to the globe, the muscles must penetrate Tenon's capsule to reach the globe. The four rectus muscles pierce this structure posterior to the equator of the eye. As they proceed forward, the muscles and their thin fibrous sheaths become invested by a sleeve-like extension of Tenon's capsule which runs with the muscle to its insertion.[11] Fine fibrous strands interconnect the muscle sheath with the investing sleeve of Tenon's capsule.

As the extraocular muscles approach the globe, the intermuscular septal planes between them fuse to posterior Tenon's capsule. After passing through Tenon's, some of these septa reform and extend as a separate layer between the muscles, just inside Tenon's capsule. They finally fuse to sclera along with Tenon's capsule about 2 mm from the corneal limbus.

Relationship of extraocular muscles to Tenon's capsule

The superior oblique tendon is covered by a delicate fibrous capsule, as well as by a reflection of posterior Tenon's capsule that extends from the globe to the trochlea. As it leaves the trochlea, the tendon travels laterally and posteriorly within this reflection of Tenon's for a distance of about 8 mm. It finally passes through Tenon's and the intermuscular septal fascia just medial to the superior rectus muscle, and anterior to the equator of the globe. As the tendon passes deep to the superior rectus muscle it establishes the same relationship with the intermuscular septa as do the rectus muscles. During surgery on the superior oblique tendon, Tenon's capsule is opened anteriorly, and the tendon is visible about 9 mm behind the medial insertion of the superior rectus muscle. Tenon's capsule overlying the latter muscle should not be incised since it forms the anterior wall of the intraconal fat compartment extending over the globe, and opening it could prolapse fat into the wound.

The inferior oblique muscle originates external to Tenon's capsule, in the extraconal compartment. Shortly after leaving its origin on the inferomedial orbital wall, the inferior oblique penetrates Tenon's capsule to enter the sub-Tenon's space. It runs within a cowel of Tenon's, crosses beneath to the inferior rectus muscle, and continues to its insertion on the posterior sclera. As it crosses the midline, the fibrous sheath of the inferior oblique becomes fused to that of the inferior rectus muscle and to a thickening in Tenon's capsule to form a central band, which is part of Lockwood's inferior suspensory ligament. As the muscle continues toward its insertion, its outer sheath surface is firmly attached to the inner surface of Tenon's capsule, and its anterior border to the intermuscular septa.

Tenon's capsule separates the globe posteriorly from the intraconal orbital fat. The anterior portion of this fat compartment is therefore bounded centrally by Tenon's capsule, and peripherally by the rectus muscles and the thin intermuscular septa between them. Tongues of intraconal fat extend forward over the globe, within the narrow wedge between the orbital part of the intermuscular septum and posterior

Tenon's. These tongues extend to about 9 or 10 mm behind the corneal limbus. During surgery on the muscle insertions, Tenon's capsule should be incised anterior to this point so as to avoid entrance into this fat compartment. Fat extruded into the surgical wound may result in significant lipogranulomatous inflammation and scarring.

The anterior suspensory systems

The anterior fascial system of the orbit is primarily related to support of the globe, Tenon's capsule, anterior orbital structures such as the lacrimal gland and superior oblique tendon, and the eyelids. It consists of a complex arrangement of well-developed fascial condensations and ligaments, as well as a more diffuse system of fibrous septa.[25] These structures include the medial and lateral "check ligaments", Lockwood's inferior ligament, Whitnall's superior suspensory ligament, the lacrimal ligaments, the suspensory ligament of the conjunctival fornix, the intermuscular septa, and the anterior orbital septal suspensory systems.

The "check ligaments" were previously believed to serve to limit and dampen ocular movement, and their elasticity thought to ensure smooth ocular rotations. However, under the active pulley hypothesis (see Chapter 3 and later in this chapter), the check ligaments are thought to be elastic suspensions of the pulley systems that actively regulate the direction of extraocular force to control ocular kinetics.[17] Under this concept, the term check ligament is probably inappropriate, although there is not yet a useful alternative.

The medial check ligament originates from the sheath of the medial rectus muscle, the medial rectus pulley, and from surrounding Tenon's capsule. It inserts along with the orbital septum and the medial horn of the levator aponeurosis onto the lacrimal and ethmoid bones. Its fibers may be interwoven with those of the posterior reflection of the orbital septum, or they may form a separate broad fibromuscular band. It may also appear as numerous fine fibromuscular wisps between the muscle sheath and the medial orbital wall.[19] The lateral check ligament is formed by a group of thin fascial connections between the lateral orbital wall and the sheath of the lateral rectus muscle and its pulley. These fibers extend over a broad area from the lateral orbital tubercle to about 14 mm posterior to the orbital rim.[30] While the function of these check ligaments is not well understood, they do not appear to limit ocular rotation.

The lacrimal ligaments are fine strands of connective tissue continuous with the interlobular septa of the lacrimal gland. They extend from the capsule of the gland to periosteum along the superolateral orbital wall. When these become lax, the lacrimal gland may prolapse from beneath the orbital rim resulting in a fullness in the lateral upper eyelid. During blepharoplasty operations, this must not be excised along with orbital fat pockets, but repositioned by suturing the investing fibrous pseudocapsule of the gland to the orbital periosteum at the superior orbital rim.

Lockwood's inferior ligament is a broad fascial sling 40–45 mm in length, 5–8 mm wide and about 1 mm thick. It is formed centrally as a connective tissue thickening in the inferior Tenon's capsule where the latter fuses with the conjoined sheaths of the inferior rectus and inferior oblique muscles. Laterally, the ligament extends as two heads. The anterior lateral head is a broad sheet that inserts onto the inferior border of the lateral canthal ligament. The posterior lateral head is a narrow band that joins the lateral retinaculum at the lateral orbital wall (Whitnall's tubercle) in company with the lateral horn of the levator aponeurosis, the lateral canthal ligament, the orbital septum, and Whitnall's ligament from the superior orbit. Medially, Lockwood's ligament blends with the sheath of Horner's muscle and with the medial check ligament, as these pass back to insert onto the posterior lacrimal crest. A superior medial head of Lockwood's ligament passes just behind the canthal angle and the medial conjunctival fornix to join the medial horn of the levator aponeurosis in company with the posterior wing of the orbital septum.

From the conjoined fascia where Lockwood's ligament crosses the inferior rectus and inferior oblique muscles, a group of connective tissue strands, termed the arcuate expansion, extends inferolaterally to insert onto the orbital rim 8–12 mm below the insertion of the lateral canthal ligament. This slip measures 9–12 mm in length and 3–4 mm in width. Hwang et al.[15] noted that in Korean cadaver specimens this structure extended medially from its attachment at Lockwood's ligament, as a tapering band of fibers passing between the orbital septum and the inferior oblique muscle to insert onto the inferior border of the medial canthal ligament. The arcuate expansion may be seen during inferior eyelid blepharoplasty procedures as a band of fascial strands separating the central from the lateral fat pockets. Its principle function is not established, but clinically at the time of lower eyelid surgery it appears that this structure can serve to limit the anteroposterior displacement of Lockwood's ligament. It may also serve to retain the inferior oblique muscle and the inferior orbital fat during downgaze, as suggested by Hwang et al.[15]

A small extension from Lockwood's ligament to the inferior rectus muscle passes backward from the central part of the ligament, and is continuous with the muscle sheath. It measures about 10 mm in length and 7 mm in width. This slip apparently may help maintain a constant topographic relationship between the inferior rectus muscle and Lockwood's ligament during downgaze, similar to that seen between Whitnall's ligament and the levator muscle/aponeurosis complex during upgaze.

The capsulopalpebral fascia is a well-defined connective tissue layer that mechanically links the lower eyelid with the downward retractor apparatus of the globe. It is composed of two distinct layers that pass forward and upward from Lockwood's ligament as dense fibrous sheets. The anterior or superficial layer is coarse and inserts onto the orbital septum and the deep fascia of the orbicularis muscle. Fingerlike extensions pass forward to insert onto the perimysium of the preseptal and pretarsal fibers of the orbicularis muscle.[16] The dense posterior layer inserts onto the inferior border of the tarsal plate. Unlike the anterior layer, the posterior layer contains clusters of smooth muscle fibers concentrated near the conjunctival fornix.[29] Together with its connections to the inferior rectus muscle sheath and pulley, the capsulopalpebral fascia serves as the major retractor of the lower eyelid during downgaze, thus maintaining a constant relationship between the lower eyelid margin and the inferior corneal limbus.[19,33] Fine fascial strands also extend from both Lockwood's ligament and the capsulopalpebral fascia to Tenon's capsule and to the conjunctiva where they form the suspensory ligaments of the inferior fornix.

Miller et al.,[34] using histochemical staining studies on thin sections through the orbit, identified bands of smooth muscle and elastin in the orbital equatorial region extending from the firmly fixed medial rectus muscle pulley to the more freely mobile fascial connections at the crossing of the inferior rectus and inferior oblique muscles. They believed these to form a single functional structure which they called the "intramedial peribulbar muscle" and stated that it would not be wrong to consider this to be a specialized part of Lockwood's ligament. It is presumed that the smooth muscle in this structure, like that in the extraocular pulleys, receives norepinephrine innervation from the superior cervical ganglion and nitric oxide innervation from the pterygopalatine ganglion, so that it has both excitatory and inhibitory control.[5] Displacement of the inferior rectus-inferior oblique complex medially could possibly have an effect on binocular alignment.

The function of Lockwood's ligament has not been clearly defined, and its designation as the inferior suspensory ligament of the orbit may be misleading. This structure is too lax to provide major global suspension. Manson et al.[33] have shown that following removal of inferior extraconal fat, the globe displaces downward, demonstrating that the fat compartment is probably more significant in global support. The complex morphology and multiple connections of Lockwood's ligament suggest a more important role in maintaining coordinated anatomic relationships during ocular movement, especially in retracting the eyelid and inferior conjunctival fornix during downgaze. It may in part also serve to stabilize the central point of horizontal ocular rotation at the point of overlap of the inferior oblique and inferior rectus muscles. Through its attachments to the orbicularis muscle, Lockwood's ligament helps create the lower eyelid crease, and therefore maintains an integrated eyelid lamellar structure during changing lid positions. It also appears to serve to limit backward displacement of inferior orbital structures.

The superior suspensory ligament of Whitnall is formed by a condensation of the fascial sheath both above and below the levator muscle, near the level at which the latter passes into its aponeurosis, just behind the superior orbital rim[46] (see Chapter 9). It inserts medially onto periosteum of the orbital wall and the adjacent suspensory system of the trochlea. Laterally, fibers of Whitnall's ligament blend with the pseudocapsule and suspensory ligaments of the lacrimal gland, and with periosteum of the superolateral orbital wall above the gland. Some fibers continue inferiorly to the retinaculum of the lateral orbital tubercle. Whitnall's ligament contributes important suspensory functions for the superior orbital fascial system. A conjoined thickening of the superior rectus muscle sheath and Whitnall's ligament extends to Tenon's capsule, and fine fibers pass to conjunctiva as the suspensory ligaments of the superior fornix. Delicate fibrous bands extend from the levator muscle in the region of Whitnall's ligament, through the interlobular septa of the preaponeurotic fat pads, to the superior orbital rim.

The function of Whitnall's ligament is complex, and is discussd further in Chapter 8. In part, it provides support to the upper eyelid and to the extensive anterior superior orbital fascial system. This includes suspension of the lacrimal gland, anterior levator muscle, Tenon's capsule, and the tendon of the superior oblique muscle. It also serves as a site of origin for Müller's sympathetic muscle in the upper lid. Just anterior to Whitnall's ligament, the horizontally oriented levator muscle is redirected to the vertically-oriented aponeurosis.[1] It also likely serves to some extent as a check ligament to upward retraction of the eyelid as originally described by Whitnall.[46] However, this functional limit is reached only with the most severe degrees of eyelid retraction due to levator or orbital fibrosis, and for the most part is clinically insignificant. An important function of Whitnall's ligament is probably to maintain the topographic relationships between various superior orbital structures during ocular movement, especially upgaze. Thus, the eyelid, the conjunctival fornix, and the lacrimal gland show coordinated vertical movements with the globe. In this regard, Whitnall's ligament is analogous to Lockwood's ligament in the inferior orbit.

The intermuscular septum

The intermuscular septum is usually depicted as a connective tissue fascial sheet extending between the rectus muscles, and enclosing the intraconal orbital space.[11,12] This fascia was first described by Motais in 1887[36] as the "common fascia of the ocular muscles" separating two distinct fat compartments, intraconal and extraconal. In reality, there is no clearly definable single intermuscular septum. Rather, there is a system of roughly circumferential and longitudinal, partially discontinuous fascial membranes that are more prominent in the plane of the rectus muscles. These membranes surround the fat lobules in the intra- and extraconal spaces forming an interconnected array of septal planes. They fill the space within the rectus muscle cone and extend between the muscles and around them to the orbital walls in a continuous fashion.[47] The septal membranes not only enclose fat lobules, but interconnect the muscle sheaths, the dura of the optic nerve, and the connective tissue suspensory septa that anchor the muscles to periorbita along the orbital walls. Therefore, the intraconal and extraconal surgical spaces are largely conceptual compartments, defined principally by the extraocular muscles. The major exceptions to this are in the posterior orbit, and in the anterior orbit where more prominent and thickened connective tissue sheets are seen interconnecting the rectus muscle pulleys. Such sheets are seen between the medial and inferior rectus muscles, between the medial and superior rectus muscles, and most prominently between the superior and lateral rectus muscles. The latter is a significant feature seen on coronal CT and MRI scans. It appears to function as part of the active pulley system of the orbit. This structure effectively separates the superolateral portion of the orbit as a distinct compartment that more anteriorly will house the orbital lobe and vessels of the lacrimal gland. More anteriorly, at the level of Whitnall's ligament, the outer layers of this septal complex merge with the lateral horn of the levator aponeurosis. The latter thickens considerably as it inserts onto the lateral retinaculum of the orbital tubercle. In this region the lateral horn of the levator aponeurosis is more consolidated and robust than its medial counterpart. This likely serves to resist the stronger forces tending to displace the globe medially. Fibrosis in this fascial layer associated with Graves' orbitopathy may in part account for the greater degree of lateral eyelid retraction seen in thyroid eye disease. The inner layers of the lateral intermuscular septal complex continue to the sheath of the lateral rectus muscle as the definitive intramuscular septum.

Shortly after consolidation of the superolateral intermuscular membrane in the mid-orbit, circumferentially aligned muscle fibers may be seen extending laterally from the edge of the levator muscle along this septal plane. Most of these fibers show cross-striations, but it appears that smooth muscle cells may be interspersed among them, as they are along many of the orbital fascial membranes. This bundle of striated and smooth fibers can reach all the way to the lateral rectus muscle, and in places may attain a thickness of nearly 1 mm. Isolated fiber bundles may even follow the lateral horn of the levator aponeurosis to its insertion into the lateral muscle pulley and the lateral retinaculum of the canthal ligament. More anteriorly, this muscular layer thins into several small fascicles that insert onto the capsule of the lacrimal gland. The function of this superolateral connective tissue layer and its muscular component remains unknown. However, in addition to its possible role in ocular motility as part of the active pulley system, it may also play some role in lacrimal secretion discharge. For now we may refer to this septal muscle layer as the *tensor intermuscularis*, a term we proposed in the first edition of this book.

As the extraocular muscles approach the globe, the intermuscular bands and septa become fused to Tenon's capsule via numerous very fine fascial slips. As the muscles continue forward, some elements of these septal sheets reform as a separate layer beneath Tenon's capsule, finally fusing with the latter near the corneal limbus.

The extraocular suspensory systems

In the anterior half of the orbit a complex system of suspensory septa connect the extraocular muscles to the orbital walls. Along the course of the superior oblique muscle and its pretrochlear tendon, encircling layers of connective tissue are joined to adjacent periorbita by extensive fascial connections. These bands form a more or less separate tubular compartment within which the oblique muscle runs from its origin to the trochlea. Anteriorly, a fascial band extends from the lower border of the trochlea and the adjacent orbital wall to insert onto Tenon's capsule medial to the insertion of the superior rectus muscle. This may serve as a check ligament against extension of the superior oblique tendon. As the posttrochlear tendon leaves the cartilaginous trochlea, it becomes surrounded by multiple fascial layers continuous with Tenon's capsule and with the sheath of the superior rectus muscle. These form an elongated cowl-like tunnel that accompanies the tendon until it reaches the sub-Tenon's space.

The medial rectus muscle lies within a complex system of septa that run predominantly craniocaudally. In the anterior half of the orbit, they perform extensive suspensory functions. Here they form thick fascial layers that surround the muscle, and pass from the sheath to periosteum of the medial and superior orbital walls. Weak connections may also extend upward to the fascia of the levator and superior rectus septal complex. This fascial system suspending the medial rectus muscle to the orbital roof is interrupted only by the passage of the superior oblique muscle and its fascial support system. Within the upper portion of the medial septal system runs the superior ophthalmic vein. At the level of the posterior globe, the superior ophthalmic vein is supported by fine fascial attachments to periorbita of the frontal bone. Medially,

the medial collateral vein lies within the vertically oriented septal complex of the medial rectus muscle.

In the inferior orbit the inferior rectus muscle has multiple, short septal connections to the orbital floor. These are especially prominent in the area around the inferior orbital fissure. Fine fascial strands interconnect the muscle with both the medial rectus and lateral rectus systems as well. Approximately 1 cm behind the orbital rim, the anchoring septa between the inferior rectus muscle and the floor are abruptly lost, as Lockwood's ligament becomes well defined. Here, the inferior rectus muscle sheath develops extensive fascial connections to the sheath of the inferior oblique as part of Lockwood's suspensory complex. Connective tissue septa extend from the latter to Tenon's capsule, the medial and lateral canthal ligaments, and into the lower eyelid.

The lateral rectus muscle has numerous strong fascial connections to periorbita along the lateral orbital wall. Only a few relatively weak fibrous septa interconnect this muscle medially to posterior Tenon's capsule and to the optic nerve sheath. Inferiorly, the lateral rectus is connected to the inferior rectus and oblique muscles via septa that extend across the inferior orbital fissure. Very strong fascial layers suspend this muscle to the orbital roof through much of its length, and to the dense septal system around the lateral side of the levator and superior rectus muscles.

The superior rectus-levator muscle complex is suspended from the orbital roof by a system of fascial connections to periorbita of the frontal bone. As the levator muscle passes into its aponeurosis, Whitnall's ligament is formed by a thickening of the levator sheath, with a thinner band inferior to the muscle, and a thicker layer superior to the muscle. This transverse collagenous band has extensive connections to the orbital walls. The aponeurosis itself is attached to the canthal ligaments through the medial and lateral horns, and to the tarsus and orbicularis muscle in the upper eyelid.

The rectus muscle pulley systems

As discussed in Chapter 3, the active pulley hypothesis as initially advocated by Miller[23] and more recently championed by Demer,[4-10] Kono,[17] Ruskell[39] and others, proposes that the elaborate suspensory system of the rectus muscles constitute pulleys through which the muscles move. Furthermore, these pulleys are capable of changing the position and direction of muscle forces coordinated with varying positions of ocular gaze. These pulleys form an encircling harness around the equator of the globe where adjacent pulleys are coupled to each other, providing inflection points along the extraocular muscle paths. In this manner they can serve as functional origins for the muscles during ocular rotation. The layered compartmentalization of extraocular muscles in which the outer orbital layer inserts onto the pulley system, and the inner global layer inserts onto the sclera via its tendon suggests that the orbital layer could modulate movement of the pulley positions, while the orbital layer influences movement of the globe in a coordinated fashion. For example, the inferior rectus pulley is coupled to the inferior oblique pulley by connective tissue bands containing heavy elastin deposits, and the orbital layer of the inferior oblique muscle inserts partially on the conjoined inferior oblique-inferior rectus pulley, partially on the temporal inferior oblique muscle sheath, and partially on the pulley of the lateral rectus muscle. The positions of all of these structures could be modified in a concerted manner to influence muscle vector forces. Likewise, the orbital layer of the superior oblique muscle exerts pull on its tendon sheath and through this on the pulley of the superior rectus muscle. The orbital surface of the muscle pulleys is thicker and presumably stiffer than the global portion and has more extensive elastin, possibly related to areas of maximum stress at inflection points.

In the mid-orbit, around the equator of the globe, a pulley ring has been described consisting of collagen laminae surrounding the extraocular muscles.[17] Elastin fibers are embedded in the collagen and along suspensory bands that connect the ring to adjacent periorbita. These and other suspensory bands provide resistance to sideslip of the muscles over the rotating globe. Smooth muscle fibers are abundant along the orbital surface of the pulley ring, the pulleys themselves, and along suspensory bands. They are associated with an intricate neural pattern including a rich sympathetic, parasympathetic, and nitroxidergic innervation suggesting a possible role in maintenance of pulley suspension stiffness, provision of slow adaptive adjustments in pulley location in order to maintain binocular alignment, and as an aid in dynamic ocular movement.[5] Along its outer or orbital surface, the pulley ring inserts into the collagen of each of the four rectus muscle pulleys. The various pulleys are also interconnected by collagenous bands to each other and to posterior Tenon's capsule.

The posterior suspensory systems

In the posterior half of the orbit the connective tissue septal system is somewhat less well-developed than in the anterior orbit. There are fewer intermuscular septa, and the extraocular muscles lie in closer proximity to the orbital walls. Thus, there is no real anatomic distinction between the intraconal and extraconal compartments.

Near the orbital apex the annulus of Zinn is fused to periorbita along the superior and medial orbital walls. Stout fascial septa pass from the inferior surface of the annulus to Müller's orbital muscle in the inferior orbital fissure. The superior oblique muscle is already supported by a sling of fibrous tissue suspended from the superomedial orbital wall. This will continue as a major feature throughout the course of this muscle. As the extraocular muscles thicken, the prominent fibrous structure of the annulus of Zinn thins rapidly, finally remaining only as several fine septa extending between the expanding muscle bellies, and merging into the muscular sheaths. Only here does a true encircling intermuscular septum exist. However, only a few millimeters more anteriorly this structure quickly passes into an irregular system of fascial septa with more prominent connections to the orbital walls and optic nerve.

Slightly more anteriorly, the superior rectus and levator muscles establish suspensory connections to the superior and superolateral orbital roof. The medial rectus muscle has some connections in this region to other orbital septa, but lacks the extensive attachments to the orbital walls seen more anteriorly. A prominent series of fascial fibers extends from the inferior rectus muscle to the smooth muscle covering the inferior orbital fissure (Müller's orbital muscle). This is continuous with similar fibers interconnecting Müller's muscle with the annulus of Zinn more posteriorly, A fibrous layer extends forward from the annulus of Zinn as a thickened sheath over the lateral and superior surface of the lateral rectus muscle. This is fused to periorbita along the superior orbital fissure. In addition, a number of septa extend from the sheath of the lateral rectus muscle to the lateral orbital wall and the region of the inferior orbital fissure. This extensive fascial system associated with the lateral rectus muscle serves to confine the muscle within its pulley fixed to the lateral wall. This muscle has the longest trajectory of any of the rectus muscles, and its course from origin to insertion tends to describe an arc around the globe, making it more susceptible to side-slip with extremes of vertical gaze shifts. The more extensive fascial suspensory system associated with this muscle helps to maintain it in a fixed relationship to the orbital wall and to the globe.

Toward the central orbit, the medial rectus fascial system establishes firm connections to the orbital roof and to the sling of the superior oblique muscle. Fine septal attachments are seen between the medial rectus and optic nerve sheaths, as well as to the inferior rectus system. Firm connections to the medial orbital wall are also established in this region. The inferior rectus muscle loses most of its attachments to Müller's muscle in the inferior orbital fissure, but establishes numerous septal connections to the medial rectus system and to the orbital floor. Somewhat more anteriorly, fibrous strands join the inferior to the lateral rectus septal complexes. The lateral rectus continues with strong connections to the orbital roof and lateral wall, as well as to the septa of the inferior rectus complex.

Extensive septa span across the upper orbit from the superior pole of the lateral rectus muscle and adjacent orbital walls to the orbital roof between the levator muscle and the superior oblique. These layers run between the optic nerve and the superior rectus muscle. They form a broad draping hammock stabilized centrally by fibers passing vertically to the optic nerve sheath and inferior rectus system. This hammock extends from the posterior orbit nearly to the globe, and in part provides support for the superior ophthalmic vein as it crosses from medial to lateral in the central 2 cm of the orbit. Smaller veins and the nasociliary nerve also run within this hammock. As these vascular and neural structures pass to the medial orbit they become supported within the vertical fascial sheets of the medial rectus system.

Orbital muscle of Müller

The orbital muscle of Müller is functionally part of the orbital connective tissue system and so is best discussed here. It represents an evolutionary vestige from earlier mammalian history. In lower mammals the bony orbit is incomplete posteriorly. The posterior orbit is separated from the temporalis fossa by a musculofascial layer containing smooth muscle. This layer functions along with the retractor bulbi muscles to regulate orbital volume and prominence of the globes. In higher primates, the bony lateral orbital wall closes with expansion of the greater sphenoid wing, likely as a means of stabilizing bifovial stereopsis and fixation by separating the orbit from the temporalis muscle as the face shortens and the cranium expands forward over the orbits. Although some authors have thought that Müller's muscle no longer has any functional significance in humans, others have suggested a limited role in vasculosympathetic control.[40] The anatomic relationships of Müller's orbital muscle in higher primates is very different from that in lower mammals, and supports the concept of venous flow regulation as a possible modified function. Also, smooth muscle fibers extend from Müller's muscle along fascial plans that blend into adjacent periorbita and into the inferior and lateral rectus muscle pulleys. Posteriorly, prominent connective tissue bands and smooth muscle fibers extend from Müller's muscle to the inferior sheath of the annulus of Zinn, suggesting that the annulus may play some role in the active orbital system through modulation of its position.

Müller's orbital muscle forms a bridge over the inferior orbital fissure, separating the orbital contents from the pterygopalatine fossa. It is composed of smooth muscle fibers roughly oriented transverse to the inferior orbital fissure. The muscle may reach 8–10 mm in thickness where its inferior fibers extend down through the inferior orbital fissure and into the pterygopalatine fossa. The orbital surface of Müller's muscle is concave, and is covered by a fascial sheath. Muscle fibers continue along fine connective tissue bands extending onto the orbital floor where they form a sheet measuring about 1 mm in thickness. They also extend toward the inferior rectus muscle for a distance of 2–3 mm before inserting onto periorbita and along some of the suspensory fibers of the inferior rectus pulley system. Along the lateral wall Müller's muscle sends a thin layer of fibers upward for 7–10 mm where they may reach to the level of the lower third of the lateral rectus muscle. Bands of fibers arise from the medial side of Müller's muscle and pass to the lateral wall forming a bridge over the inferior fissure, enclosing the zygomatic nerve and venous channels from the inferior ophthalmic vein. In places, fibers from Müller's muscle extend into the orbit as multiple finger-like projections that insert onto fascial septa of the inferior rectus and lateral rectus suspensory complexes. Posteriorly, a stout connective tissue band extends from the lower border of the annulus of Zinn to the capsule surrounding Müller's muscle. At the orbital apex, near the entrance of the inferior orbital fissure, the inferior ophthalmic vein breaks up into several large venous sinuses between the annulus of Zinn and Müller's muscle. Smooth muscle fibers extend between and around these sinuses forming a U-shaped cup that may compress them upward against the annulus of Zinn. The anatomic relationship suggests a possible role for this smooth muscle in modulating orbital hemodynamics. Müller's muscle fibers continue along these venous channels backward through the base of the superior orbital fissure onto the floor and lateral wall of the cavernous sinus.[37]

Inferiorly, Müller's muscle forms the roof of the pterygopalatine fossa.[45] Prominent fibers from the temporalis muscle on the lateral side of the fossa insert onto the sheath of Müller's muscle. Just how these contribute to the physiology of the inferior orbit remains to be determined. Small collateral branches from the maxillary artery pierce Müller's muscle to reach the orbit. They anastomose with the inferior muscular branch of the ophthalmic artery. Numerous larger venous channels from the inferior ophthalmic vein pass through the muscle to the pterygoid venous plexus. The zygomatic nerve, a branch from the maxillary division of the trigeminal, arises in the pterygopalatine fossa and penetrates Müller's muscle through a prominent canal along the sphenoid bone en route to the lateral orbital wall. A number of fine nerve branches from maxillary artery sympathetic plexus in the pterygopalatine ganglion pass into and end within the Müller's muscle, and appear to supply its sympathetic innervation.[37,40]

The function of Müller's muscle in humans is not clear. Its insignificant contribution to orbital wall surface makes it unlikely that it can directly alter orbital volume as in lower mammals. However, the intimate relationship between its muscular fibers and branches of the inferior ophthalmic vein, the inferior venous sinus at the orbital apex, and its extension into the cavernous sinus, all suggest a possible influence on autonomically mediated vascular dynamics. The fascial connections between this muscle and the inferior orbital fascial septa, the annulus of Zinn, and with fibers of the temporalis muscle remain unexplained. Investigations will be needed to determine whether Müller's muscle can modulate the vertical position of the annulus, and, if so, whether this can have any effect on extraocular muscle vector moments.

Clinical correlations

The extensive fascial septal planes of the orbit provide an intricate interconnected system that unites many structures, limits movement, and maintains order within a constantly shifting, dynamic environment. If it were not for these septal membranes, the semi-fluid orbital fat lobules would quickly redistribute themselves, as may be seen following enucleation or extensive orbital surgery when the fascial system is disrupted. These septa also support delicate structures, such as veins and nerves, and provide pathways along which fluid may drain forward to the eyelid lymphatics or backward to the cavernous sinus.

The distinct septal system for each of the extraocular muscles provides a broad area of support and helps maintain the functional relationships between them during complex ocular movements. Although the two globes are directed forward in primary gaze, the axes of the muscle cones are oriented posteromedially at about 22.5° to the sagittal plane. This angular relationship would result in significant positional shifts of muscle vector alignments and of forces during ocular rotation. The septal system allows for a more constant vector force orientation in all positions of gaze. Similar morphologic adaptations to minimize vector shifts in muscular force have been described elsewhere, for example in the masticatory apparatus of elephants and their relatives.[31]

In the orbit, Koornneef[18] has demonstrated the importance of the connective tissue septal systems in producing motility restriction following trauma. Restrictive ophthalmoplegia after orbital floor fracture is often not the result of direct incarceration of the inferior rectus muscle in the bony fragments. Rather, it frequently results from herniation of orbital fat and entrapment of connective tissue septa into the fracture site, with traction on the muscle sheaths through its complex septal connections.[18]

The orbital deformities following some surgery may result from loss of supporting septa, and emphasizes the interconnection of the entire system. During orbital decompression surgery, removal of large sections of the orbital walls results in changes in position of the supporting slings to the extraocular muscles, the globe, and orbital soft tissues. The result is a change in position of the eye, usually downward and inward, and alterations in the degree and direction of motility restriction. Reduction in proptosis is related mostly to volume loss in the intraconal fat pads as the muscles spread peripherally. Increased motility restriction may follow orbital decompression due to shifting of fibrosed fascial compartments, alterations in the position of muscle pulleys, and redistribution of muscle tension. Koornneef[18,19] emphasized the importance of opening the entire periorbita in order to more evenly relax the orbital contents.

During enucleation surgery alterations in the fascial and pulley systems are extensive, and can result in major anatomical deformities. While some authors have advocated the closure of posterior Tenon's capsule over an implant, this becomes highly disruptive to the fascial suspensory systems when extraocular muscles are also attached to the implant. The reason is that the EOM's pass from the orbit through Tenon's capsule to reach the globe (or implant), so that they are anatomically "inside" Tenon's, whereas pulling up Tenon's between the rectus muscles to close over the implant places the implant "outside" or behind Tenon's capsule. Since Tenon's and the muscle sheaths are intimately involved in the muscle pulley and suspension apparatus, this procedure results in a gross distortion of these structures. While there are no comprehensive studies on how these structural alterations affect eyelid position, cosmesis, and implant motility, nevertheless at least theoretically they would seem to have a major impact on orbital anatomy and function. Damage to, or removal of, anterior extraconal fat alone does not significantly alter global position, but may contribute to the formation of the superior sulcus deformity frequently seen in the anophthalmic socket,[33] or in overly aggressive upper eyelid blepharoplasties.

The fascial system is related to a number of clinical phenomena. In Graves' orbitopathy motility restriction has been thought to result from fibrosis in the extraocular muscles.

However, it is more likely associated with hypertrophy of fascial septa resulting from chronic orbital inflammation.[26] This thickening of septal planes can be seen during surgery, and is responsible for the often observed failure of fat to prolapse following orbital decompression procedures, even when periorbita is widely opened. Recession of the upper eyelid in such patients frequently fails to correct retraction even after complete disinsertion of the levator aponeurosis and extirpation of Müller's tarsal muscle. Careful dissection of hypertrophied fascial tissue between conjunctiva and Whitnall's ligament, the lacrimal gland, the horns of the aponeurosis, and the canthal tendons is often necessary to reposition the eyelids.

The orbital congestion seen as an early clinical sign in Graves' orbitopathy is related to alterations in orbital vascular dynamics. The major venous channels lie within the septal planes, and in the case of the superior ophthalmic vein runs between the superior orbital fascial hammock the superior rectus muscle.[19,23] Fibrosis of this septal layer and even minimal enlargement or inflammation of the superior rectus muscle can compress the vein,[14] which serves as a major blood drainage reservoir in the orbit. Also, Müller's orbital muscle in the inferior orbital fissure may modulate venous outflow in the inferior orbit. If hypertrophy in this muscle occurs as is often seen for Müller's supratarsal muscle, then reduced venous outflow to the pterygopalatine venous plexus might contribute to orbital vascular congestion.

Orbital hemorrhage is usually of little permanent consequence, but in some individuals, particularly the young, compartmentalization of blood within septal pockets adjacent to the optic nerve may result in significant visual loss due to compression from compartment syndrome. This phenomenon may be related to the extent and thickness of these septal planes.

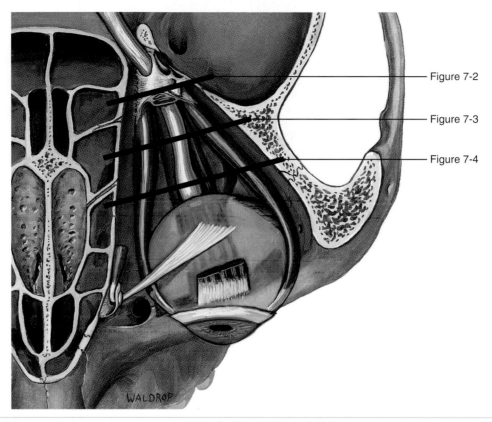

Figure 7-1 Orbital fascial connective tissue system, cross-section planes for Figures 7-2 through 7-4.

Figure 7-2

Figure 7-3

Figure 7-4

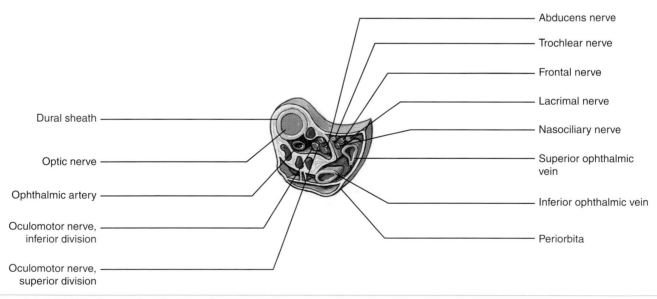

Dural sheath

Optic nerve

Ophthalmic artery

Oculomotor nerve, inferior division

Oculomotor nerve, superior division

Abducens nerve

Trochlear nerve

Frontal nerve

Lacrimal nerve

Nasociliary nerve

Superior ophthalmic vein

Inferior ophthalmic vein

Periorbita

Figure 7-2 Orbital fascial system, frontal section, orbital apex.

119

Frontal nerve

Nasociliary nerve

Trochlear nerve

Ophthalmic artery

Zygomatic nerve

Oculomotor nerve, superior division

Periorbita

Lacrimal nerve

Superior orbital fissure

Abducens nerve

Oculomotor nerve, inferior division

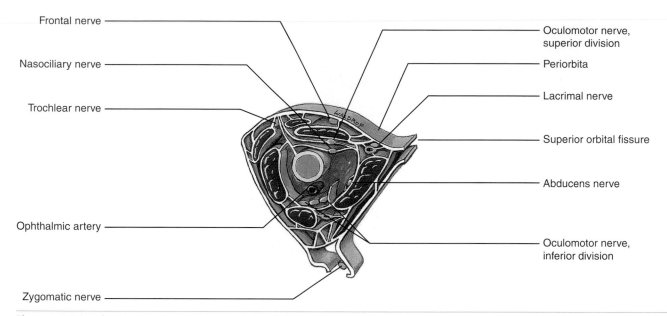

Figure 7-3 Orbital fascial system, frontal section, posterior orbit.

Frontal nerve

Periorbita

Ophthalmic artery

Nasociliary nerve

Oculomotor nerve, branch to medial rectus muscle

Oculomotor nerve, branch to inferior rectus muscle

Zygomatic nerve

Oculomotor nerve branch to superior rectus muscle

Superior ophthalmic vein

Lacrimal nerve

Abducens nerve

Inferior ophthalmic vein

Oculomotor nerve, branch to inferior oblique muscle

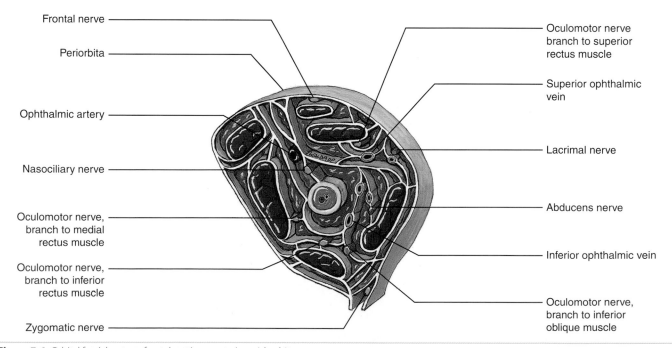

Figure 7-4 Orbital fascial system, frontal section, posterior mid-orbit.

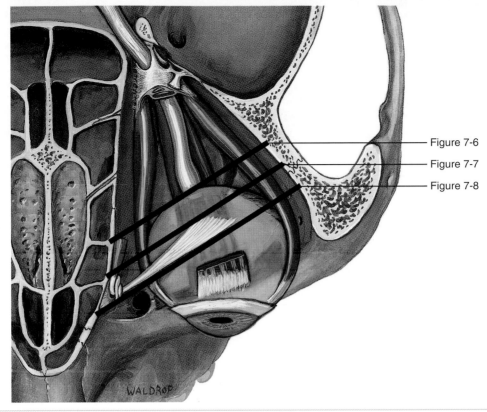

Figure 7-5 Orbital fascial connective tissue system, cross-section planes for Figures 7-6 through 7-8.

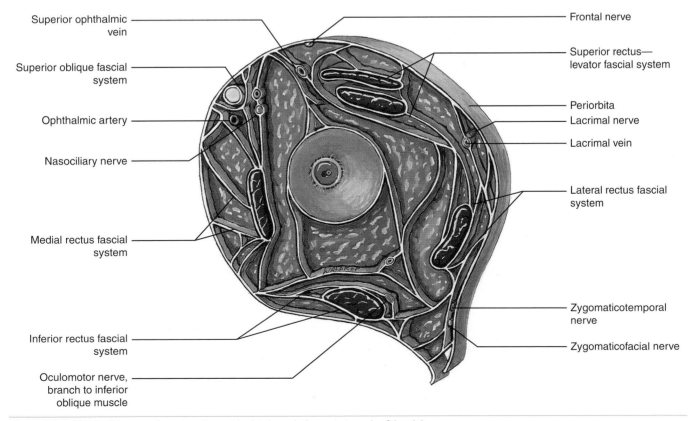

Figure 7-6 Orbital fascial system, frontal section, mid-orbit through the posterior pole of the globe.

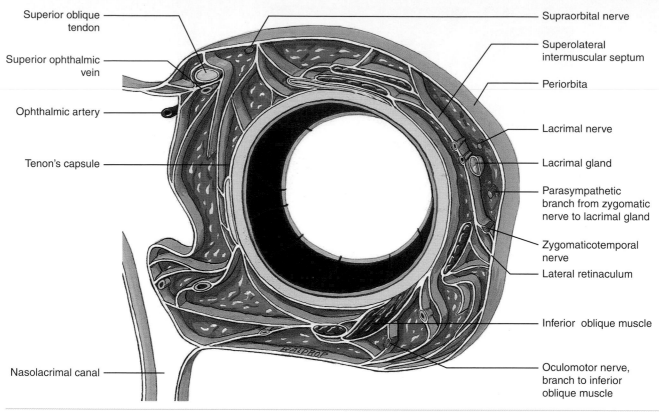

Superior oblique tendon

Superior ophthalmic vein

Ophthalmic artery

Tenon's capsule

Nasolacrimal canal

Supraorbital nerve

Superolateral intermuscular septum

Periorbita

Lacrimal nerve

Lacrimal gland

Parasympathetic branch from zygomatic nerve to lacrimal gland

Zygomaticotemporal nerve

Lateral retinaculum

Inferior oblique muscle

Oculomotor nerve, branch to inferior oblique muscle

Figure 7-7 Orbital fascial system, frontal section, anterior mid-orbit through the globe.

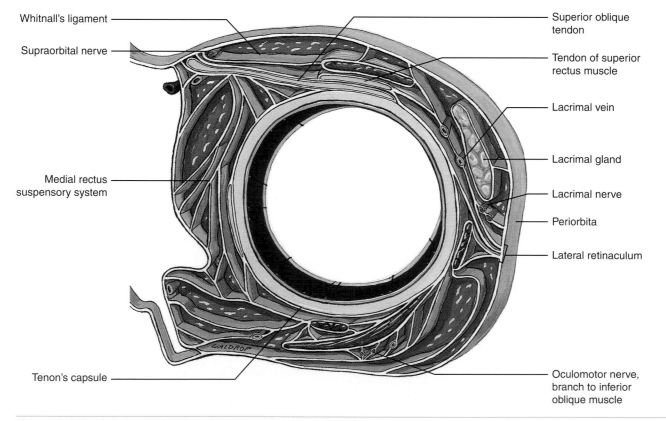

Whitnall's ligament

Supraorbital nerve

Medial rectus suspensory system

Tenon's capsule

Superior oblique tendon

Tendon of superior rectus muscle

Lacrimal vein

Lacrimal gland

Lacrimal nerve

Periorbita

Lateral retinaculum

Oculomotor nerve, branch to inferior oblique muscle

Figure 7-8 Orbital fascial system, frontal section, anterior orbit through the mid-globe.

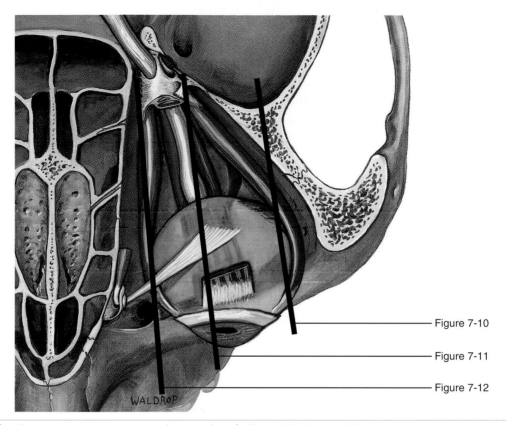

Figure 7-10

Figure 7-11

Figure 7-12

Figure 7-9 Orbital fascial connective tissue system, sagittal-section planes for Figures 7-10 through 7-12.

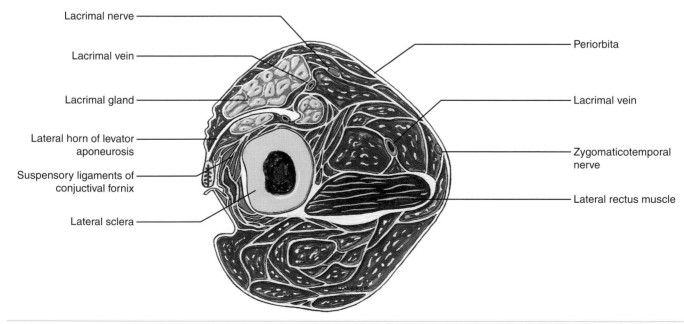

Lacrimal nerve

Lacrimal vein

Lacrimal gland

Lateral horn of levator aponeurosis

Suspensory ligaments of conjuctival fornix

Lateral sclera

Periorbita

Lacrimal vein

Zygomaticotemporal nerve

Lateral rectus muscle

Figure 7-10 Orbital fascial system, sagittal section, lateral orbit.

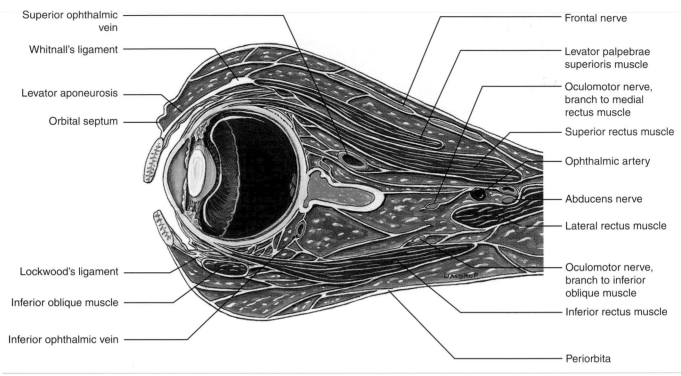

Superior ophthalmic vein

Whitnall's ligament

Levator aponeurosis

Orbital septum

Lockwood's ligament

Inferior oblique muscle

Inferior ophthalmic vein

Frontal nerve

Levator palpebrae superioris muscle

Oculomotor nerve, branch to medial rectus muscle

Superior rectus muscle

Ophthalmic artery

Abducens nerve

Lateral rectus muscle

Oculomotor nerve, branch to inferior oblique muscle

Inferior rectus muscle

Periorbita

Figure 7-11 Orbital fascial system, sagittal section, mid-orbit.

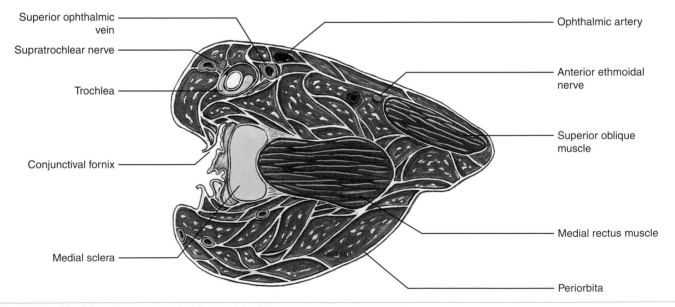

Superior ophthalmic vein

Supratrochlear nerve

Trochlea

Conjunctival fornix

Medial sclera

Ophthalmic artery

Anterior ethmoidal nerve

Superior oblique muscle

Medial rectus muscle

Periorbita

Figure 7-12 Orbital fascial system, sagittal section, medial orbit.

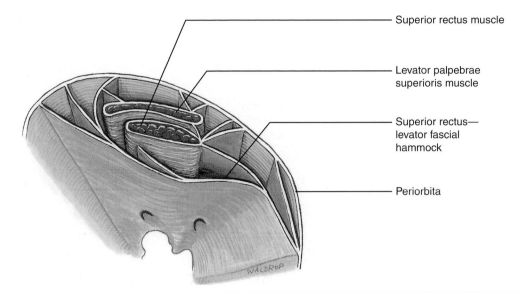

Superior rectus muscle

Levator palpebrae superioris muscle

Superior rectus— levator fascial hammock

Periorbita

Figure 7-13 Orbital fascial system, 3D reconstruction, superior rectus-levator muscle suspensory system.

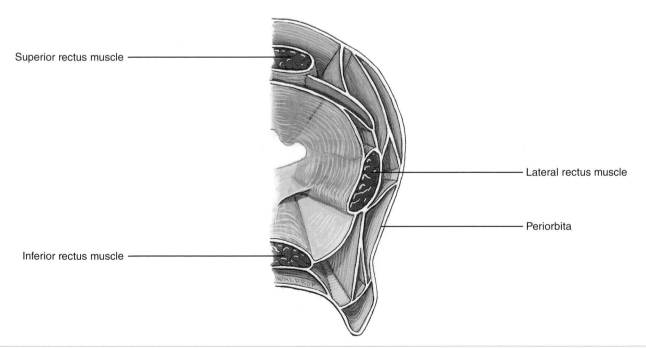

Superior rectus muscle

Lateral rectus muscle

Periorbita

Inferior rectus muscle

Figure 7-14 Orbital fascial system, 3D reconstruction, lateral rectus muscle suspensory system.

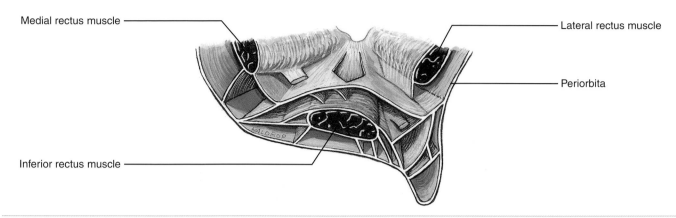

Medial rectus muscle

Lateral rectus muscle

Periorbita

Inferior rectus muscle

Figure 7-15 Orbital fascial system, reconstruction, inferior rectus system.

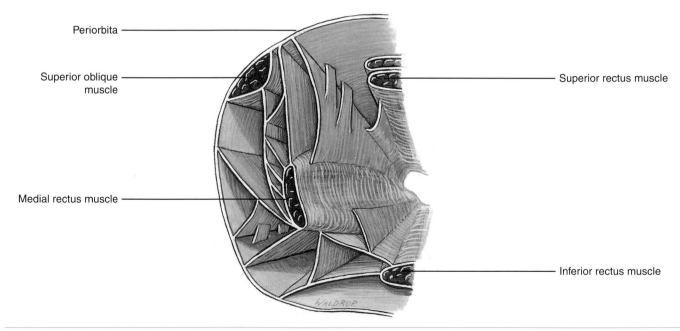

Periorbita

Superior oblique muscle

Superior rectus muscle

Medial rectus muscle

Inferior rectus muscle

Figure 7-16 Orbital fascial system, 3D reconstruction, medial rectus muscle suspensory system.

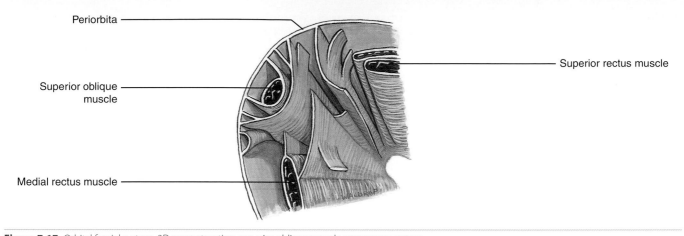

Periorbita

Superior oblique muscle

Medial rectus muscle

Superior rectus muscle

Figure 7-17 Orbital fascial system, 3D reconstruction, superior oblique muscle suspensory system.

References

1. Anderson RL, Dixon RS: The role of Whitnall's ligament in ptosis surgery. *Arch Ophthalmol* 97:705, 1979.

2. Bergin MP: A spatial reconstruction of the orbital vascular pattern in relation with the connective tissue system. *Acta Morphol Neerl -Scand* 20:117, 1982.

3. Bremond-Gignac D, Copin H, Cussenot O, et al: Anatomic histologic and mesoscopic study of the adipose tissue of the orbit. *Surg Radiol Anat* 26:297, 2004.

4. Demer JL, Oh SY, Poukens V: Evidence for active control of rectus extraocular muscle pulleys. *Invest Ophthalmol Vis Sci* 41:1280, 2000.

5. Demer JL, Poukens V, Miller JM, Micevych P: Innervation of extraocular pulley smooth muscle in monkeys and humans. *Invest Ophthalmol Vis Sci* 38:1774, 1997.

6. Demer JL: Active pulley system: magnetic resonance imaging of rectus muscle paths in tertiary gazes. *Invest Ophthalmol Vis Sci* 43:2179, 2002.

7. Demer JL: Current concepts of mechanical and neuralfactors in ocular motility. *Curr Opin Neurol* 19:4, 2006.

8. Demer JL: Gillies Lecture: ocular motility in a time of paradigm shift. *Clin Exp Ophthalmol* 34:822, 2006.

9. Demer JL: Mechanics of the orbita. *Dev Ophthalmol* 40:132, 2007.

10. Demer JL: The orbital pulley system: a revolution in concepts of orbital anatomy. *Ann NY Acad Sci* 956:17, 2002.

11. Doxanas MJ, Anderson RL: *Clinical Orbital Anatomy*. Baltimore, Williams & Williams. 1984, p 80.

12. Ducasse A: L'orbite. In: Chevrel JP (ed), *Anatomie Clinique. Tète et Cou*. Paris, Springer, 1995, p 91.

13. Gola R, Carreau JP, Faissal A: The adipose tissue of the orbit. Anatomic classification, therapeutic deductions. *Rev Stomatol Chir Maxilofac* 96:123, 1995.

14. Hudson HL, Levin L, Feldon SE: Graves exophthalmos unrelated to extraocular muscle enlargement. *Ophthalmology* 98:1495, 1991.

15. Hwang K, Choi HG, Nam YS, Kim DJ: Anatomy of arcuate expansion of capsulopalpebral fascia. *J Craniofac Surg* 21:239, 2010.

16. Kakizaki H, Chan WO, Madge SN, et al: Lower eyelid retractors in Caucasians. *Ophthalmology* 116:1402, 2009.

17. Kono R, Poukens V, Demer JL: Quantitative analysis of the structure of the human extraocular muscle pulley system. *Invest Ophthal Vis Sci* 43:2923, 2002.

18. Koornneef L: Eyelid and orbital fascial attachments and their clinical significance. *Eye* 2:130, 1988.

19. Koornneef L: A new anatomical approach to the human orbit. *Mod Probl Ophthalmol* 14:49, 1975.

20. Koornneef L: Details of the orbital connective tissue system in the adult. In: Korrnneef L (ed), *Spatial Aspects of Orbital Musculo-Fibrous Tissue in Man*. Amsterdam, Swets & Zeitlinger B.V., 1977.

21. Koornneef L: New insights into the human orbit connective tissue. *Arch Ophthalmol* 95:1269, 1977.

22. Koornneef L: Orbital septa: anatomy and function. *Ophthalmology* 86:876, 1979.

23. Koornneef L: *Spatial Aspects of Orbital Musculo-Fibrous Tissue in Man: A New Anatomical and Histological Approach*. Amsterdam, Swets & Zeitlinger, 1977, p 890.

24. Koornneef L: The architecture of the musculo-fibrous apparatus in the human orbit. *Acta Morphol Neerl -Scand* 15:35, 1977.

25. Koornneef L: The development of the connective tissue in the human orbit. *Acta Morphol Neerl -Scand* 14:263, 1976.

26. Kronish JW, Gonnering RS, Dortzbach RK, et al: The pathophysiology of the anophthalmic socket. Part I. Analysis of orbital blood flow. *Ophthal Plast Reconstr Surg* 6:77, 1990.

27. Kronish JW, Gonnering RS, Dortzbach RK, et al: The pathophysiology of the anophthalmic socket. Part II. Analysis of orbital fat. *Ophthal Plast Reconstr Surg* 6:88, 1990.

28. Lang J, Reiter W: Topographie des Orbitainhaltes Teil II: Über die Kammerung des Corpus adiposum orbitae. *Neurochirurgia* 34:1, 1991.

29. Lim W-K, Rajendran K, Choo C-T: Microscopic anatomy of the lower eyelid in Asians. *Ophthal Plast Reconstr Surg* 20:207, 2004.

30. Lockwood CB: The anatomy of the muscles, ligaments, fascia of the orbit. *J Anat Physiol* 20:1, 1886.

31. Maglio VJ: Origin and evolution of the Elephantidae. *Trans Amer Phil Soc ns*, 63:1, 1973.

32. Mann I: *The Development of the Human Eye*. 3rd ed. New York, Grune and Stratton, 1964.

33. Manson PN, Clifford C, Su CT, et al: Mechanisms of global support and posttraumatic enophthalmos: I. The anatomy of the ligament sling and its relationship to intramuscular cone orbital fat. *Plast Reconstr Surg* 77:193, 1986.

34. Miller JM, Demer JL, Poukens V, et al: Extraocular connective tissue architecture. *J Vision* 3:240, 2003.

35. Miller JM, Robins D: Extraocular muscle sideslip and orbital geometry in monkeys. *Vis Res* 27: 381, 1987.

36. Motais E: *L'appareil moteur de l'homme er des vertebras*. Paris, Delalaye et Lecrosnier, p 303.

37. Rodriguez Vazquez JF, Merida Velasco JR, Jimenez Collado J: Orbital muscle of Muller: observations on human fetuses measuring 35–150 mm. *Acta Anat* 139:300, 1990.

38. Rohrich RJ, Ahmad J, Hamawy AH, Pessa JE: Is intraorbital fat extraorbital? Results of cross-sectional anatomy of the lower eyelid fat pads. *Aesth Surg J* 29:189, 2009.

39. Ruskell GL, Kjellevold Haugen IB, Bruenech JR, van der Werf F: Double insertions of extraocular rectus muscles in humans and the pulley theory. *J Anat* 206:295, 2005.

40. Ruskell GL: The orbital branches of the pterygopalatine ganglion and their relationship with internal carotid branches in primates. *J Anat* 106:323, 1970.

41. Sires BS, Lemke BN, Dortzbach RK, Gonnering RS: Characterization of human orbital fat and connective tissue. *Ophthal Plast Reconstr Surg* 14:403, 1998.

42. Sires BS, Saari JC, Garwin GG, et al: The color difference in orbital fat. *Arch Ophthalmol* 119:868, 2001.

43. Snyder C: An operation designated "the extirpation of the eye". *Arch Ophthalmol* 74:429, 1965.

44. Tenon JR: *Mémoires et observations sur l'anatomie, la pathologie et la chirurgie, et principalement sur l'organe de l'oeil*. Paris, Méquignon, 1806, p 193.

45. Warwick R: *Eugene Wolff's Anatomy of the Eye and Orbit*. 7th ed., Philadelphia, WB Saunders, 1976.

46. Whitnall SE: *The Anatomy of the Human Orbit and Accessory Organs of Vision*. Milford H (ed), London, Oxford University Press, 1932, p 146.

47. Wolfram-Gabel R, Kahn JL: Adipose body of the orbit. *Clin Anat* 15:186, 2002.

CHAPTER 8

The Eyelids and Anterior Orbit

The eyelids form a soft-tissue barrier that protects the globe and anterior entrance to the orbit. The orbital septum separates the orbit from the eyelid and represents the anterior-most orbital structure. All structures anterior to the orbital septum are technically in the eyelid. The orbicularis muscle and palpebral skin are usually considered as part of the eyelid. However, anatomically this distinction is rather difficult to support since, as discussed below, the orbital septum does not extend the full length of the eyelid. The septum does not extend over the tarsus, and in the medial canthal region, it has several separated layers, so that it cannot be used as a convenient division between the orbit and eyelid in these locations. While it may be useful to think about the septum as separating the orbit and eyelid, physiologically the eyelid, with all of its layers from skin to conjunctiva, forms a single anatomic and functional complex. Many of its structures, for example in the upper lid the levator aponeurosis, Müller's supratarsal muscle, and the preaponeurotic fat pockets, bridge the boundary between orbit and eyelid. Therefore, any topographic division between these two compartments is rather arbitrary.

The eyelids serve an important function by protecting the globe. They provide important elements to the precorneal tear film, and help distribute these layers evenly over the surface of the eye. Together with the lacrimal drainage apparatus, the eyelids collect and propel tears to the medial canthus, where they are removed to the nose. The eyelashes sweep air-borne particles from in front of the eye, and the constant voluntary and reflex movements of the eyelids protect the cornea from injury and glare.

Soft tissue layers and spaces

The face and scalp are arranged in concentric tissue layers, which, although variable in detail from one part of the head to another, still follow a single basic pattern.[107] This pattern consists of five basic layers: skin, subcutaneous tissue, superficial musculoaponeurotic layer, loose areolar tissue, and the deep fascia and periosteum. The skin and subcutaneous layers are basically the same over the entire face and scalp, except for thickness. The musculoaponeurotic layer is attached to the skin and subcutaneous layers by fine connective tissue bands called retinaculi cutis fibers. Over the scalp and forehead, the musculoaponeurotic layer is formed by the galea aponeurotica and its muscular components, the occipitalis and frontalis muscles. Here, the skin, subcutaneous layer, and galea form a single functional unit that is mobile over

the underlying loose and relatively avascular areolar tissue layer. Elevation of flaps on the forehead and scalp are usually developed in this subgaleal areolar tissue plane.

Over the mid-cheek, the musculoaponeurotic layer includes the intrinsic muscles of facial mobility, and here it is referred to as the superficial musculoaponeurotic system or SMAS. These intrinsic muscles have a limited attachment to the underlying periosteum, but firm attachments to the overlying skin. The sub-SMAS areolar layer contains a series of retaining ligaments, such as the orbicularis and zygomatic retaining ligaments, that suspend overlying tissues to the facial skeleton.[46] Between these ligaments are a series of glide planes that allow for mobility of the facial tissues.[138] These glide planes are bounded above by the inferior fascia of the SMAS, and below by the periosteum.

The eyebrows

Embryology

The superficial muscles of the head develop as mesodermal laminae beginning at the second branchial arch.[47,49] The orbicularis, corrugator, depressor supercilii, and procerus muscles develop from the infraorbital lamina, while the frontalis muscle develops from the temporal lamina. As these laminae join above the eye they form the interdigitating muscular structure of the brow. Beginning at the 8–10 week stage of fetal development primary hair germs are seen in the regions of the brow, upper lip, and chin. Among non-human mammals, these regions contain longer thicker tactile hairs called vibrissae. Primitive hair germs start as a focal crowding of basal cell nuclei in the fetal epidermis. As the basal cell germ enlarges it becomes asymmetric and extends obliquely downward as a solid column. The advancing tip becomes concave and encloses an aggregate of mesodermal cells that later differentiates to form the papilla, matrix, and root sheath layers of the hair bulb. Melanocytes are seen between the epithelial cells in the lower portion of the bulb, and the outer mesodermal cells differentiate to form a connective tissue sheath. The epithelial cord opens centrally and two swellings appear in its posterior wall. The upper swelling differentiates into a sebaceous gland, and the lower one into the attachment site for the future arector pili muscle. No new hair follicles are formed after birth.

The adult eyebrow

Although the eyebrows are technically part of the forehead and scalp, and not the eyelids, they are considered here because of their important functional and surgical relationships to the lids. Their mobility is part of the system of facial expression so important in primate evolution. The eyebrows are situated over the bony superior orbital rims, at the junction between the upper eyelid and the forehead. They extend from just above the trochlear fossa medially, nearly to the frontozygomatic suture line laterally. The flattened and generally hairless glabellar region separates the two eyebrows in the midline. Above the brows, the forehead is covered by skin that becomes thinner more cephalad and thicker closer to the eyebrows. The eyebrow consists of thickened skin overlying the supraorbital torus, from which it is separated by a prominent fat pad. This skin supports short, course eyebrow hairs that emerge from the skin surface at an oblique angle. Medially these hairs may be directed upward, centrally more downward, and laterally they are usually directed horizontally and laterally. These changing orientations are important to note during direct brow elevations with resection of skin just above the brow line, because truncating the brow follicles will result in loss of cilia and exposure of the scar.

The eyebrow is capable of a wide range of movement, averaging 1 cm downward and 2.5 cm or greater upward.[29] Excursion is more extensive in the medial portion of the brow. These complex movements are provided by the interdigitation of five striated muscles that insert partially along the brow—the frontalis, procerus, depressor supercilii, corrugator supercilii, and orbicularis oculi muscles. All are innervated by the seventh cranial, or facial, nerve. The frontalis muscle fibers are oriented vertically on the forehead and form the anterior belly of the occipitofrontalis musculofascial complex that forms the epicranius. The latter includes two flat muscle masses, the frontalis muscle anteriorly and the occipitalis muscle posteriorly. Over the scalp the muscular stratum is represented by the galea aponeurotica. The galea forms the thick superficial fascia of the scalp that invests the frontalis and occipitalis muscles on either end, and carries a rich supply of blood vessels and nerves. The galea covers the upper scalp between the occipitalis and frontalis muscles. It invests these muscles posteriorly and anteriorly, and continues centrally as a short prolongation between the left and right segments of the frontalis muscle bellies. On either side the galea fuses to the superficial temporal fusion line. Here it loses its aponeurotic character and then continues downward over the temporalis muscle as the superficial temporal fascia. The galea is firmly attached to the overlying skin by a firm, dense adipose layer, and is separated from the underlying pericranium (cranial periosteum) by a loose areolar fascial cleft that allows for mobility of the scalp. At 8–10 cm above the orbital rim, the galea from the scalp splits into superficial and deep layers that surround the forehead muscles.[94] The deep layer of the galea extends below the frontalis muscle and fuses to periosteum 8–10 mm above the orbital rim. The superficial layer continues downward over the front of the frontalis muscle to the orbital rim, where it inserts onto a fusion line, the arcus marginalis, along the margin of the orbital rim. From the arcus marginalis, the anterior galea continues downward into the upper eyelid, where it continues as the anterior layer of the orbital septum.

Frontalis muscle

The frontalis muscle is usually considered to be part of the epicranius, or occipitofrontalis muscle that includes the occipitalis muscle posteriorly and the frontalis muscle anteriorly, with the galea aponeurotica joining the two portions. The frontalis muscle has no bony attachments. Rather, its proximal fibers originate from the galea aponeurotica at about the level of the coronal suture line and extend toward the supraorbital rim. On the lateral side, frontalis muscle fibers extend slightly more cephalad than on the medial border.[88] The muscle belly is surrounded by layers of the galea, anteriorly by the thin superficial layer and posteriorly by the thicker deep layer. The frontalis muscle is paired, with a distinct midline separation. Its medial fibers blend with those of the procerus muscle. More laterally, under the brow, frontalis fibers interdigitate with the corrugator and orbital portion of the orbicularis muscles. The frontalis muscle does not extend laterally beyond the junction of the middle and lateral thirds of the brow, so that the lateral brow lacks an elevator. Because of this the lateral brow is under the depressor influence of the lateral orbicularis muscle.[29] This results in progressive lateral brow ptosis with age, and is the rationale of using botulinum toxin into the lateral orbicularis muscle to help elevate the lateral brow.

The superficial fascia over the forehead and brows is relatively thin, so that the skin is closely applied to the superficial galea over the frontalis muscle by fibrous septa that extend through the galea and superficial fat to the dermis. Transverse forehead wrinkles, perpendicular to the frontalis muscle, are related to very thick zones of vertical fibrous septa.[29,142] The frontalis muscle is separated from the periosteum by a fat pocket in the deep fascia of the forehead. This has been referred to as the sub-brow fat pad or the superior retro-orbicularis oculi fat pocket (ROOF).[20,111] It extends from the supraorbital notch medially to the temporal ligamentous adhesion laterally. This fat pad measures approximately 1 cm vertically and is 5 mm in thickness. It lies within a split in the deep galea, and is analogous to the fat pad between the superficial and deep temporal fascial layers over the temple. The ROOF helps cushion the brow during movement. Not uncommonly the ROOF may continue into the upper eyelid through the orbicularis retaining ligament, where it extends downward within the postorbicular fascial plane, anterior to the orbital septum and behind the orbicularis muscle.[30] In some individuals, fat lobules may extend very deep into the eyelid proper and be confused with the preaponeurotic fat pockets. A second split is present in the deepest layer of the galea beneath the brow, and ends just above the orbital rim where the deep galea finally fuses to periosteum.[29] This serves as a deep glide plane for the lower forehead and brow.

The frontalis muscle elevates the brow, and together with the occipitalis belly, tightens the scalp and provides mobility of the skin along the temples. Brow elevation may be transmitted through other tissues to serve as an accessory retractor of the eyelid. This function is learned early in patients with congenital or acquired blepharoptosis, and is the basis for the frontalis suspension operations used to repair poor-function upper eyelid ptosis. Because of this contribution to eyelid elevation it is essential to mechanically immobilize the frontalis muscle during preoperative evaluation of levator muscle function in ptosis patients.

With progressive stretching of supraorbital tissues, loss of frontalis muscle tone, and disruption of attachments to both superficial and deep fascial layers, brow ptosis may be a prominent feature of the aging face. Because deeper fascial attachments are particularly sparse over the lateral orbital rim, and because the frontalis muscle does not extend to the lateral edge of the brow, eyebrow ptosis is frequently more prominent temporally. A more important factor relating to temporal brow ptosis is the structure of the orbicularis retaining ligaments (see below) which are longer and less rigid laterally, and therefore prone to age-related laxity. Brow ptosis may be repaired by direct elevation with resection of skin from just above the brow cilia, through a temporal hairline or mid forehead incision, or through a coronal forehead elevation.[122] During repair of brow ptosis, except in cases of frontalis paralysis, the muscle should not usually be fixed to the underlying periosteum, as this will severely limit brow mobility. Also, for adequate brow elevation, the orbicularis muscle retaining ligaments may be divided to allow for maximum mobility and redraping of the skin.

Procerus muscle

The procerus muscle is a small pyramidal slip closely related to the frontalis muscle complex. It arises by tendinous fibers from the periosteum of the lower portion of the nasal bone, the perichondrium of the upper lateral nasal cartilage, and from the aponeurosis of the transverse nasalis muscle.[96] The medial portions of each procerus muscle often fuse in the midline with its contralateral counterpart, forming a single central belly over the nasal dorsum.[29] The muscle then passes vertically between the brows and separates into its paired heads which interdigitate with the medial border of the frontalis muscle. Distally, the procerus muscle is said to insert onto the dermis of the skin over the lower forehead, between the frontalis muscles. However, Daniel and Landon[29] found in their dissections that the procerus extended high onto the mid forehead.

Contraction of the procerus muscle draws the medial angle of the brow downward and produces transverse wrinkles over the nasal bridge. Recent studies demonstrated that the procerus muscle is supplied by a nerve from the buccal branch of the facial nerve,[65,113] after having received a contribution from the zygomatic branch.[18] This nerve courses inferomedially around the orbicularis muscle and between the nasion and medial canthal angle, and has been termed the angular nerve.[18] Injection of botulinum toxin for reduction of glabellar folds should take the placement of this innervation into consideration. During coronal brow elevation procedures, reduction of cosmetically objectionable glabellar folds often requires cutting of the procerus muscles. In patients with essential blepharospasm the procerus is usually involved so that this muscle must be extirpated during myectomy procedures or weakened with chemodenervation.

Depressor supercilii muscle

The depressor supercilii muscle was previously thought to be part of the orbicularis muscle.[94] However, most anatomists now consider this as a distinct muscle separate from the corrugator, procerus, and orbicularis muscles.[1,25,29,70] It arises from the frontal process of the maxillary bone near the edge of the medial orbital rim, about 8–10 mm above the medial canthal ligament, and 2–5 mm below the frontomaxillary suture line. It usually arises as two distinct heads, with the angular vessels passing between the heads. The muscle passes deep to the lateral edge of the procerus muscle, and over the origin of the corrugator muscle to insert into the dermis about 13–15 mm directly above the canthal ligament.

Corrugator supercilii muscle

The corrugator supercilii muscle forms a coarse pyramidal band of fibers beneath the main portion of the frontalis muscle complex, and the medial orbicularis muscle.[16] It arises from a broad base at the medial end of the frontal bone at the superomedial orbital rim, about 10 mm above the medial canthal ligament. Here some of its fibers blend with the deep portion of the preseptal orbicularis muscle. Park et al.[118] reported the corrugator muscle to arise as 3–4 vertically oriented long, narrow rectangular bands that run parallel to each other to their points of insertion. However, most reports show the muscle to arise as a single muscle mass which then divides into two heads—oblique and transverse. The oblique head runs superiorly and slightly laterally along the junction of the palpebral and orbital fibers of the orbicularis muscle. It interdigitates through the frontalis and orbicularis muscles, and inserts into dermis along the medial eyebrow near the insertion of the depressor supercilii. This head of the corrugator, along with the depressor supercilii, the procerus, and the medial slip of the orbital portion of the orbicularis muscle, act to depress the medial brow.[89,90]

The larger transverse head of the corrugator muscle passes laterally and slightly superiorly. It divides into 6–8 discrete fiber bundles that run immediately beneath the orbital portion of the orbicularis muscle, and within the galeal fat pad between the deep layers of the subfrontalis galea. These slips insert into the deep fascia of the frontalis and orbicularis muscles along the central, and less commonly the lateral, one-third of the brow, about 4 cm lateral to the midline.[71] In this region the deep fascia is composed of several distinct layers, and corrugator muscle fibers may be seen to interdigitate among them. Muscle fibers may sometimes extend far laterally to the lateral third of the brow. Nerve supply is from the facial nerve, largely through the temporal branches, but with some contribution from the zygomatic and buccal branches.[18] The temporal branches innervate the transverse head. These fibers lay 1 cm lateral to the supraorbital foramen, and vary from 3–25 mm above the orbital rim.[66] They can be injured during direct brow elevation surgical procedures. The angular nerve, from the buccal branch of the facial nerve, passes below the lower eyelid and medial to the medial canthus, to innervate the oblique head of the corrugator muscle and the procerus muscles. Contraction of the corrugator muscle pulls the brow medially and downward, and produces vertical glabellar folds. Several cases of congenital agenesis of the corrugator muscle have been described.[4]

The eyelids

Embryology

The upper and lower eyelids develop from mesenchymal folds above and below the optic cup beginning during the 8–12 mm (4–5-week) embryonic stages.[131] The connective tissue within these folds is believed to be of neural crest origin.[93,95] These folds are the frontonasal (paranasal) and maxillary (visceral) processes, and are continuous anteriorly with folds forming the boundaries of the nasal pit. The mesenchyme within these folds differentiates into several tissues; tarsus posteriorly, and orbital septum anteriorly. During the second month of gestation these mesenchymal folds proliferate, beginning at the future lateral canthus.[115] These folds move toward each other by differential growth,[8] and elongate medially. Blood vessels and macrophages enter the folds during the third month.[8] Rudiments of the orbicularis muscle develop from mesenchyme of the second visceral arch, and migrate into the lids during the 10th week of fetal life. Nerve fibers enter the eyelids at this time, primarily associated with motor endings on conjunctival vascular elements and within the orbicularis muscle.[102] The levator muscle develops from orbital mesenchymal tissue, differentiating from the primordial superior rectus muscle. Its aponeurosis migrates into the eyelid, eventually establishing contact with the anterior tarsus and orbicularis muscle. The enlarging eyelid folds finally make contact along their margins during the 45 mm (10th week) fetal stage, and temporarily fuse by desmosomes, thus isolating the eyes from amniotic fluid.[7]

Beginning in the 40 mm (10-week) stage the first cilia appear in the surface epithelium along the eyelid margins. The hair follicles form as proliferating epithelial cells and penetrate, along with their basal laminae, into the underlying mesenchyme. Mucus-secreting goblet cells are seen in the conjunctiva beginning at the 52 mm (11-week) fetal stage. Meibomian glands first appear as epithelial buds during the 80 mm (13-week) stage, and glands of Moll and Zeiss are seen between the 80 and 100 mm (13–15-week) stages associated with the developing cilia.

The fused eyelids begin to separate along their anterior margins during the 150–170 mm (5th month) stages. The posterior margin follows shortly thereafter, during the 180 mm stage. This dysjunction results through disruption of the desmosome epithelial bridges, possibly related to holocrine production of lipids in the developing meibomian glands.[8] Separation is complete by about the 200 mm (25-week) stage. Failure of complete separation results in varying degrees of ankyloblepharon.

The adult eyelid

In the young adult the interpalpebral fissure measures 10 to 11 mm in vertical height, but with advancing years the upper eyelid assumes a more ptotic position, resulting in a fissure of only about 8–10 mm. The horizontal length of the fissure is 30–31 mm, and is achieved by the age of about 15 years.[60] The upper and lower eyelids meet medially and laterally at an angle of approximately 60°. Laterally, this canthal angle rests against the globe, but medially it is displaced away from the globe about 5–6 mm. Within this medial space, called the lacus lacrimalis, are a fleshy mound, the caruncle, and a fold of conjunctiva lateral to it called the plica semilunaris. The interpalpebral fissure is usually inclined slightly upward at its lateral end, such that the lateral canthal angle is about 2–3 mm higher than the medial canthal angle. In primary position of gaze, the upper eyelid margin usually lies at the superior corneal limbus in children and 1.5–2.0 mm below

it in the adult. The lower eyelid margin rests at the inferior corneal limbus. The upper eyelid marginal contour reaches its highest point just nasal to the pupil. These relationships should be kept in mind during ptosis repair or eyelid reconstructions.

The margin of each eyelid is about 2 mm thick. Posteriorly, the marginal tarsal surface is covered with conjunctival epithelium, interrupted by the meibomian gland orifices. Anteriorly, the margin is covered with cutaneous epidermis from which emerge the eyelashes. Separating these two regions is a faint linear zone, sometimes forming a slight sulcus. This is the gray line, which is the marginal projection of the pars ciliaris of Riolan's muscle (see below).

The upper eyelid crease is a horizontal indentation caused by attachments of superficial levator aponeurotic fibers into orbicularis intermuscular septa and subcutaneous tissue. It lies about 8–11 mm above the eyelid margin centrally. Medially, the crease is generally lower, about 4–5 mm from the lid margin. Laterally, it lies about 5–6 mm above the margin. In non-Asian eyelids, this crease should be reformed during ptosis or blepharoplasty surgery to maintain normal cosmetic appearance, and to prevent downward displacement of preaponeurotic fat or overhang of eyelid skin. In the Asian eyelid, the upper lid crease is typically less well developed due to the more distal attachment of the orbital septum onto the levator aponeurosis. This relationship allows the preaponeurotic fat to prolapse further into the eyelid, and prevents the anterior attachments of the levator aponeurosis into the orbicularis interfascicular septa.

A similar, but less well defined crease is present in the lower eyelid. It serves to retract the eyelid marginal skin downward with depression of the globe. Congenital absence of this crease results in epiblepharon, where the marginal eyelid skin rolls upward during downgaze and mechanically pushes the lashes inward against the cornea. This should not be confused with the rare occurrence of congenital lower eyelid entropion.[139] Correction of epiblepharon is by surgical reformation of the eyelid crease,[72] or placement of full-thickness eyelid sutures. Internal reformation of a disrupted crease following any lower eyelid surgery in which a skin-muscle flap is elevated will avoid postoperative secondary epiblepharon.

Orbicularis oculi muscle

The orbicularis oculi is a complex periocular striated muscle sheet that lies just below the skin and is an integral component of the superficial musculoaponeurotic system (SMAS). The SMAS is that part of the superficial fascia of the head and neck which covers the midface. It is continuous superiorly with the galea aponeurotica over the forehead, and laterally with the temporoparietal or superficial temporal fascia over the temporal fossa. Inferiorly, the SMAS is continuous with the platysma of the neck and lower face. The SMAS invests the muscles of facial expression, and separates the subcutaneous fat into two layers, a superficial and deep layer. It is connected to the overlying dermis by fibrous septa that extend through the superficial fat layer. Motor nerves to the facial muscles lie just inferior to the SMAS.

The orbicularis muscle is separated from the overlying dermis by a fibroadipose layer that forms the upper layer of the investing galea in the upper eyelid and the SMAS in the lower eyelid.[106] This is 4–6 mm thick just beneath the brow, but tapers to less than 0.1 mm in thickness in the pretarsal portion of the eyelids. Thick fibrous septa extend from the dermis through this layer, and merge with the interfascicular sheaths and epimysium of the orbicularis muscle fibers. These help maintain the skin and muscle as a single lamellar anatomic unit. Histologically, the orbicularis muscle consists of striated fibers that run parallel to the eyelid margins. The bundles are compact and separated by collagenous septa.

The orbicularis muscle is divided anatomically into four segments, three contiguous and one separate. The contiguous parts are the orbital, preseptal, and pretarsal portions of the orbicularis, and the separate part is the muscle of Riolan. The orbital portion of the orbicularis muscle overlies the bony orbital rims. It arises from insertions on the frontal process of the maxillary bone in front of the anterior lacrimal crest, from the orbital process of the frontal bone, and from the common medial canthal ligament. A medial slip of this muscle passes superficial to the depressor supercilii and the origin of the corrugator supercilii, and inserts onto the dermis at the medial brow.[90] The major bundle of fibers passes around the orbital rim to form a continuous ellipse without interruption at the lateral palpebral commissure. These fibers insert medially just below their points of origin. They are innervated by the temporal and zygomatic branches of the facial nerve, and serve as a sphincter of the eyelids.

The palpebral portion of the orbicularis muscle overlies the mobile eyelid from the orbital rims to the eyelid margins. The muscle fibers sweep circumferentially around each eyelid as a half ellipse, fixed medially and laterally at the canthal ligaments. Although this portion forms a single anatomic unit in each eyelid, it is customarily further divided topographically into two parts, the preseptal and pretarsal orbicularis.

The preseptal part is positioned over the orbital septum in both upper and lower eyelids, and its fibers originate perpendicularly along the upper and lower borders of the medial canthal ligament. The inferior preseptal muscle arises as a single head from the entire length of the common ligament. Posterior muscle fibers may be seen to attach to dense collagen fibers that insert onto the upper portion of the lacrimal sac.[145] The preseptal muscle arises by two heads in the upper lid. The anterior or superficial head is the more prominent, arising as a broad sheet from the upper surface of the common canthal ligament. The posterior head arises from the superior limb, and to a lesser extent from the posterior limb of the canthal ligament. The superior limb of the medial canthal ligament is fused to the fundus of the lacrimal sac by a layer of fibrovascular fascia so that on contraction, this deep head of the preseptal muscle pulls the sac laterally, thus contributing to the lacrimal pump mechanism (see Chapter 9). Fibers of the upper and lower preseptal muscles arc around the eyelids and interdigitate laterally along the lateral horizontal raphé. This structure may be indistinct in the majority of individuals, however. A few deep slips, primarily from the inferior preseptal muscle, extend backward to merge with the lateral canthal ligament. From its orientation, the preseptal orbicularis muscle appears to function largely in counteracting opposing tone in the retractors of the eyelids by distally displacing the levator aponeurosis and capsulopalpebral fascia. Secondarily, it likely contributes to the lacrimal pump mechanism at the level of the lacrimal sac.

The pretarsal orbicularis muscle overlies the tarsal plates. Its fibers in both upper and lower eyelids are attached to the medial canthal ligament via separate superficial and deep heads. The superficial head runs from the medial canthus and maintains its position anterior to the crura of the canthal ligament. As it passes over the ampulla of the canaliculi the muscle thickens to form a C-shaped cuff of muscle fibers that invest the canaliculus anteriorly, superiorly, and inferiorly. Contractions of these fibers compress and fold the canaliculi, and aid in the lacrimal pump mechanism (see Chapter 9). The superficial heads of the pretarsal orbicularis muscle extend across the eyelid to finally insert onto the lateral canthal ligament at a shallow angle, nearly parallel to the horizontal plane.

Medially, the deep heads of the pretarsal orbicularis muscle emerge from the superficial heads in the region where the latter thicken to partially invest the canaliculi. These fibers pass medially around the superior and inferior crura of the canthal ligament along with the canaliculi, remaining in intimate contact with the posterior surface of latter to the level of the common canaliculus. Thus, the canaliculi, for part or all of their lengths are nearly completely surrounded by muscle fibers of the superficial and deep heads of the pretarsal orbicularis muscle. Near the common canaliculus, the deep heads fuse and join with the muscles of Riolan running along the eyelid margins. Together, these fibers form a prominent bundle known as Horner's muscle that runs just behind the posterior limb of the canthal ligament. Shinohara et al.[133] observed that lateral to the medial canthal angle fibers from Horner's muscle arise from short fascicles along the eyelid margins, at least some of which presumably are Riolan's muscle fibers. Ahl et al.[3] observed that most of Horner's muscle fibers attach directly to the anterior surface of the tarsal plates, but in some cadavers it was continuous with fibers from the muscle of Riolan and the pretarsal orbicularis muscle. Horner's muscle attains a thickness of about 2.5 mm and a vertical height of 6 mm. As it passes backward, its fibers surround the medial third of the canaliculi just before they merge into the common canaliculus. Some of its fibers also fuse with the posterior limb of the medial canthal ligament that immediately overlies the fundus of the lacrimal sac, but they do not insert onto the sac.[145] Where the common canaliculus pierces the posterior limb of the ligament *en route* to the lacrimal sac, Horner's muscle fibers attach to its upper and lower surface.[3] Horner's muscle continues posteriorly to its point of insertion onto periosteum of the posterior lacrimal crest, immediately behind the posterior limb of the medial canthal ligament. Some fibers continue more posteriorly for a distance of 3–5 mm along the medial orbital wall. *En route* to the posterior crest several other structures join the posterior limb of the canthal ligament and the sheath of Horner's muscle. Together these form a retinaculum, analogous to the well described lateral retinaculum. They include the medial horn of the levator aponeurosis, the posterior layer of the orbital septum, and the medial check ligament. Horner's muscle helps maintain the posterior position of the canthal angle, and tightens the eyelids against the globe during eyelid closure. It may also contribute to the lacrimal pump mechanism through its relationship with the canaliculi, and by its insertions onto the posterior limb of the canthal ligament, and through the latter to the lacrimal sac. Reconstruction in the medial canthal region must take these functional relationships into consideration. Adequate orbicularis muscle tone is essential for proper eyelid apposition to the cornea, as well as for functioning of a normal lacrimal drainage.

Laterally, the pretarsal orbicularis muscle fibers from the upper and lower eyelids usually interdigitate along the surface of the lateral canthal ligament and the lateral horizontal raphé. There has been some controversy as to the presence of a true raphé. Some studies have failed to identify a tendinous intercalation between the upper and lower orbicularis muscles at the lateral canthus, and observed only a smooth continuous array of muscle fibers around the lateral angle.[54,80] Others have described an intercalation of muscle fibers forming a raphé beneath the skin and over the lateral canthal ligament.[68] The definition of the term raphé is broad and encompasses a wide variety of anatomic unions between two bilateral structures, so that it's application in the human eyelid, while of only nomenclatural significance and of no functional consequence, seems appropriate. Loose fibrous bands extend from the raphé to the lateral canthal ligament where they help maintain appropriate vector alignments of the muscle around the lateral curvature of the globe. Some fibers also extend anteriorly to the deep fascia of the subcutaneous tissue to help maintain the lateral canthal contour.

Muscle of Riolan

A distinct bundle of muscle fibers is present along the lid margin and is anatomically separated from the pretarsal orbicularis. This was originally described by Riolan as a single bundle along the free eyelid margin, between the tarsus and the orbicularis muscle.[126] Klodt[87A] described the microscopic features of this muscle and noted a distinct bundle of fibers located behind the meibomian glands. Virchow[140] later reported that Riolan's muscle was actually composed of two separate components: the larger pars ciliaris or pars marginalis originally described by Riolan, and the pars subtarsalis which corresponds to the fibers noted by Klodt. Wulc et al.[144] demonstrated that the pars ciliaris component actually corresponds to the gray line seen clinically along the eyelid margin.

The muscle of Riolan shows a very complex structure. The major portion, or pars ciliaris, runs parallel to the eyelid margin as a thin bundle of striated muscle fibers between the tarsal plate and the pretarsal orbicularis muscle, separated by a space containing the eyelash follicles. The individual muscle fibers are small, averaging about 30 μm in diameter.[100] In this regard they resemble the extraocular muscles. In their banding characteristics and neuromuscular junctions they do not differ from other skeletal muscles. The muscle of Riolan arises laterally from the deep surface of the pretarsal orbicularis muscle near the junction of the tarsal plate and lateral canthal ligament, but some fibers can be seen extending from the lateral canthal ligament and even from the lateral rectus muscle pulley system fascia.[83] Medially, the main superficial portion of the muscle of Riolan inserts around the puncta and ampullae of the lacrimal drainage system. Deeper fibers pass posterior to the canaliculi for a short distance before they finally blend into the deep or posterior heads of the pretarsal orbicularis (Horner's muscle).[100]

Unlike the rest of the orbicularis muscle whose fibers run circumferentially around the eyelids, some fibers in the muscle of Riolan along the tarsal border are arranged in very short bundles that run in various directions. Along the eyelid margins these can extend over the marginal surface of tarsus between the latter and the overlying conjunctiva, and occasionally even subconjunctivally onto the palpebral surface of the eyelid for a short distance. This is the portion previously referred to as the pars subtarsalis. In addition, prominent fine bundles joining the pars ciliaris and pars subtarsalis lie perpendicular to the lid surface between and around the lash follicles, penetrating into the fibrocollagenous substance of the tarsus. Here, minute bundles of muscle fibers surround the acini and ductules of the Meibomian glands. This third bundle was proposed as the pars fascicularis by Lipham et al.[100] These fiber bundles may help rotate the lashes toward the eyelid margin during closure. It is unclear whether these can also play any role in discharging glandular contents during blinking.

The postorbicular fascial plane

The postorbicular fascial plane is an avascular loose areolar layer between the orbicularis muscle and the orbital septum-levator aponeurosis fascial complex. It extends to the eyelid margin where it blends with the gray line. This plane is an important surgical reference. Within the lid it allows bloodless dissection and identification of the underlying orbital septum. On the eyelid margin, the gray line marks the approximate anatomic separation of the anterior skin-muscle lamella from the posterior tarso-conjunctiva lamella. This fascial space is also responsible for the easy accumulation of fluid and blood in the eyelid following surgery or trauma.

The postorbicular fascial plane is best defined beneath the pretarsal portion of the orbicularis muscle. Under the preseptal portion, this plane becomes more complex and contains a thin layer of fibroadipose tissue continuous with the deep brow fat pad (ROOF).[108] This tissue layer ends at about the level of the eyelid crease. Within it thin fibrous sheets extend from the epimysium of the orbicularis muscle and also directly from the interfascicular sheaths; these sheets pass through the fibroadipose layer as interconnected planes, and finally merge with superficial fibers of the orbital septum. This loose connective tissue plane allows some degree of slippage between the muscle and underlying orbital septum, while at the same time it maintains an integrated lamellar structure. Disruption of these fibrous connections during eyelid surgery is responsible for the secondary epiblepharon that may be seen following elevation of a lower eyelid myocutaneous flap, or overhang of the anterior lamella in the upper lid following ptosis, blepharoplasty, and other upper eyelid surgery. Fixation of the orbicularis muscle to the underlying septum or levator aponeurosis should be reestablished with a few interrupted sutures prior to closure in order to reform the integrated lamellar unit.

Clinical correlations

Dysfunction of the orbicularis muscle may be seen from numerous etiologies. Mechanical restriction may be seen with scarring from trauma or surgical repair. This may result in a deficient blink or various eyelid malpositions.

Benign essential blepharospasm is a focal cranial dystonia of uncertain etiology. It typically affects older individuals and is characterized by involuntary contractions of the orbicularis, procerus, and corrugator muscles. Spasms may be brief, simulating rapid eyelid blinking, or more sustained, resulting in functional blindness.[38] Symptoms are often worse during periods of stress, ocular surface irritation, and increased sensory input, such as bright lights. While the cause remains unknown, evidence suggests a neurotransmitter/receptor defect at the level of the basal ganglia. There is no cure, but symptoms can often be minimized by peripheral chemodenervation with botulinum toxin.

Hemifacial spasm is a unilateral condition seen in older individuals and characterized by tonic and clonic spasms of facial muscles in the distribution of the ipsilateral facial nerve. In most cases it is caused by a vascular compression of the seventh nerve at its exit root in the cerebellopontine angle. Surgical decompression of the seventh nerve can achieve a cure in many cases, but most often symptoms are controlled with peripheral chemodenervation using botulinum toxin.

Myokymia is a benign condition characterized by involuntary spontaneous localized twitching of a few superficial muscle bundles within a muscle. It often involves the lower eyelid, and less commonly the upper eyelid. The condition is exacerbated by caffeine, stress, anxiety, and lack of sleep. It is typically of short duration, and spontaneously resolves with 3–4 weeks.

Bell's palsy is an idiopathic, unilateral, paralysis of the seventh cranial nerve. It is characterized by weakness of the facial muscles on one side. The etiology is unknown, but thought to be inflammatory, perhaps in response to a virus. Swelling of the nerve within the temporal bone canal causes a compressive neuropathy. It is usually self-limited and resolves spontaneously, but may be permanent in some cases.

Myasthenia gravis is a chronic autoimmune disorder manifest by varying degrees of striated skeletal muscle weakness. It can affect the facial and eyelid muscles. Autoantibodies block the acetylcholine receptors at the neuromuscular junction, preventing muscle contraction.

The orbital septum

The orbital septum is a fibrous, multilayered membrane anatomically beginning at the arcus marginalis along the orbital rim. Contrary to conventional teaching, the septum is not a separate structure, but is continuous with other layers on the forehead and within the orbit. The inner layers of the septum are anterior continuations of the orbital fascial layers that contribute to the periorbita. At the arcus marginalis the periorbita separates into its component layers, with periosteum continuing over the frontal bone of the forehead, and the orbital fascial layers extending downward into the eyelid as the posterior layers of the orbital septum. The orbital septum, therefore, is the anteriormost septal sheet of the orbital fascial system, and therefore defines the anterior limit of the orbit. The anterior layer of the septum is formed by the deep galea from the forehead, which initially fuses to the arcus marginalis and then continues inferiorly as the anterior surface of the septum. The multilayered structure of the orbital septum is easily noted in most individuals during upper eyelid surgery.

Kakizaki et al.[79] noted that, at least in the Asian eyelid, the orbital septum in both the upper and lower eyelid is reinforced on its posterior surface by distinct thickenings, or "ligaments." In the upper eyelid they originate from around the trochlea, and course inferolaterally to the lateral orbital rim. These are denser in their lateral aspect. In the lower eyelid these ligaments arise from the posterior lacrimal crest and are more densely concentrated medially. The function of these structures is not clear, but they may serve to reinforce lines of tension within the septum.

Within the upper eyelid, the septum forms a nearly continuous layer that separates the anterior eyelid lamellae from the posterior lamellae and from the deeper orbital structures. It is interrupted only at the medial orbital rim where separations are present for passage of muscular and neurovascular structures. From the superior arcus marginalis the septum passes inferiorly between the orbicularis muscle and the preaponeurotic fat pockets. Distally, the septum is loosely joined to the levator aponeurosis. The point of insertion is usually about 3–5 mm above the tarsal plate, but may be quite variable, occasionally as much as 10–15 mm. Hwang et al.[63] showed that in the Asian eyelid a posterior layer of the septum wraps around the distal preaponeurotic fat pad and is then reflected upward along the surface of the aponeurosis and continues up to Whitnall's ligament. According to this finding, the preaponeurotic fat is completely enclosed within a thin layer of orbital septum, rather than lying between the septum and the aponeurosis, at least in the Asian eyelids they examined. The more anterior layers of the septum gradually interdigitate distally with those of the levator aponeurosis.[12]

In the Caucasian eyelid Rein et al.[124] reported that after fusing with the aponeurosis, the anterior layer of the septum continues to extend downward over the distal aponeurosis and along the anterior tarsal surface. They called this the 'septal extension' and noted fibrous connections from the aponeurosis passing through this membrane to the overlying orbicularis muscle and skin. They followed the earlier suggestion by Putterman and Urist[123] that tucking this layer during ptosis repair could result in operative failure. This membrane may be the same structure previously described by some authors as the tendon of Muller's muscle.

In the lower eyelid the orbital septum originates from the arcus marginalis of the inferior orbital rim. Medially, the septum arises just inside the rim, whereas laterally it is attached just outside and inferior to the rim.[77] As in the upper lid, the septum is composed of several layers of connective tissue continuous with the fascial membranes of the periorbita, and the deep fascia of the maxillary bone. The septum fuses with the anterior layer of the capsuloplapebral fascia 3–5 mm below the inferior border of the tarsus. The common fascial sheet then inserts onto the inferior tarsal edge.[11,23,58]

Medially the anatomy of the orbital septum is more complex. Here the septum divides into several layers and has an intimate relationship with the lacrimal drainage system. In the lower eyelid the anterior septal layer inserts onto the anterior lacrimal crest, and onto the inferior border of the fibrous medial canthal ligament. A posterior layer separates and passes posteriorly around the lacrimal sac. It is fused to periorbita along the orbital opening of the nasolacrimal duct, and also to the fascia of the lower lacrimal sac. In the upper eyelid an anterior layer of the orbital septum inserts onto the superior limb of the medial canthal ligament and onto the orbital process of the maxillary bone. Here it encloses the lacrimal sac fossa anteriorly, and is interrupted along the canthal ligament for penetration of Horner's muscle. Thus, the anterior layer of the septum forms an anterior fibrous wall to the lacrimal sac fossa. A thicker intermediate septal layer separates from the anterior layer and passes backward around the lacrimal sac in both upper and lower eyelids. It inserts along the posterior crus of the canthal ligament and onto the posterior lacrimal crest, just in front of Horner's muscle.

The anterior and intermediate layers of the orbital septum effectively isolate the lacrimal sac and duct within their own fascial compartment, separate from the eyelid and orbit.

The walls of this compartment are interrupted only along the canthal ligament where the canaliculi enter, and at the entrance to the bony nasolacrimal canal. A very thin posterior layer of the septum separates from the intermediate layers and lies immediately behind Horner's muscle. It inserts as a sheet onto periorbita behind the posterior lacrimal crest.

Laterally, the orbital septum passes slightly behind the bony orbital rim where it inserts onto the lateral canthal ligament, and the lateral retinaculum at the orbital tubercle in company with the lateral horn of the levator aponeurosis.[2]

Immediately behind the orbital septum are the yellowish preaponeurotic fat pockets, which help in its identification during surgery. However, as mentioned above, the sub-brow fat pad may extend into the eyelid within the postorbicular fascial plane, and this can be confused with the preaponeurotic fat pockets. In this case, the orbital septum could be misidentified as the levator aponeurosis. Attempted advancement of this septal layer will result in significant lagophthalmos and corneal exposure.[34] These anatomical relationships are important to note, since advancement of the levator aponeurosis or capsulopalpebral fascia without first separating the septum can cause a tethering of the lid to the orbital rim with resultant eyelid retraction. Also, the orbital septum should not be closed, either during eyelid surgery, or during repair of trauma, since this carries the risk of inadvertent shortening and lagophthalmos.

In younger individuals the orbital septum may form a thick fascial layer that is readily identified at surgery. In older patients, and in younger individuals as a familial trait, the septum may be a flimsy, transparent film through which orbital fat pockets easily herniate. At surgery, the septum can usually be identified by pulling it distally and noting the firm resistance against its bony attachments.

The preaponeurotic fat pockets

The preaponeurotic fat pockets in the upper eyelid, and the precapsulopalpebral fat pockets in the lower eyelid are anterior extensions of extraconal orbital fat. However, these pockets are surrounded by thin fibrous sheaths that are forward extensions of the anterior orbital septal system that separate the eyelid fat pockets from the deeper orbital fat lobules. Within the limiting sheath surrounding the entire fat pocket, each of the individual lobules is surrounded by secondary interlobular septa. Very fine septal bands interconnect these sheaths with the overlying orbital septum and with the underlying levator aponeurosis or capsulopalpebral fascia. These eyelid fat pockets are surgically important landmarks and they help identify a plane immediately anterior to the major eyelid retractors. In the upper eyelid these fat pockets lie just in front of the levator aponeurosis, a relationship that is essential to remember during eyelid surgery under general anesthesia, or in traumatized eyelids. With weakening and redundancy of the orbital septum, the fat pockets bulge forward, producing the puffy and baggy eyelids seen commonly in the elderly, or as a familial trait in some younger individuals.

The distinction of the individual fat pockets in upper and lower eyelids has been questioned. However, several studies have demonstrated septal compartmentalization that can restrict dye diffusion.[7,14,134,143] In the upper eyelid there are usually two major fat pockets, a medial and a central one, that are separated by fascial connections continuous with the trochlea and superior orbital fascial systems. Each pocket is covered anteriorly by a thin capsule loosely adherent to the underlying levator aponeurosis. The medial pocket is whiter in color, and contains thicker, more abundant interlobular septa. The central pocket is larger and fills the middle half of the upper eyelid. The orbital septum is situated anterior to the fat lobules, separate from the interlobular septa. During blepharoplasty or ptosis operations in which fat is to be removed, these capsules must be opened to allow the fat to freely prolapse forward. However, when fat is not resected, these capsules should be preserved intact to prevent loose fat lobules from extending downward between the aponeurosis and orbicularis muscle, thereby "orientalizing" the eyelid. Establishment of a connective tissue barrier by surgically reforming the lid crease will prevent such displacement. The lacrimal gland is located laterally in the upper eyelid, just under the orbital rim. Normally it is not visible during eyelid surgery. However, when its fascial support system becomes lax, the lacrimal gland may prolapse downward beneath the bony rim, where it can easily be mistaken for a lateral fat pocket. Its lobulated structure, firmer texture, and pinker color distinguish it as a gland. Occasionally a thin fat layer is present behind the orbital septum in the lateral upper eyelid, seen in 21% of normal individuals.[119] It is a lateral extension of the central pocket and often extends over the surface of the lacrimal gland. The interlobular fascial membranes may fuse with the capsule of the lacrimal gland making distinction more difficult. It is important to recognize this fat layer during blepharoplasty surgery in order to dissect it from the gland.

In the lower eyelid, three fat pockets are continuous with the extraconal orbital fat compartments, but separated by fibrous septa continuous with the orbital connective tissue system. The central and lateral pockets are separated by a connective tissue extension from Lockwood's ligament called the arcuate expansion. The latter runs inferolaterally from the fusion zone joining Lockwood's ligament and the capsulopalpebral fascia to the inferolateral orbital rim. The lateral fat pocket may be multiple, which explains the frequent residual lateral lid bulge following blepharoplasty surgery. The central and medial fat pockets are separated by the inferior oblique muscle and its fascial system. In individuals with more prominent eyes, the inferior oblique muscle can be located at the orbital rim or even anterior to it, so care must be exercised to avoid injury to this structure during lower eyelid surgery.

As noted above, the orbital septum inserts onto the zygomatic bone inferolaterally just outside the orbital rim. A small fat lobule extension from the lateral precapsulopalpebral pocket in the lower eyelid spills over the rim in this region and also extends upward between the orbital septum and the lateral canthal ligament. This has been referred to as Eisler's pocket.

Despite the traditional description of fat pockets in the lower eyelid, there is considerable variation in compartmentalization, from three to only a single fat pocket.[77,114] An encapsulated pretarsal fat compartment has also been described laterally between the tarsus and orbicularis muscle, outside and above the orbital septum. This can contribute to the lateral bulk of the eyelid just below the eyelashes.[77] Rohrich et al.[127] recently demonstrated the isolation of the lower eyelid fat pads from deeper orbital fat. They found the eyelid fat pockets posteriorly to be separated from deep orbital extra-conal and intraconal fat by distinct fascial membranes. These membranes were located at the level of the globe equator, closely associated with the previously described rectus muscle pulleys (see Chapter 3). Rohrich et al. termed them the "circumferential intraorbital retaining ligament".

Levator palpebrae superioris muscle

In the upper eyelid the levator palpebrae superioris muscle arises from the lesser sphenoid wing just above the annulus of Zinn, superolateral to the optic canal. The muscle is about 36 mm in length.[95] At its origin it measures about 4 mm in width, and widens to 8 mm in the mid-orbit. As it passes forward it remains in close approximation to the superior rectus muscle. Unlike the rectus muscles, the levator muscle does not show the layered structure of orbital and global fibers, but is rather uniform throughout its width. Fibrous strands of the superior fascial system extend between the levator and superior rectus muscles. These are most prominent along the lateral and especially along the medial sides of the muscles, and become stronger more anteriorly.[95] Along the anterior third of the levator muscle, posterior to Whitnall's ligament, a thin sheet of fibrous tissue separates and interconnects the levator muscle sheath with the superior rectus muscle.[69] More anteriorly this becomes thicker until it completely envelopes the levator, fusing with a similar covering around the superior rectus muscle. Hwang et al.[69] referred to this as the "conjoint fascial sheath". This possibly acts as a check ligament that allows for coordinated movement of the upper eyelid with changes in vertical ocular gaze position. Fibrous attachments also run downward about 2 mm from this structure to the superior conjunctival fornix forming the forniceal suspensory ligaments.

Just behind the superior orbital rim the levator muscle widens to about 18 mm. Kakizaki et al.[78] noted that in its distal portion the levator muscle divided into two layers, superior and inferior, separated by connective tissue. The superior layer continued into the levator aponeurosis, but the inferior layer passed into Müller's smooth muscle. At this point a variably thickened condensation is seen within the muscle sheath around the levator muscle. This structure runs horizontally across the superior orbit and attaches medially to the fascia around the trochlea, and laterally onto the capsule of the lacrimal gland and periosteum of the frontal bone. This condensation is firmly adherent to the levator muscle sheath along its medial and lateral surfaces, but is only loosely attached centrally. It forms the superior transverse orbital ligament of Whitnall (see Chapter 7). A thin, often diaphanous, fascial sheet passes from Whitnall's ligament, downward around the preaponeurotic fat pockets, and then upward again to insert onto the superior orbital rim.[95] As its fibers pass around and through the preaponeurotic fat pockets, it fuses to the interlobular septa. This structure may work along with the septal layer noted above to retract the fat pockets upward during upgaze, to prevent bulking of eyelid tissue. The sometimes disappointing results obtained following ptosis repair, with a bulky upper eyelid, may result from disruption of these fascial sheets during dissection of fat lobules from the surface of the aponeurosis.

The superior suspensory ligament of Whitnall is formed by a condensation of the fascial sheath around the levator muscle, near the level at which the latter passes into its aponeurosis, just behind the superior orbital rim. It usually appears as a prominent white fibrous band. Lim et al.[98] noted that this structure was weekly developed or undifferentiated in 40% of their cadaver specimens. Although this might have been an age-related phenomenon since the average age of their sample was 66.8 years, nevertheless we have noted a poorly developed or unrecognizable ligament in many patients at the time of ptosis surgery. Codère et al.[22] noted that Whitnall's ligament consisted of an inferior and a superior component that completely invested the levator muscle. Ettl et al.[43] confirmed that Whitnall's ligament consisted of two distinct layers; a transverse layer below the levator muscle that is part of the conjoined fascia between the levator and superior rectus muscles, and a superior transverse ligament. They reported that the latter inserts medially onto periosteum of the orbital wall and the adjacent suspensory system of the trochlea. It also extends to the medial horn of the levator aponeurosis and to the pulley of the medial rectus muscle. Laterally, weak fibers of Whitnall's ligament blend with the capsule and suspensory ligaments of the lacrimal gland, and also with periosteum of the superolateral orbital wall above the gland. Some fibers continue inferiorly to the retinaculum of the lateral orbital tubercle and to the lateral rectus muscle pulley system. Whitnall's ligament contributes important suspensory functions for the superior orbital fascial system. Delicate fibrous bands extend from the levator muscle in the region of Whitnall's ligament, through the interlobular septa of the preaponeurotic fat pockets, to the superior orbital rim.

The exact role of Whitnall's ligament has been a matter of some controversy. However, it appears to provide some support for the fascial system that maintains spatial relationships between a variety of anatomic structures in the superior orbit. Although it has been suggested that this structure serves to redirect vector forces of the levator muscle from horizontal in the orbit to vertical in the eyelid,[11] Whitnall's ligament is usually very lax under normal physiologic conditions, and it seems unlikely that this structure can provide more than minimal supporting function.[95] There is some evidence that the globe provides a more important pivotal vector for redirection of levator forces to the eyelids.[135] This would explain the frequent occurrence of ptosis, superior sulcus deformity, and superior orbital volume loss following enucleation procedures. From its anatomic relationships, Whitnall's ligament appears to function as a hammock sling supporting the levator aponeurosis, but allowing it to swing anteriorly and posteriorly. Surface coil MRI studies have also shown that Whitnall's ligament is not situated at the apex of curvature where the levator muscle and aponeurosis change vector from horizontal to vertical, suggesting that it does not provide a true suspensory pulley function as was previously thought.[44] Whitnall's ligament may also serve as a check ligament against posterior excursion of the levator muscle, and through its connecting ligaments, of the superior rectus muscle, and the conjunctival fornix. Whitnall's ligament usually remains lax during eyelid closure, but with significant amounts of aponeurotic advancements it may result in some degree of lagophthalmos. During ptosis repair, cutting of this structure results in marked prolapse of the levator muscle and, therefore requires significantly more resection than would otherwise be necessary.[11] The supra-Whitnall's levator muscle resection procedure, with advancement of the muscle over Whitnall's ligament to the tarsus, preserves the fascial relationship in the superior orbit, and minimizes the amount of muscle to be resected.[40] If at all possible, this ligament should never be cut.

At Whitnall's ligament the levator muscle passes into its fibrous aponeurosis. Whitnall's forms as a thickening of the levator sheath both above and below the muscle, but the superior portion is the more prominent.[75] Both the upper and lower components are composed of collagenous fibers, elastic fibers and smooth muscle fibers.[97] Levator muscle fibers continue between these two ligamentous layers before passing completely into the aponeurosis. This transition is variable, and striated levator muscle fibers may continue for some distance below Whitnall's ligament. In such cases these muscle fibers lie beneath a thin and attenuated connective tissue layer, and may occasionally extend all the way to the tarsal plate. These muscle fibers can be seen to superficially interdigitate with the connective tissue layer anteriorly, and with Müller's supratarsal muscle posteriorly.

From Whitnall's ligament, the aponeurosis continues downward some 14–20 mm to its insertions.[10] Kakizaki et al.[81] have reported that in the Asian upper eyelid the levator aponeurosis consists of two distinct layers, with the anterior layer being thicker than the posterior layer. Both layers contain smooth muscle fibers, but most are concentrated in the posterior layer. The authors hypothesized that tension in the two layers may be regulated independently. They suggested that the anterior layer functions primarily to exert traction on the heavy preaponeurotic fat pad, elevating it with eyelid elevation, and the posterior layer was thought to be the major retractor of the eyelid. In the Caucasian upper eyelid, with rare exceptions, the aponeurosis consists of only a single layer, but with smooth muscle fibers still concentrated along the posterior surface.[76]

Inferior to Whitnall's ligament the aponeurosis is adherent to the underlying Müller's muscle by a loose connective tissue layer that can be dissected during ptosis and eyelid recession procedures.[58] This plane frequently contains spotty collections of fat that may be adherent to the aponeurosis, or infiltrated into Müller's muscle.[15,95,141] Occasionally, this fat layer may be so extensive as to be mistaken for the preaponeurotic fat pocket. Anteriorly, the aponeurosis is separated from the orbital septum by the preaponeurotic fat pockets, and from orbicularis muscle just above the tarsus by the postorbicular areolar tissue layer.

In some individuals the aponeurosis thins abruptly beginning 2–3 mm above the tarsus, and continues inferiorly as a thin translucent membrane that sends slips to the overlying orbicularis muscle. At this transition point, the distal edge of the thicker aponeurosis may appear as a sharp line. Below this line the peripheral arterial arcade and Müller's muscle can be seen through the more distal translucent aponeurotic membrane.[13] In such cases, it may appear that the aponeurosis is disinserted even though this thin anterior layer remains intact onto the tarsal face. However, in our experience this is an inconsistent feature.

Contrary to previous teaching, only a small percentage of the terminal fibers of the aponeurosis inserts directly onto tarsus. These insertions occur mainly along the lower two-thirds of the anterior tarsal surface, but are most firmly attached at about 3–5 mm above the eyelid margin.[10,23,98,137] Additional aponeurotic fibers insert into the pretarsal fascia that forms a thickened bundle along the lower 3–4 mm of the tarsus. Beginning 2–3 mm above the upper edge of

tarsus the aponeurosis sends numerous delicate interconnecting slips forward and downward to insert onto the interfascicular septa of the pretarsal orbicularis muscle. Some continue through the muscle to fuse with fibers of the subcutaneous fascia. These multilayered slips maintain the close approximation of the skin, muscle, aponeurosis, and tarsal lamellae, thus integrating the distal eyelid as a single functional unit and contributing to the formation of the Caucasian upper eyelid crease. Similar slips are found in the Asian double eyelid.[21] The major forces of retraction exerted by the levator appear to be to the anterior skin-muscle lamella rather than directly to the tarsus. The direct connections between the levator and orbicularis muscle may be related to their antagonistic relationship. On elevation of the lid, these slips retract skin and muscle to prevent overhang. The upper limit of these conjoined layers is marked by the upper eyelid crease. With stretching or disinsertion of the aponeurosis, the lower segments of these slips may become disrupted. In this case, upward retraction of the aponeurosis-orbital septum fascial complex exerts traction on the orbicularis muscle and skin through the more superior septum-to-orbicularis fascial connections, resulting in an apparent upward displacement of the eyelid crease. In a recent report by Lim et al.,[98] in older Korean cadaver specimens only a few fibers from the aponeurosis insert onto the overlying skin, with most fibers strongly attached to the lower 3 mm of the tarsal plate. This likely represents a racial and/or age-related difference.

As the levator aponeurosis passes into the eyelid from Whitnall's ligament it broadens to form the medial and lateral "horns." The lateral horn is stronger and far more complex. It differentiates from the superficial layers of the superolateral intermuscular septal layers that extend from the levator muscle to the lateral rectus fascial system, at about the level of the posterior globe (see Chapter 7). This structure forms a prominent fibrous sheet that indents the posterior aspect of the lacrimal gland, forming its orbital and palpebral lobes. It also separates the lacrimal gland fossa from the rest of the orbit, so that the gland sits within its own fascial compartment, bounded by the frontal and zygomatic bones laterally and the lateral horn medially. The lateral horn inserts through numerous slips onto the lateral orbital tubercle of the zygomatic bone, at the lateral retinaculum. Just before inserting, it fuses with fibers of the capsulopalpebral fascia from the lower eyelid.

The medial horn of the levator aponeurosis is less well-developed. It blends with the intermediate layer of the orbital septum, and inserts onto the posterior crus of the medial canthal ligament and the posterior lacrimal crest. Together, the medial and lateral horns serve an important function in distributing the forces of the levator muscle along the aponeurosis such that the central eyelid elevates maximally, while the more peripheral portions move progressively less. They also hold the upper eyelid in firm contact with the globe when the eye is opened. The horns are usually cut during eyelid recession procedures for eyelid retraction. During aponeurotic advancement procedures for ptosis repair, the central aponeurosis should be shortened with preservation of the horns. With large advancements, however, the horns may become redundant, and lose there supporting function. When the lids have normal orbicularis muscle tone, this is of little significance. However, when there is significant horizontal eyelid laxity, and when the aponeurosis is maximally advanced or the levator muscle is resected in combination with cutting of the horns, tarsal kinking and ectropion may result. This is avoided by advancing the levator muscle over Whitnall's ligament to tarsus with preservation of the aponeurosis and the horns in their normal configuration. During any eyelid surgery, the horns of the aponeurosis must not be confused with the slightly more superior attachments of Whitnall's ligament.

The capsulopalpebral fascia

In the lower eyelid the capsulopalpebral fascia is analogous to the levator aponeurosis in the upper eyelid. It is a fibrous sheet arising from Lockwood's ligament and from the sheaths around the inferior rectus and inferior oblique muscles (see Chapter 7). It passes upward and generally fuses with fibers of the orbital septum about 4.0–5.5 mm below the tarsal plate, closer on the medial side than on the lateral side.[67] From this junction, a common fascial sheet continues upward and inserts onto the lower border of tarsus. Fine fibrous slips pass forward from this fascial sheet to the orbicularis interfascicular septa and subcutaneous tissue, forming the lower eyelid crease. This unites the anterior and posterior lamellae into a single functional unit.[35] A medial head extends from the capsulopalpebral fascia to insert onto the medial canthal ligament. It continues under Horner's muscle to insert onto the posterior lacrimal crest.[82]

Müller's tarsal sympathetic muscles

Smooth muscles innervated by the sympathetic nervous system are present in both upper and lower eyelid. In the upper eyelid, the supratarsal muscle of Müller originates abruptly from the under surface of the levator muscle just anterior to Whitnall's ligament.[92] Here, striated muscle fibers in the inferior layer of the levator muscle and Müller's smooth muscle fibers may superficially interdigitate for several millimeters below the ligament. Müller's muscle runs downward, posterior to the levator aponeurosis, to which it is loosely adherent. It measures 8–12 mm in length, 0.5–1.0 mm in thickness, and spans across nearly the width of the tarsus. Smooth muscle fibers are interspersed with connective tissue, adipose cells, and numerous small vascular elements. Medially and laterally, smooth muscle fibers extend along fascial septa to the medial and lateral rectus muscle pulley systems.[109] A thin layer of fibrovascular tissue lies between Müller's muscle and conjunctiva, and between it and the levator aponeurosis.[23] Müller's muscle inserts onto the anterior edge of the superior tarsal border via a zone of dense connective tissue that fuses with collagen fibers of the tarsus.[92] This zone measures 0.5–2.5 mm in length and is about 0.1–0.5 mm in thickness. A thin fibrofatty elastic fascia, termed the pretarsal fascia, has been described extending from Müller's muscle surrounding the peripheral vascular arcade, and proceeding down along the anterior surface of the tarsus, separate from the levator aponeurosis. Haramoto et al.[57] proposed a dual elastic suspension system for the eyelid, with the elastic component of the aponeurosis mainly suspending the pretarsal structures, and the pretarsal fascia of Muller's muscle suspending the tarsus.

In the lower eyelid, smooth muscle fibers are present along the posterior surface of the capsulopalpebral fascia a short distance distal to Lockwood's ligament. They form a very thin, variably discontinuous sheet of muscle adherent to the posterior surface of the capsulopalpebral fascia. Muscle fibers extend upward from Lockwood's ligament and usually end 2–5 mm below the tarsal plate. Occasionally, smooth muscle fibers may extend all the way to the inferior border of tarsus.[59]

The accessory retractor muscles of Müller in the upper and lower eyelids are innervated by sympathetic nerve fibers derived from the paravertebral sympathetic chain, via the internal carotid plexus. Their course to the eyelids is not well understood, and probably lie along multiple pathways. They appear to reach their targets primarily along the orbital sensory nerves,[24] the levator muscle, and less so along the orbital arterial system.[103]

Matsuo[104,105] showed that stretching of Müller's muscle evokes electromyographic detection of involuntary contraction of the ipsilateral levator muscle. He suggested that Müller's muscle acts as a large serial muscle spindle of the levator muscle. According to this hypothesis, voluntary phasic contraction of the levator muscle during initial eye opening can evoke an afferent impulse to the mesencephalic trigeminal nucleus, with subsequent stimulation of the central caudal nucleus of the oculomotor nuclear complex. This leads to involuntary contraction of the ipsilateral or bilateral levator muscles in the form of a continuous stretch reflex. Thus, involuntary tonic contraction of the levator muscle to keep the palpebral fissures open may require traction on the mechanoreceptor mechanism of the Müller muscle by way of this reflex arc.

Clinical correlations of eyelid retractors

The most common cause of adult acquired ptosis is involutional thinning and stretching of the aponeurosis. Less frequently, the aponeurosis may show spontaneous local areas of dehiscence, or rarely even frank disinsertion from the tarsal plate.[11,74] In most cases of apparent disinsertion, it is more likely that the aponeurosis is so attenuated as to be missing along its lower edge, and therefore appear disinserted. Compensatory disinsertion or attenuation may be seen in patients with proptosis, such as in severe Graves' orbitopathy, resulting from forced eyelid closure in the presence of chord length tarso-ligamentous to globe disparity.[45] In all cases of eyelid ptosis, repair is directed at the source of pathology by shortening or reattaching the aponeurosis to tarsus.[11,39,40,74] Ptosis following cataract or other ocular surgeries may be seen in up to 13% of cases.[5,117] It is commonly believed to result from attenuation of the levator aponeurosis from manipulation of the superior rectus and levator muscles.[99] The degree of ptosis is significantly reduced if traction is restricted to the superior rectus muscle, and not transmitted through the superior conjunctiva and sub-Tenon's fascia,[101] or if a traction suture is not used at all.[17] Tension on the superior conjunctiva and Tenon's capsule exerts tension on the superior suspensory ligament of the conjunctival fornix, and through this structure, to the levator aponeurosis. Combined with the use of an eyelid speculum, excessive traction is exerted on the upper eyelid retractors, and may result in aponeurotic dehiscence or stretching.

In myogenic cases of upper eyelid ptosis where the levator muscle shows reduced function, it may not be possible to elevate the lid by shortening the aponeurosis. In these patients, resection of the levator muscle above Whitnall's ligament may use useful. When levator muscle function is poor to absent (less than 4 mm) it may be necessary to suspend the eyelid to the frontalis muscle using a sling material, such as a silicone rod or fascia lata.[36]

Following trauma to the eyelids, prolapse of orbital fat into the wound occurs with lacerations of the orbital septum. The septum should not be repaired, since this frequently causes shortening of this structure, with resultant lagophthalmos. With horizontal eyelid lacerations the presentation of orbital fat suggests deep eyelid injury to the level of the orbit, and should alert the clinician to the possibility of aponeurotic injury. Levator function is easily tested by asking the patient to look upward. Lacerations or disinsertions should be repaired primarily, if possible.

Entropion and ectropion are among the most common acquired lower eyelid malpositions.[73] These frequently result from involutional stretching of the capsulopalpebral fascia, horizontal laxity of the tarsus or canthal ligaments, or both.[35] As an added anatomic complexity, loss of posterior lamellar fixation of the preseptal orbicularis muscle may allow these fibers to ride up over the tarsus to the lid margin, resulting in an-epiblepharon-like "entropion". The relative contributions of these various factors will determine the exact nature of the eyelid malposition. Surgical repair should attempt to correct the specific anatomic defects.

Disruption of sympathetic innervation to Müller muscles, anywhere from its origin in the hypothalmus to its terminal postsynaptic branches in the eyelids, results in a form of Horner's syndrome. This is characterized by the classic triad of ptosis, miosis, and ipsilateral anhidrosis of the face. Specific clinical findings vary according to the location of the lesion along the polysynaptic pathway. The upper eyelid ptosis and elevation of the lower eyelid result from loss of sympathetic smooth muscle tone and accessory eyelid retraction. The existence of Horner's ptosis raises an interesting question as to the relationships between the levator aponeurosis and Müller's muscle in upper eyelid elevation. If under normal physiologic conditions the aponeurosis provides the major retracting force, as is generally accepted, then paresis of Müller's muscle would not be expected to produce ptosis. Horner's-induced ptosis implies that this sympathetic muscle is responsible for at least some elevation of the lid in normal situations. If this is true, then the aponeurosis must be relatively lax under normal physiologic states. However, involutional ptosis is a common phenomenon, generally attributed to aponeurotic stretching, and less frequently to frank disinsertion. However, inadvertent disinsertion of the aponeurosis during eyelid surgery does not usually result in immediate ptosis. Clearly, retraction of the upper eyelid is a more complex phenomenon than has been believed in the past, and appears to function as a cooperative dynamic interplay between the levator and its aponeurosis, and Müller's muscle. The exact roles of each in this process remains to be elucidated.

Overstimulation of Müller's sympathetic muscles may contribute in small part to eyelid retraction seen in Graves' orbitopathy. At surgery it is not uncommon to find this muscle somewhat thickened and hypertrophied. However, cicatricial shortening of the levator and Müller's muscles may play an equal or more significant role. In eyelids that cannot lengthen to accommodate advancing proptosis, retraction and lagophthalmos will result from chord length disparity between the tarso-ligamentous length of the lids and that of the anterior ocular surface.[93] Correction of upper eyelid retraction requires extirpation, division, or recession of Müller's muscle, and in about 60–65% of patients this will have to be combined with recession of the levator aponeurosis as well[19] Forward advancement of the lateral orbital wall may displace the tarso-ligamentous band to better accommodate the anterior ocular surface.[144]

Tarsal plates

The tarsal plates consist of dense fibrous tissue approximately 1.0–1.5 mm thick that give structural integrity to the eyelids.[53] Each measures about 25 mm in horizontal length, and is gently curved to conform to the contour of the anterior globe. The central vertical height of the tarsal plate is 8–12 mm in the upper eyelid, and 3.5–5.0 mm in the lower eyelid. The mean height of the upper tarsus is somewhat less in Asian eyelids (9.2 mm) than in Caucasians (11.3 mm).[54] Medially and laterally the tarsal plates taper to 2 mm in height as they pass into the canthal ligaments. As these tarsal plates approach the canthal ligaments they broaden slightly toward the margin, and narrow toward the proximal surface, thus assuming a more triangular cross-section. Within each tarsus are the Meibomian glands, approximately 25 in the upper lid and 20 in the lower lid. These are holocrine-secreting sebaceous glands not associated with lash follicles. Each gland is multilobulated and empties into a central ductule that opens onto the posterior eyelid margin behind the gray line. They produce the lipid layer of the precorneal tear film. Meibomian glands are innervated by sympathetic and sensory nerves, as well as by parasympathetic fibers, similar to the lacrimal glands.[91]

Although the Meibomian glands are not usually associated with lash cilia, they may occasionally revert to a pilosebaceous structural unit.[12] In congenital distichiasis, and in acquired distichiasis associated with chronic inflammatory diseases, the posteriorly situated ectopic cilia arise from the region of the Meibomian gland orifices. This may represent a regressive metaplasia of a specialized sebaceous gland back to a pilosebaceous unit.[33]

Obstruction of the Meibomian gland ductules by lipid and cellular debris, or by abnormalities of keratinization[56] may result in lipogranulomatous inflammation and frank infection, and the clinical manifestations of chalazion.[34]

Canthal ligaments

The terms canthal ligament and canthal tendon are used interchangeably in the medical literature without any medical justification. A tendon is a fibrous connective tissue structure that unites bone or cartilage to bone or cartilage. A ligament is a connective tissue structure that unites muscle to bone or cartilage. In the eyelids fibrous connective tissue bands join the medial and lateral tarsal plates to the adjacent orbital bones, forming the medial and lateral commissures or angles. Since the tarsus is neither muscle, cartilage, nor bone, both the terms tendon and ligament are technically inappropriate. Nevertheless, the tarsus is a structural component of the eyelid, functionally and anatomically, if not structurally, and therefore analogous to cartilage and bone. We therefore prefer use of the term ligament for the canthal suspensory structures. This is also the preferred term recommended in the current issue of Terminologica Anatomica.

Medially the tarsal plates pass into fibrous bands that form the crura of the medial canthal ligament. These lie between the orbicularis muscle anteriorly and the conjunctiva posteriorly. The superior and inferior crura of the medial canthal ligament fuse to form a stout common ligament that inserts via three limbs. The anterior or superficial limb passes medially where it initially measures about 1.5–2.5 mm wide and 1–2 mm thick. As it approaches the medial orbital rim the ligament fans out to a vertical width of about 3–5 mm and attains an anteroposterior thickness of 3–4 mm. The anterior limb is about 8–10 mm in length and inserts onto the orbital process of the maxillary bone in front of, and above the anterior lacrimal crest. It provides the major support for the medial canthal angle. The posterior limb of the medial canthal ligament arises from the common ligament near the junction of the superior and inferior crura, and passes between the canaliculi. As it extends along the posterolateral side of the lacrimal sac it is fused to the latter by a layer of fibrovascular fascia. As the posterior limb extends backward, it fans out to form a broad thin sheet about 1 mm in thickness and 6–10 mm in vertical width. This inserts onto the posterior lacrimal crest just in front of Horner's muscle. The posterior limb directs the vector forces of the canthal angle backward in order to maintain close approximation of the eyelids with the globe.

The superior limb of the medial canthal ligament arises as a broad arc of fibers from both the anterior and posterior limbs. It passes upward 7–10 mm where it inserts onto the orbital process of the frontal bone. The posterior head of the preseptal orbicularis muscle inserts onto this limb and the unit forms the soft-tissue roof of the lacrimal sac fossa. This tendinous extension may function to provide vertical support to the canthal angle,[9] but also appears to play a significant role in the lacrimal pump mechanism. The medial canthal ligament is clearly a complex structure with many interrelated functions. Replacement of an adequate substitute is important in reconstructive procedures. This is especially true in the lower eyelid where vertical support is necessary to oppose the forces of gravity.

Laterally the tarsal plates pass into less well developed fibrous strands that become the crura of the lateral canthal ligament. Contrary to some earlier views, the lateral canthal ligament is a distinct entity separate from the orbicularis muscle, and can easily be followed on histologic sections. The crura unite to form the common ligament with superficial and deep components. The superficial component is continuous with the overlying orbital septum, and measures about 1 mm in thickness, 3–4 mm in width, and is approximately 9–10 mm in length.[68] It inserts onto periosteum of the lateral orbital rim. The posterior or deep component arises from the lateral edges of the tarsal plates. It measures about 6–7 mm in width, but broadens to about 9 mm as it approaches the zygomatic bone where it inserts onto the lateral orbital tubercle of Whitnall about 2.5–3.0 mm inside the lateral bony rim. The inferior border of the ligamentous insertion extends downward somewhat where it provides a countervailing vector to upper eyelid retraction. Along its superior border, the deep component of the lateral canthal ligament is contiguous with the lateral horn of the levator aponeurosis. Together they form a broad tendinous insertion onto Whitnall's tubercle about 6–10 mm in width, and extending upward to within 4.5 mm from the frontozygomatic

suture line.[52] Insertion of these fibers extends posteriorly along the lateral orbital wall, where it blends with strands of the lateral check ligament from the sheath of the lateral rectus muscle. This tripartite tendinous complex continues posteriorly for some distance as each of its contributing elements successively drop out. The lateral canthal ligament fibers end 5 mm inside the orbital rim. Fibers from the lateral check ligament end about 4.0–6.5 mm from the rim, and those from the lateral horn of the aponeurosis continue to about 8.5 mm from the rim. The fibrous connections between the check ligament, the lateral rectus pulley, and the lateral canthal ligament serves to displace the canthal angle laterally on extreme lateral gaze, analogous to retraction of the lids during upgaze and downgaze.[52,83,130] Several other ligamentous structures insert onto the lateral tubercle and, along with the lateral canthal ligament complex, form the lateral retinaculum. These are the lateral fibers of Whitnall's superior suspensory ligament, and the lateral portion of Lockwood's inferior suspensory ligament. Together, these structures make up the lateral palpebral complex.[6]

Anteriorly, fibers from the orbital septum of both upper and lower lids extend to, and blend with, superficial fibers of the lateral canthal ligament just lateral to the insertion of the pretarsal orbicularis muscle. The thickened septum then separates from the canthal ligament and continues to the lateral rim where it inserts at the arcus marginalis. Thus, the canthal ligament does have a "functional" anterior limb as described by Couly et al.[28] In this region, as the ligament passes toward the orbital tubercle, and the thickened septum continues to the orbital rim, a small lobule of fat from the precapsulopalpebral pocket extends upward between the septum and ligament. This is Eisler's pocket as described by Kestenbaum.[85] It provides a bursa-like surface and appears to allow some independent movement of the ligament and septum during eyelid motility, especially on lateral gaze.

The free portion of the lateral canthal ligament between eyelid and insertion is a rather flimsy structure. With advancing age it frequently becomes redundant, causing laxity of the lower eyelid. Reformation of lateral canthal support is important in reconstruction of the lower eyelid or in the correction of involutional ectropion. It is important to maintain proper anatomic alignment of the lids by attaching the ligament or its substitute to periosteum inside the orbital rim in order to prevent canthal angle dystopia.

Conjunctiva

The conjunctiva is a mucous membrane that covers the posterior surface of the eyelids and the anterior pericorneal surface of the globe. The palpebral portion is closely applied to the posterior surface of the tarsal plate and the sympathetic tarsal muscle of Müller. It is continuous around the fornices where it joins the bulbar conjunctiva. The superior fornix is located about 10 mm above the superior corneal limbus. A suspensory ligament consisting of fibrous tissue and smooth muscle arises from the conjoined tendon of the levator and superior rectus muscles and Whitnall's ligament, and inserts onto the apex of the superior fornix. This serves to elevate this loose conjunctival tissue with supraduction of the globe. The inferior fornix lies about 8 mm below the inferior corneal limbus, and is supported by a suspensory ligament that arises from Lockwood's ligament. This lies immediately behind the capsulopalpebral fascia and the infratarsal sympathetic muscle, and serves to pull the fornix downward with infraduction of the globe. During certain eyelid procedures, these suspensory structures may be cut, and therefore should be reconstructed with sutures passed from the conjunctiva through the levator aponeurosis or capsulopalpebral fascia in order to prevent conjunctival prolapse.

Histologically the conjunctiva consists of an epithelium with several layers of stratified columnar cells and underlying lamina propria of loose connective tissue. Near the cornea this changes to stratified epithelial cells that are continuous with the corneal epithelium. Goblet cells are present in the epithelium. Small accessory lacrimal glands are located within the connective tissue of the conjunctiva. A submucosa of fine connective tissue fibers contains a rich supply of lymphocytes and lymphatic vessels. Blood vessels and sensory nerves are located within the deeper layers of this submucosal zone.

At the medial canthal angle is a small mound of tissue, the caruncle. This consists of modified skin containing fine hairs, sebaceous glands, and sweat glands. Unlike skin, however, it is nonkeratinized, and contains accessory lacrimal gland elements. Just lateral to the caruncle is a vertical fold of conjunctiva, the plica semilunaris. The submucosa contains adipose cells and smooth muscle fibers resembling the nictitating membrane of lower vertebrates. This likely represents a vestigial remnant of the nictitating membrane that has been modified to allow enough horizontal slack at the shallow medial fornix for rotation of the globe.

Nerves to the eyelids

As discussed in Chapter 4, motor nerves to the orbicularis muscle derive from the facial nerve (VII), mainly through its temporal and zygomatic branches. The motor root of the facial nerve exits the braincase at the stylomastoid foramen, and continues anteriorly through the parotid gland, across the external carotid artery, and divides into two divisions, an upper temporofacial division and a lower cervicofacial division. The upper division further subdivides into the temporal, zygomatic, and buccal branches. The temporal branch runs within the temporoparietal fascia over the zygomatic arch. It divides into three to four branches beginning about 7 cm lateral to and 2 cm below the lateral canthal angle. Each branch runs medially and ends in 3–6 terminal twigs in the orbital portion of the orbicularis muscle, between 1.5–3.5 cm above the level of the canthal angles.[62] The zygomatic branch of the temporofacial division crosses the zygomatic arch deep to the facial muscles. As it approaches the lateral canthus it becomes more superficial to innervate the lower half of the orbicularis muscle.

The lower cervicofacial division gives rise to the mandibular and cervical branches, innervating muscles of the lower face and neck. There is variation in branching pattern, and in some individuals extensive anastomoses interconnect all these peripheral branches.

The sensory nerves to the eyelids derive from the ophthalmic and maxillary divisions of the trigeminal nerve. Sensory input from the upper eyelid passes to the ophthalmic division, primarily through its main terminal branches, the supraorbital, supratrochlear, and lacrimal nerves. The infratrochlear nerve receives sensory information from the extreme medial portion of both upper and lower eyelids. The zygomaticotemporal branch of the infraorbital nerve innervates the lateral portion of the upper eyelid and temple. These last two branches also innervate portions of the adjacent brow, forehead and nasal bridge. The lower eyelid sends sensory impulses to the maxillary division via the infraorbital nerve. The zygomaticofacial branch from the infraorbital nerve innervates the lateral portion of the lower lid and portions of the upper lateral cheek.

Vascular supply of the eyelids

Vascular supply to the eyelids is extensive (see Chapter 5). The eyelids receive their major blood supply through the ophthalmic artery, with some contribution from the external carotid system via the facial vessels.[42] Both the anterior and posterior eyelid lamellae receive blood through the vascular palpebral arcades.[84] The medial palpebral artery arises as the terminal branch of the ophthalmic artery. It exits the orbit beneath the trochlea and enters the eyelid just above the medial canthal ligament. Here it gives rise to a marginal arcade that runs horizontally about 2 mm from the eyelid margin between the orbicularis muscle and the tarsus. A peripheral arcade extends along the upper border of tarsus between the levator aponeurosis and Müller's muscle.[32] The palpebral arcades anastomose laterally with the superior lateral palpebral vessel from the lacrimal artery.

A larger inferior branch from the medial palpebral artery passes beneath the medial canthal ligament and enters the lower eyelid. It gives off a branch to the lacrimal sac and divides into a marginal and sometimes a peripheral arcade that continues horizontally to the lateral inferior palpebral artery. The marginal and peripheral arcades in each lid are interconnected by small tortuous branches that course anterior and posterior to the orbicularis muscle and the tarsal plate. Some branches extend to the overlying skin. Anastomotic connections pass from the anterior ciliary arteries through the conjunctiva to the palpebral arcades. Feeders to these arcades must be preserved in eyelid reconstructive procedures whenever possible. Vessels in the anterior eyelid lamellae also freely anastomose with the external carotid arterial system through the periocular branches of the transverse facial, superficial temporal, and angular arteries. Along the eyebrow, two arterial arcades run parallel to the supraorbital rim, anterior and posterior to the orbital portion of the orbicularis muscle. These anastomose laterally with the superficial temporal artery via the frontal branch, the zygomaticotemporal artery and the transverse facial artery, and medially with the supratrochlear artery. These periorbital arcades give off vertical branches that anastomose with the palpebral arcades.

Venous drainage from the eyelids begin as small superficial vessels draining the forehead and glabellar region. These coalesce into the supratrochlear and supraorbital veins that anastomose medially with each other, and with the angular and anterior facial veins that drain into the external jugular venous system. A transverse branch of the supraorbital vein runs along the orbital rim to anastomose laterally with the superficial temporal vein. The supraorbital and supratrochlear veins penetrate the orbital septum in the superior and superomedial orbit respectively to form the superior oph-thalmic vein that runs posteriorly to the cavernous sinus (see Chapter 6). An irregular interconnecting network of veins run from the supraorbital vein and the superior venous arcade to the superior palpebral vein running along the upper border of the brow. Branches from the facial and angular veins form a similar network in the lower eyelid that runs to the inferior palpebral vein along the lower border of the inferior tarsus.

Lymphatic drainage from the eyelids is extensive, but is restricted to the region anterior to the orbital septum. Eyelid lymphatics have been divided into a superficial pretarsal plexus and a deep post tarsal plexus that are interconnected through a subconjunctival network.[31] Using histochemi-cal techniques, Cook et al. confirmed the superficial plexus, but could not identify the post tarsal plexus.[26] The superfi-cial plexus was shown to have two compartmentalized com-ponents; a superficial preorbicularis plexus composed of many tortuous and linear lymphatic vessels situated in the epidermal and subcutaneous tissues between the skin and orbicularis muscle, and a similar postorbicularis (pretarsal) component.

Lymphatics from the eyelids drain into two groups of ves-sels. The lateral two-thirds of the upper eyelid and the lateral one-third of the lower eyelid drain inferior and lateral into the deep and superficial parotid and submandibular nodes, and then into the deep cervical nodes. Drainage from the medial one-third of the upper eyelid and the medial two-thirds of the lower eyelid is medially and inferiorly into the submaxillary lymph nodes and then into the anterior cervi-cal nodes.[27] More recent studies suggest that this classic con-cept of lymphatic drainage may not be completely correct and that drainage may be less precisely defined (see Chapter 6). Extensive excision of subcutaneous eyelid tissues or deep incisions in the inferolateral eyelid area may result in persis-tent lymphedema due to disruption of these vessels.

Periorbital facial anatomy

Superficial musculoaponeurotic system (SMAS)

The superficial musculoaponeurotic system or SMAS repre-sents the superficial fibromuscular fascial layer of the face and neck. This layer helps distribute forces of the facial mus-cles to the overlying dermis. While this global anatomic layer is very extensive and covers a large expanse of the face, neck, and scalp, regional differentiation and anatomic relation-ships have been used to nominally distinguish specific por-tions. In our usage the SMAS proper covers the malar region under the lower eyelid and over the cheek and the zygomatic eminence. Superiorly, the SMAS becomes continuous with the galea aponeurotica of the forehead which invests the frontalis muscle and extends over the forehead.[107] Laterally, the SMAS extends over the parotid gland where it is closely applied to the thin superficial parotid fascia, which is some-times considered as part of the SMAS. Inferiorly, the SMAS passes over the chin and neck where it is continuous with the platysma muscle. Superotemporally, the SMAS is often described as fusing along the posterior edge of the lateral orbital rim where it transitions into the superficial tempo-ral fascia covering the temporalis muscle. The latter contains the superficial temporal artery and facial nerve. However,

Gosain et al.[55] did not find any direct continuation between the SMAS and the temporoparietal fascia.

In the midface the SMAS invests the superficial mimetic muscles including the orbicularis muscle, the zygomaticus muscles, and the levator labii superioris muscle. It plays an important functional role in facial movement, containing the tendon fibers of the facial muscles that attach to the overlying dermis. These muscles have only a limited attach-ment to the underlying facial skeleton. Histologically the SMAS is distinct from the subcutaneous fat and has been described as having two layers. A deep layer of horizontal septa, containing collagen and elastic fibers, surrounds lob-ules of fat cells and underlies the facial muscles. It forms an areolar tissue layer just above the periosteum that helps provide a glide plane for movement of facial muscles. In sev-eral places retaining ligaments connect this and more super-ficial layers of the SMAS to the underlying periosteum. A more superficial layer of the SMAS has vertical septa con-nected to the overlying dermis and forms a superficial archi-tecture of rectangular lobules of fat cells.[50] A contrary view was taken by Yousif et al.[146] who argued that this superfi-cial fascial-fatty layer is actually distinct from the underlying SMAS, and that this layer thickens in the midface to create the superficial malar fat pad. It thins out superiorly, finally disappearing near the orbital rim so that in the lower eyelid the orbicularis muscle lies in direct contact with the dermis, without an intervening fat layer. The eyelid is the only place in the face where the SMAS and facial muscles are not cov-ered by a layer of fat.

Retaining ligaments

The periorbital region has an extensive arrangement of liga-mentous connections related to tissue compartmentalization and movement of overlying tissues. The superficial facial fas-cia or SMAS receives the insertions of those facial muscles that originate from bone (e.g. the zygomaticus major), and envelopes others that have no bony attachments (e.g. the orbicularis muscle). A fibrofatty layer is present above the SMAS through which fibrous septa extend to the skin. Deep ligamentous attachments pass from the SMAS to the perios-teum. These connections help define the amount and direc-tion of movement of overlying skin and muscle planes.[10] Moss et al.[110] introduced terms to clearly define these liga-mentous attachments. *True ligaments* were considered to be similar to skeletal ligaments being discrete cylindrical col-lections of fibrous tissue. They allow the greatest latitude of movement in all directions. Current definition of ligaments includes not only bone attachments but also cutaneous attachments.[136] In the face, these ligaments arise from deep fascia or periosteum and insert onto the undersurface of the SMAS, and then from the SMAS into the overlying dermis via the retinacula cutis. *Septa* were defined as linear fibrous walls extending between deep fascia or periosteum and the SMAS. Because of some confusion surrounding this term we prefer the use of the older term, *fusion line* or *fusion zone*, such as the superior temporal fusion line. These ligamentous attach-ments allow movement only perpendicular to the zone of attachment. *Adhesions* were defined as diffuse low density fibrous attachments between periosteum or deep fascia, and the superficial fascia. This structure restricts movement in all directions.

In the periorbital region there are a number of ligamentous structures of anatomic and surgical importance. The arcus marginalis is a septal ligamentous fusion line that extends circumferentially around the orbit along the bony rim. It serves for the attachment of the deep and superficial galea from the forehead, and periorbita from the orbital walls. The orbital septum extends from the arcus marginalis into the eyelids and represents continuations of the galea and orbital fascial septa.

At the superotemporal orbital rim the temporal ligamentous adhesion (TLA), also known as the temporal or orbital ligament, suspends the deep galea at the junction of the middle and lateral brow. It is situated about 10 mm from the orbital rim and measures about 15 mm horizontally by 20 mm vertically.[110] Three ligamentous structures radiate from the TLA. The superior temporal fusion line runs superiorly along the superior temporal ridge of the skull. This serves as the attachment zone for the galea medially and the superficial temporal fascia laterally. The inferior temporal fusion line runs obliquely over the temporal fascia from the TLA toward the external auditory meatus. It connects the deep and superficial temporal fascial layers over the temporalis muscle. The supraorbital ligamentous adhesion is a wide adhesion zone that runs horizontally from the TLA to the origin of the corrugator muscle. It extends from about 6 mm above the orbital rim, superiorly for a distance of about 2–4 cm,[110] and attaches the deep galea beneath the sub-brow fat pad and glide plane to the frontal bone.

The orbicularis retaining ligament (ORL) or fusion zone (periorbital septum of Moss et al.[110]) lies about 2–3 mm outside the orbital rim and runs from the origin of the corrugator muscle at the superomedial corner of the orbit, laterally and circumferentially around the orbit to end at the inferomedial corner of the orbit near the base of the anterior lacrimal crest.[51] Ligamentous attachments pass from periosteum to the deep fascia of the orbicularis muscle, that is the deep galea underlying the superior orbicularis and the SMAS underlying the lateral and inferior orbicularis. There are two areas where the ORL widens to provide a stronger adhesion zone. The larger one is located at the lateral orbital rim and has been called the lateral orbital thickening. It measures about 7 mm by 10 mm and is situated just superolateral to the insertion of the lateral canthal ligament. Muzaffar et al.[112] noted that this lateral thickening formed a single anatomic unit along with the lateral palpebral raphé of the orbicularis muscle and the deep head of the lateral canthal ligament at its insertion onto the lateral orbital tubercle.[48] They also described a lateral expansion from the lateral orbital thickening along the deep temporal fascia that seems to be similar to the inferior temporal fusion line described by Moss et al.[110] A smaller zone of adhesion along the ORL is located at the superolateral orbital rim above the zyomaticofrontal suture.

Inferiorly, below the orbital rim, the ORL fuses to the deep facial fascia (SMAS) underlying the orbicularis muscle and overlying the suborbicularis oculi fat pad (SOOF) Here it forms the cephalad boundary of the prezygomatic glide plane space.[112] The retaining ligaments are shorter and more taut medially where they provide greater support to the lower lid, whereas laterally they are longer and more lax.[51] In the lateral and central portion of the inferior orbital rim, the ORL thickens to provide a greater area of adhesion to the malar region. This is the same structure described by Kikkawa et al.,[87] and termed the orbitomalar ligament between the inferior orbital rim and fanning out through the orbicularis muscle to insert on the dermis of the malar skin.

The zygomatic ligaments originate near the inferior border of the zygomatic arch, just behind the insertion of the zygomticus minor muscle and 4.5 cm anterior to the tragus. They attach to dermis of the skin serving as an anchoring point,[46] and help to suspend the lateral cheek. Release of these ligaments is important in facelift procedures.[116] Laxity of the retaining ligaments is partially responsible for midface ptosis and decent of the malar fat pad as an aging phenomenon. Release of the zygomatic and orbicularis retaining ligaments allows for complete mobilization of the lateral cheek and orbicularis muscle for mid-cheek elevation in ectropion repair procedures.

Facial fat pads

The face is characterized by the presence of multilayered fat pads that are important for dynamic movement of overlying tissues. These can be divided into three basic layers, each further divided into a number of distinct compartments. There is considerable confusion and disagreement in the literature concerning the number of distinct fat pads and their terminology, so that a comprehensive understanding can be difficult. Nevertheless, we have distilled these into a simple interpretation necessary for understanding periorbital anatomy.

Immediately beneath the dermis over the face and forehead is the subcutaneous fat, a thin layer that is distinct from the underlying superficial fat layer. It varies in thickness, being thickest over the cheek and absent in the eyelids. Beneath the subcutaneous fat, the facial fat is present in two distinct layers. A superficial fat layer composed of several distinct pockets lies anterior to the SMAS, galea, and superficial temporal fascia. A deep fat layer is situated beneath the SMAS and its peripheral components, and lies, between it and the underlying periosteum. The superficial layer in the cheek is broadly referred to as the premalar fat pocket. It is traversed by numerous thin *retinaculi cutis* fibers most densely concentrated along the orbital rim. The malar fat pocket is further divided into three pockets.[129] The nasolabial malar fat pocket lies medial to the nasolabial fold, along the side of the nose. Beneath it the SMAS is thin or absent, and a scaffolding of fibrous septa pass through this fat pocket to the dermis. The medial cheek malar fat pocket is bounded medially by the nasolabial fold and middle cheek ligament, and extends superiorly to the inferior orbital rim. This becomes thickened over the zygoma where it forms the prominent malar fat pouch. Laxity of the SMAS and anterior fascial layers results in decent of the malar fat pocket with aging. The lateral malar fat pocket lies along the lateral orbital rim and extends over the anterior portion of the superficial temporal fascia.

The deep facial fat pockets lie posterior to the SMAS and its equivalent components elsewhere on the cranium.[37] On the cheek the sub-orbicularis oculi fat pad (SOOF) sits below the inferior orbital rim and medial to the nasolabial cheek ligament.[64] Using a dye diffusion technique Rohrich et al.[128] showed that the sub-orbicularis fat in the cheek was composed of two distinct areas, a medial component over the cheek along the lower orbital rim, and a lateral component extending from the lateral canthus to the temporal fat pocket. The SOOF is bounded superiorly by the orbicularis retaining ligament which separates it from the eyelid. It is more compact than orbital fat and laterally it is traversed by numerous fine bands of connective tissue fibers that form the diffuse coarse zygomatic ligaments between the orbicularis muscle and periosteum of the zygomatic bone.[48]

The aging face

Craniofacial growth was traditionally thought to end in early adulthood except for minor degenerative changes. The concept that the facial skeleton was in a state of continual change was introduced by Humphrey in 1858,[61] and later elaborated upon by Enlow,[41] who developed the idea of growth fields. According to this concept the frontonasal bones lay down new bone and drift forward while the midfacial skeleton resorbs and shows gradual posterior drift. Pessa[120] and Pessa et al.[121] concurred, presenting a theoretical model called Lambro's algorithm which postulated that the facial skeleton showed a gradual rotation around the orbit, such that the forehead rotates anteriorly and slightly inferiorly while the midface rotates posteriorly and slightly superiorly. This ontogenetic change in some sense reflects and continues the phylogenetic evolutionary changes seen in primate evolution. Shaw et al.[132] found that with aging the orbital aperture increased in the superomedial and inferolateral directions along with a flattening of the glabellar-maxillary angle. These changes in the facial skeleton with aging cause the bony angles of the face to become more acute, with resultant changes in soft-tissue support structures of the midface.[125]

Concomitant with loss of bony projection, aging changes occur in the facial soft-tissues, beginning in the third decade of life. Aging of the skin occurs both from intrinsic genetic mechanisms and from environmental exposure, primarily UV light.[86] Smoking may have a deleterious effect on skin aging by disrupting its microvasculature. The dermis loses collagen and elastin, and ground substance is replaced by fibrous tissue. The rate of cell renewal decreases. These changes result in skin laxity and the formation of creases perpendicular to the direction of muscle tension. Dry skin results from loss of sebaceous glands, and hyperpigmentation occurs from increased melanin. Skin wrinkles and folds advance with progressive skin laxity.

The superficial and deep fat pads of the face undergo changes that alter facial contour. The superficial subcutaneous fat layer shows gradual loss of volume, whereas in the discontinuous deep pockets fat depots accumulate from reduced metabolism and hormonal changes.[86] The orbicularis and zygomatic retaining ligaments become lax resulting in progressive descent of the adjacent fat pockets and overlying skin. The soft tissue pockets droop more between the retaining ligaments, presenting as folds. Inferior migration of malar tissues is especially prominent adjacent to the nasolabial line of fixation resulting in deepening of the nasolabial fold. The thicker portion of cheek skin and subcutaneous layers descend from the orbital rim to the malar eminence. The thinner eyelid skin comes to lie over the orbital rim. As the orbital septum becomes lax, preaponeurotic fat prolapses into the lower eyelid, eventually draping over the orbital rim. This causes loss of the smooth contour of the youthful lid-cheek junction. Laxity of the superior orbicularis retaining ligaments causes general brow and glabellar descent, but is more pronounced laterally so that lateral pronounced brow ptosis is seen as a progressive aging phenomenon.

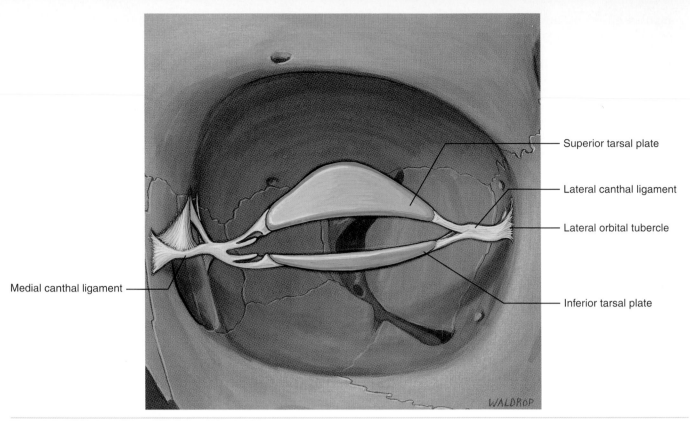

Superior tarsal plate

Lateral canthal ligament

Lateral orbital tubercle

Inferior tarsal plate

Medial canthal ligament

WALDROP

Figure 8-1 Tarsal plates with medial and lateral canthal ligaments.

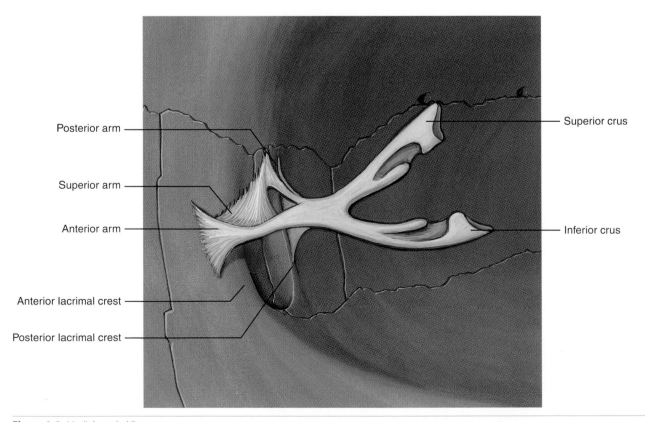

Posterior arm

Superior arm

Anterior arm

Anterior lacrimal crest

Posterior lacrimal crest

Superior crus

Inferior crus

Figure 8-2 Medial canthal ligament.

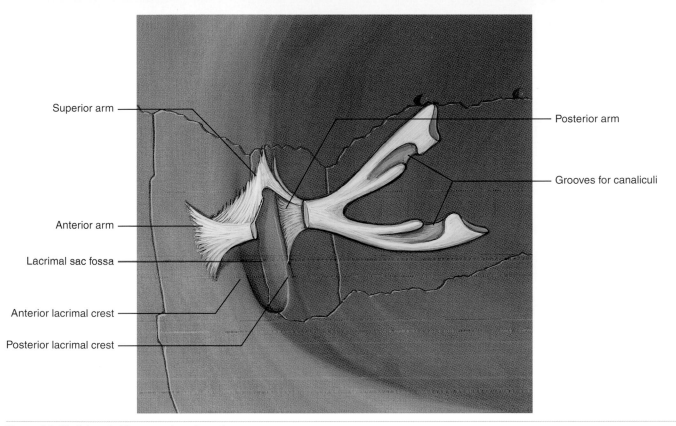

Superior arm

Anterior arm

Lacrimal sac fossa

Anterior lacrimal crest

Posterior lacrimal crest

Posterior arm

Grooves for canaliculi

Figure 8-3 Medial canthal ligament, deep dissection.

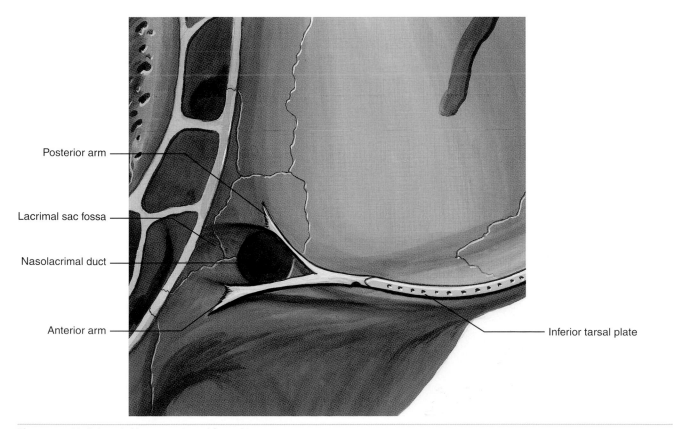

Posterior arm

Lacrimal sac fossa

Nasolacrimal duct

Anterior arm

Inferior tarsal plate

Figure 8-4 Medial canthal ligament, viewed from above.

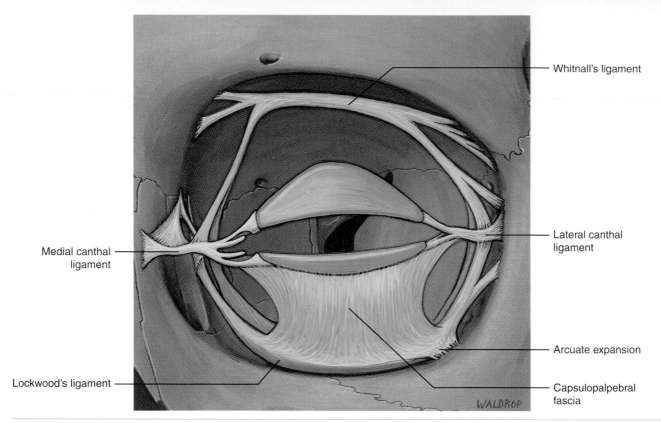

Figure 8-5 Anterior fascial support system with Whitnall's and Lockwood's ligaments.

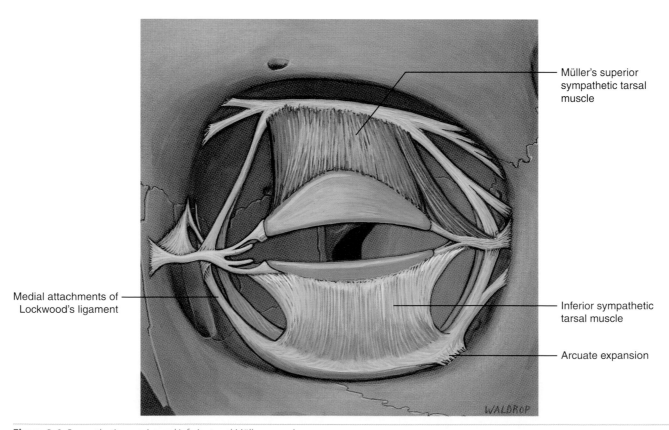

Figure 8-6 Sympathetic superior and inferior tarsal Müllers muscles.

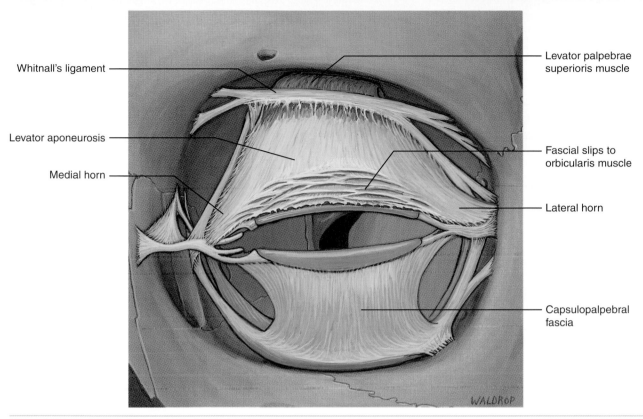

Whitnall's ligament

Levator aponeurosis

Medial horn

Levator palpebrae
superioris muscle

Fascial slips to
orbicularis muscle

Lateral horn

Capsulopalpebral
fascia

Figure 8-7 Levator aponeurosis and capsulopalpebral fascia.

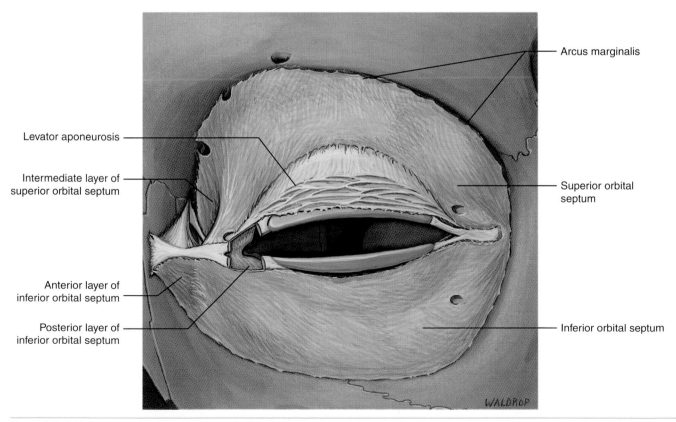

Levator aponeurosis

Intermediate layer of
superior orbital septum

Anterior layer of
inferior orbital septum

Posterior layer of
inferior orbital septum

Arcus marginalis

Superior orbital
septum

Inferior orbital septum

Figure 8-8 Orbital septum.

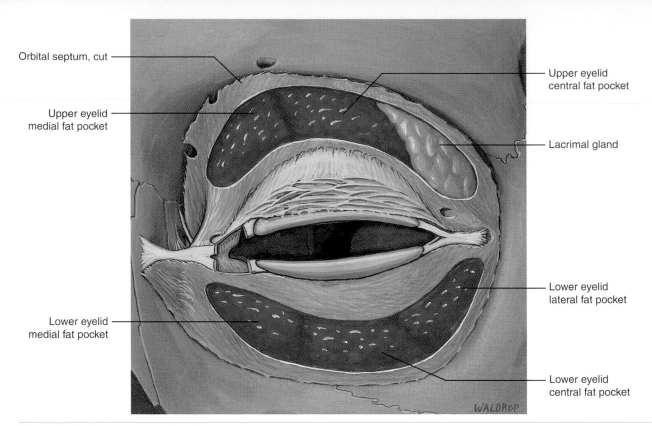

Orbital septum, cut

Upper eyelid medial fat pocket

Upper eyelid central fat pocket

Lacrimal gland

Lower eyelid medial fat pocket

Lower eyelid lateral fat pocket

Lower eyelid central fat pocket

Figure 8-9 Eyelid preaponeurotic fat pockets.

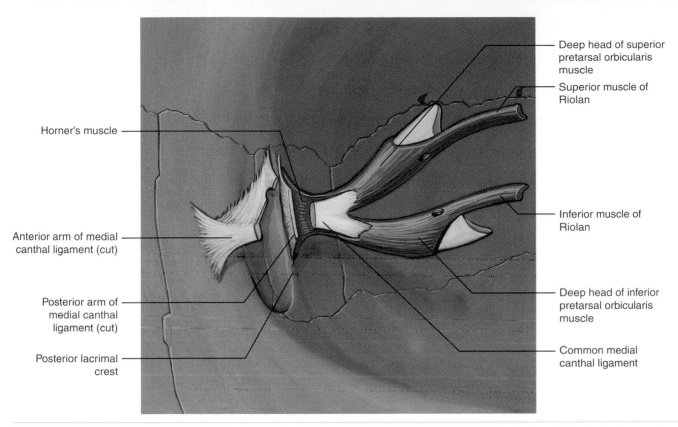

Horner's muscle

Anterior arm of medial canthal ligament (cut)

Posterior arm of medial canthal ligament (cut)

Posterior lacrimal crest

Deep head of superior pretarsal orbicularis muscle

Superior muscle of Riolan

Inferior muscle of Riolan

Deep head of inferior pretarsal orbicularis muscle

Common medial canthal ligament

Figure 8-10 Deep pretarsal orbicularis and Horner's muscles.

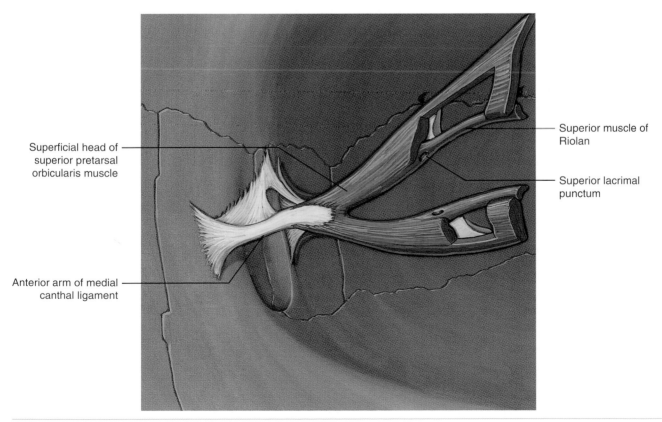

Superficial head of superior pretarsal orbicularis muscle

Anterior arm of medial canthal ligament

Superior muscle of Riolan

Superior lacrimal punctum

Figure 8-11 Superficial pretarsal orbicularis muscle and the muscles of Riolan.

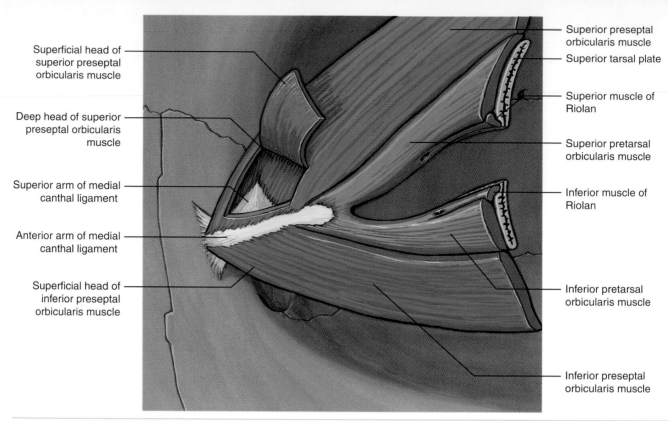

Superior preseptal orbicularis muscle

Superior tarsal plate

Superior muscle of Riolan

Superior pretarsal orbicularis muscle

Inferior muscle of Riolan

Inferior pretarsal orbicularis muscle

Inferior preseptal orbicularis muscle

Superficial head of superior preseptal orbicularis muscle

Deep head of superior preseptal orbicularis muscle

Superior arm of medial canthal ligament

Anterior arm of medial canthal ligament

Superficial head of inferior preseptal orbicularis muscle

Figure 8-12 Superficial and deep preseptal orbicularis muscles.

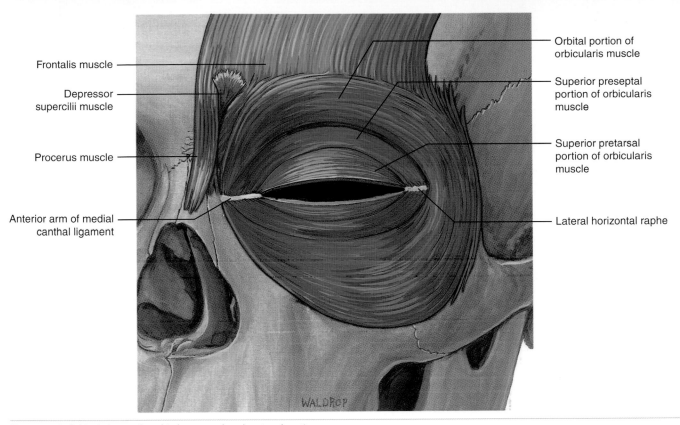

Frontalis muscle

Depressor supercilii muscle

Procerus muscle

Anterior arm of medial canthal ligament

Orbital portion of orbicularis muscle

Superior preseptal portion of orbicularis muscle

Superior pretarsal portion of orbicularis muscle

Lateral horizontal raphe

WALDROP

Figure 8-13 Orbicularis muscle, orbital, preseptal, and pretarsal portions.

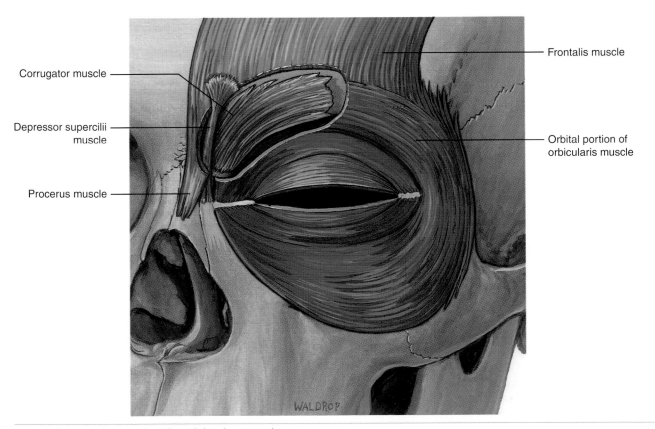

Corrugator muscle

Depressor supercilii muscle

Procerus muscle

Frontalis muscle

Orbital portion of orbicularis muscle

WALDROP

Figure 8-14 Orbicularis muscle with medial eyebrow muscles.

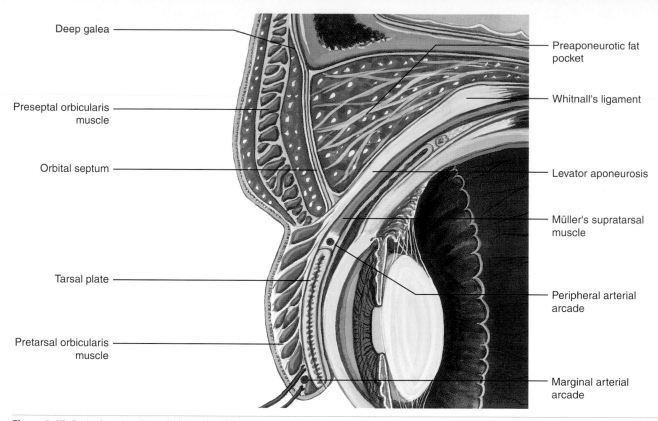

Deep galea

Preseptal orbicularis muscle

Orbital septum

Tarsal plate

Pretarsal orbicularis muscle

Preaponeurotic fat pocket

Whitnall's ligament

Levator aponeurosis

Müller's supratarsal muscle

Peripheral arterial arcade

Marginal arterial arcade

Figure 8-15 Sagittal section through the mid-eyelid.

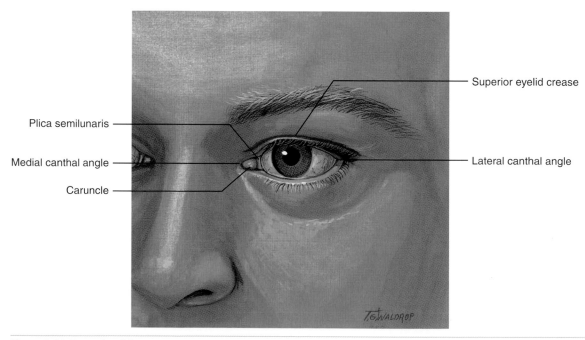

Plica semilunaris

Medial canthal angle

Caruncle

Superior eyelid crease

Lateral canthal angle

Figure 8-16 External eyelid anatomy.

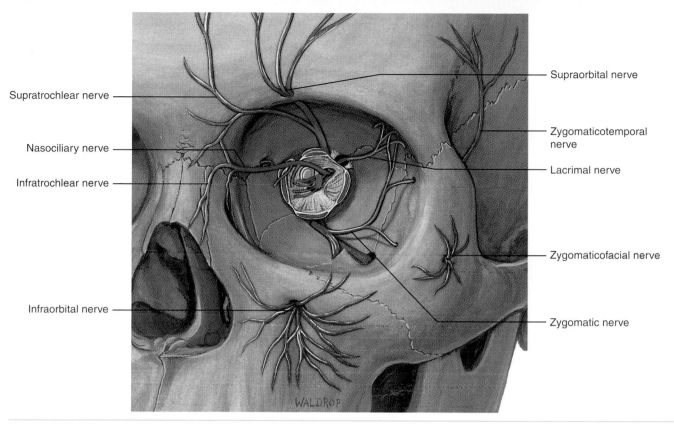

Supratrochlear nerve

Nasociliary nerve

Infratrochlear nerve

Infraorbital nerve

Supraorbital nerve

Zygomaticotemporal nerve

Lacrimal nerve

Zygomaticofacial nerve

Zygomatic nerve

Figure 8-17 Eyelid sensory nerves, cranial nerve V1 and V2.

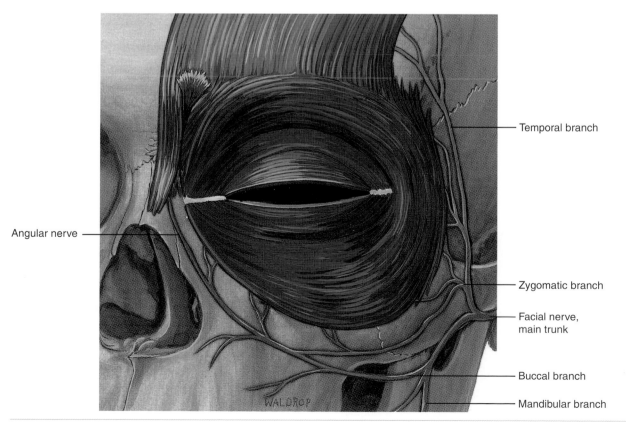

Angular nerve

Temporal branch

Zygomatic branch

Facial nerve, main trunk

Buccal branch

Mandibular branch

Figure 8-18 Eyelid motor nerves, cranial nerve VII.

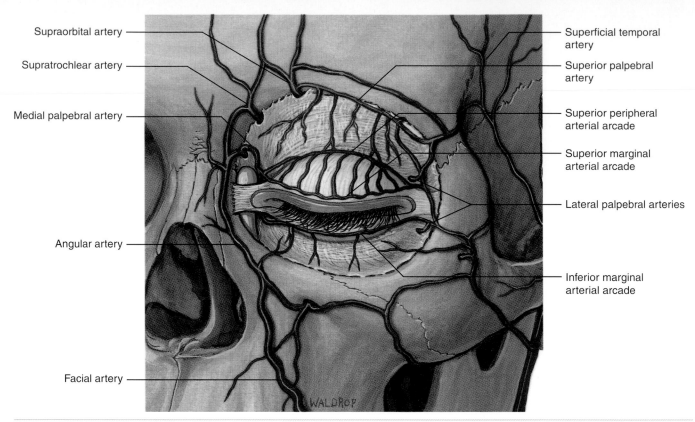

Figure 8-19 Eyelid arterial supply.

Supraorbital artery

Supratrochlear artery

Medial palpebral artery

Angular artery

Facial artery

Superficial temporal artery

Superior palpebral artery

Superior peripheral arterial arcade

Superior marginal arterial arcade

Lateral palpebral arteries

Inferior marginal arterial arcade

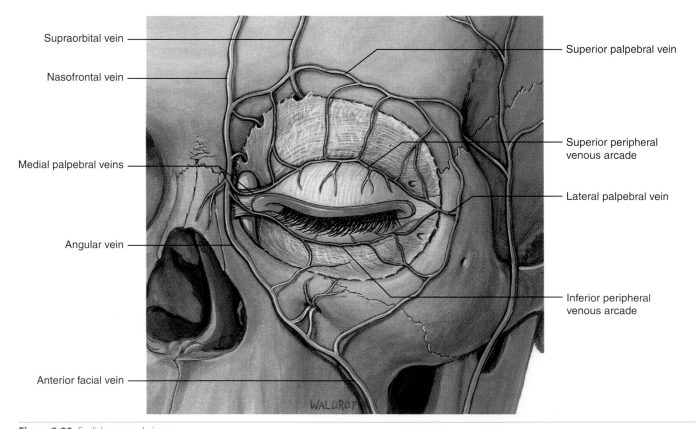

Figure 8-20 Eyelid venous drainage.

Supraorbital vein

Nasofrontal vein

Medial palpebral veins

Angular vein

Anterior facial vein

Superior palpebral vein

Superior peripheral venous arcade

Lateral palpebral vein

Inferior peripheral venous arcade

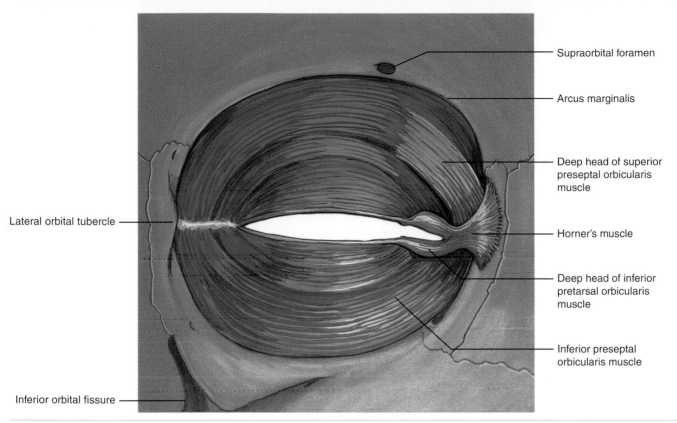

Supraorbital foramen

Arcus marginalis

Deep head of superior preseptal orbicularis muscle

Horner's muscle

Deep head of inferior pretarsal orbicularis muscle

Inferior preseptal orbicularis muscle

Lateral orbital tubercle

Inferior orbital fissure

Figure 8-21 Orbicularis muscle, internal orbital view.

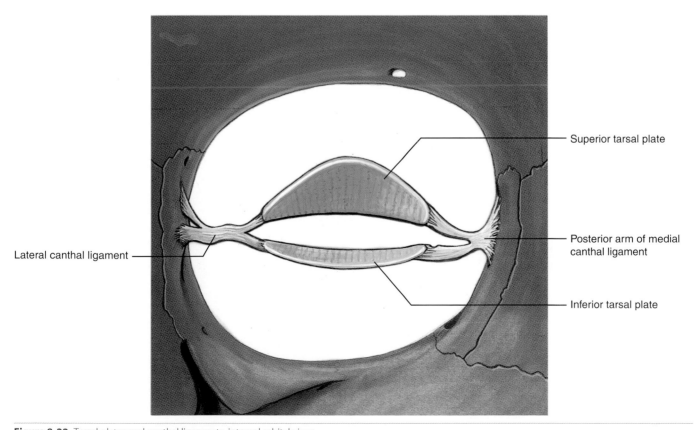

Superior tarsal plate

Posterior arm of medial canthal ligament

Inferior tarsal plate

Lateral canthal ligament

Figure 8-22 Tarsal plates and canthal ligaments, internal orbital view.

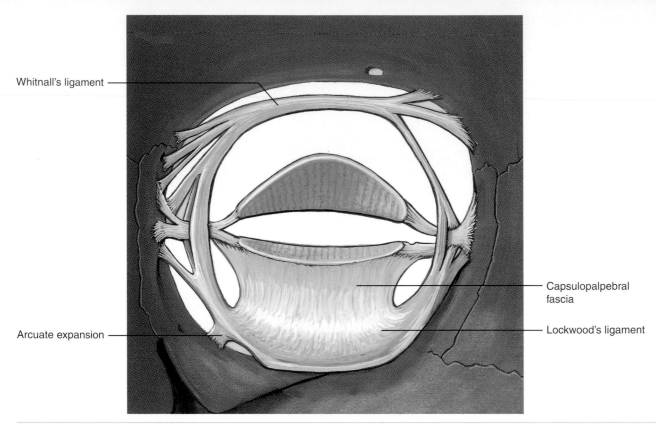

Whitnall's ligament

Capsulopalpebral fascia

Arcuate expansion

Lockwood's ligament

Figure 8-23 Anterior orbital and eyelid fascial support, internal orbital view.

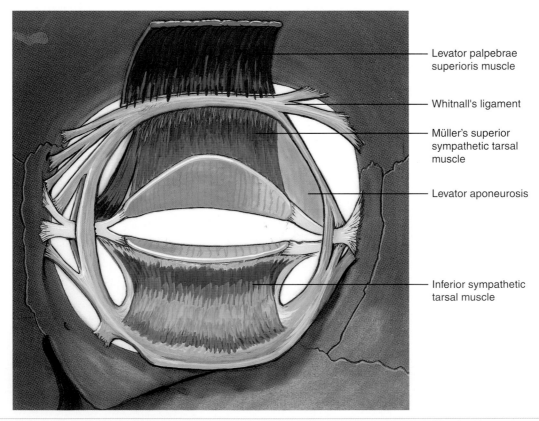

Levator palpebrae superioris muscle

Whitnall's ligament

Müller's superior sympathetic tarsal muscle

Levator aponeurosis

Inferior sympathetic tarsal muscle

Figure 8-24 Levator aponeurosis and Müller's tarsal muscles, interior orbital view.

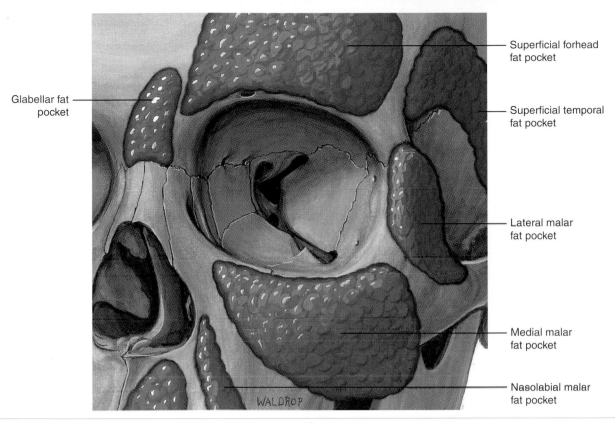

Glabellar fat pocket

Superficial forhead fat pocket

Superficial temporal fat pocket

Lateral malar fat pocket

Medial malar fat pocket

Nasolabial malar fat pocket

Figure 8-25 Superficial facial fat pockets, situated anterior to the SMAS and facial muscle.

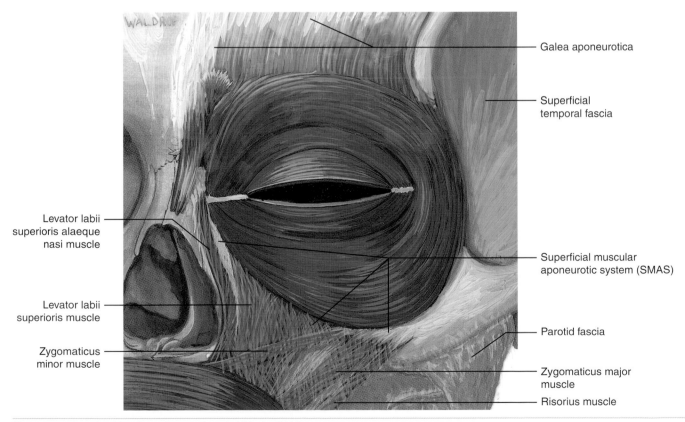

Galea aponeurotica

Superficial temporal fascia

Levator labii superioris alaeque nasi muscle

Levator labii superioris muscle

Zygomaticus minor muscle

Superficial muscular aponeurotic system (SMAS)

Parotid fascia

Zygomaticus major muscle

Risorius muscle

Figure 8-26 Periorbital facial muscles, enveloped within the SMAS.

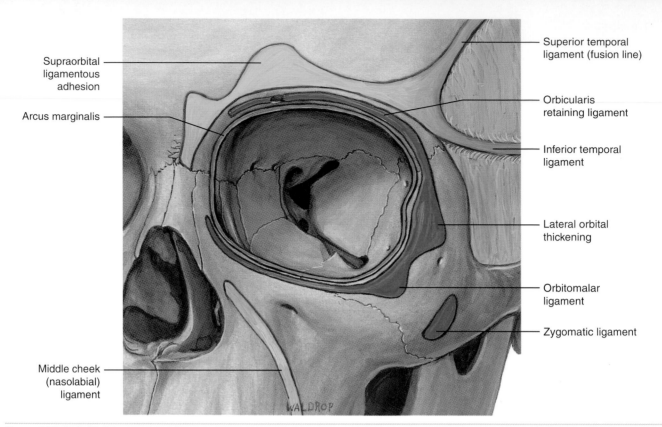

Supraorbital ligamentous adhesion

Arcus marginalis

Middle cheek (nasolabial) ligament

Superior temporal ligament (fusion line)

Orbicularis retaining ligament

Inferior temporal ligament

Lateral orbital thickening

Orbitomalar ligament

Zygomatic ligament

Figure 8-27 Periorbital deep retaining ligaments.

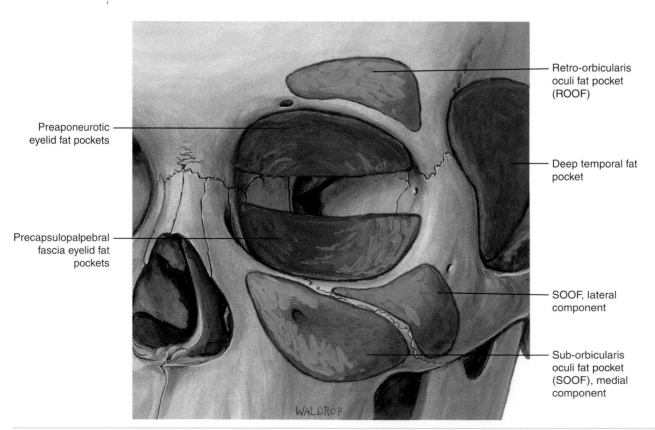

Preaponeurotic eyelid fat pockets

Precapsulopalpebral fascia eyelid fat pockets

Retro-orbicularis oculi fat pocket (ROOF)

Deep temporal fat pocket

SOOF, lateral component

Sub-orbicularis oculi fat pocket (SOOF), medial component

Figure 8-28 Deep facial fat pockets, situated posterior to the SMAS.

References

1. Abramo AC: Anatomy of the forehead muscles: The basis of the endoscopic approach in forehead rhytidoplasty. *Plast Reconstr Surg* 95:1170, 1995.

2. Aguilar GL, Nelson C: Eyelid and anterior orbital anatomy. In: Hornblass A (ed): *Oculoplastic, Orbital, and Reconstructive Surgery.* Baltimore, Williams and Wilkins, 1989, p 7.

3. Ahl NC, Hill JC: Horner's muscle and the lacrimal system. *Arch Ophthalmol* 100:488, 1982.

4. Alfonso I, Miranda F, Reeves-Garcia J, et al: Agenesis of the corrugator supercilii: A benign condition. *J Child Neurol* 25:383, 2010.

5. Alpar JJ: Acquired ptosis following cataract and glaucoma surgery. *Glaucoma* 4:66, 1982.

6. Anatassov GE, Damme PA: Evaluation of the anatomic position of the lateral canthal ligament: Clinical implications and guidelines. *J Craniofac Surg* 7:429, 1996.

7. Andersen H, Ehlers N, Matthiessen ME, Claessen MH: Histochemistry and development of the human eyelids. II. A cytochemical and electron microscopical study. *Acta Ophthalmol* 45:288, 1967.

8. Andersen H, Ehlers N, Matthiessen ME: Histochemistry and development of the human eyelids. *Acta Ophthalmol* 43:642, 1965.

9. Anderson RL: The medial canthal tendon branches out. *Arch Ophthalmol* 95:2951, 1977.

10. Anderson RL, Beard C: The levator aponeurosis. Attachments and their clinical significance. *Arch Ophthalmol* 95:1437, 1977.

11. Anderson RL, Dixon RS: The role of Whitnall's ligament in ptosis surgery. *Arch Ophthalmol* 97:705, 1979.

12. Anderson RL, Harvey JT: Lid splitting and posterior lamellar cryosurgery for congenital and acquired distichiasis. *Arch Ophthalmol* 99:631, 1981.

13. Bang YH, Park SH, Kim JH, et al: The role of Müller's muscle reconsidered. *Plast Reconstr Surg* 101:1200, 1998.

14. Barker DE: Dye injection studies of orbital fat compartments. *Plast Reconstr Surg* 59:82, 1977.

15. Bartley GB, Waller RR: Retroaponeurotic fat. *(Letter) Am J Ophthalmol* 107:301, 1989.

16. Bartolin C, Lao J: The corrugator supercilii muscle. A review. *Morphologie* 92:145, 2008.

17. Bullock JD: Prevention of post-cataract extraction ptosis. *Arch Ophthalmol* 104:972, 1986.

18. Caminer D, Newman M, Boyd J: Angular nerve: New insights on innervation of the corrugator supercilii and procerus muscles. *J Plast Reconstr Aesthet Surg* 59:366, 2009.

19. Chalfin J, Putterman AM: Müller's muscle excision and levator muscle resection in retracted upper lid. Treatment of thyroid related retractions. *Arch Ophthalmol* 97:1487, 1979.

20. Charpy A: Le coussinet adipeux du sourcil. *Bibl Anat* 19:47, 1909.

21. Cheng J, Xu F-Z: Anatomic microstructure of the upper eyelid in the Oriental double eyelid. *Plast Reconstr Surg* 107:1665, 2001.

22. Codère F, Tucker NA, Renaldi B: The anatomy of Whitnall ligament. *Ophthalmology* 102:2016, 1995.

23. Collin JR, Beard C, Wood I: Experimental and clinical data on the insertion of the levator palpebrae superioris muscle. *Am J Ophthalmol* 85:792, 1978.

24. Collin JR, Beard C, Wood I: Terminal course of nerve supply to Müller's muscle in the rhesus monkey and its clinical significance. *Am J Ophthalmol* 87:23446, 1979.

25. Cooke BE, Lucarelli MJ, Lemke BN: Depressor supercilii muscle. *Ophthal Plast Reconstr Surg* 17:404, 2001.

26. Cook BE, Lucarelli MJ, Lemke BN, et al: Eyelid lymphatics I. *Ophthal Plast Reconstr Surg* 18:18, 2002.

27. Cook BE, Lucarelli MJ, Lemke BN, et al: Eyelid lymphatics II. *Ophthal Plast Reconstr Surg* 18:99, 2002.

28. Couly G, Hureau J, Tessier P: The anatomy of the external palpebral ligament in man. *J Maxillofac Surg* 4:195, 1976.

29. Daniel RK, Landon B: Endoscopic forehead lift: Anatomic basis. *Aesthet Surg J* 17:97, 1997.

30. Delmer H: Anatomie descriptive du tiers moyen de la face. *Ann Chirurg Plast Esthet* 54:399, 2009.

31. Dewey KW: A contribution to the study of the lymphatic system of the eye. *Anat Rec* 19:125, 1920.

32. DiFrancesco LM, Codner MA, McCord CD: Upper eyelid reconstruction. *Plast Reconstr Surg* 114:98e, 2004.

33. Doxanas MT, Anderson RL: *Clinical Orbital Anatomy.* Baltimore, Williams and Wilkins, 1984.

34. Doxanas MT, Green WR, Arentsen JJ, Elas FJ: Lid lesions of childhood: A histopathologic survey at the Wilmer Institute (1923-1974). *J Pediatr Ophthalmol* 13:7, 1976.

35. Dryden RM, Leibsohn J, Wobig J: Senile entropion: Pathogenesis and treatment. *Arch Ophthalmol* 96:1883, 1978.

36. Dryden RM, Flemming JC, Quickert MH: Levator transposition and frontalis sling procedure in severe unilateral ptosis and the paradoxically innervated levator. *Arch Ophthalmol* 100:462, 1982.

37. Dumont T, Simon E, Stricker M, et al: La graisse de la face: Anatomie descriptive et fonctionnelle à partir d'une revue de la literature et de dissections de dix hémifaces. *Ann Chirurg Plast Esthet* 52:51, 2007.

38. Dutton JJ, Buckley EG: Botulinum toxin in the management of blepharospasm. *Arch Neurol* 43:380, 1986.

39. Dutton JJ: *The Evaluation and Management of Ptosis: A Color Atlas and Practical Guide.* Singapore, PG Publishing, LTD, 1989.

40. Dutton JJ: *Atlas of Ophthalmic Surgery.* Vol II. Oculoplastic, Lacrimal, and Orbital Surgery. St. Louis, CV Mosby, 1992.

41. Enlow DH: *The Human Face: An Account of the Postnatal Growth and development of the Craniofacial Skeleton.* New York, NY, Harper and Row, 1968.

42. Erdogmus S, Govsa F: The arterial anatomy of the eyelid: Importance for reconstructive and aesthetic surgery. *J Plast Reconstr Aesthet Surg* 60:241, 2007.

43. Ettle A, Priglinger S, Kramer J, Korrnneef L: Functional anatomy of the levator palpebrae superioris muscle and its connective tissue system. *Br J Ophthalmol* 80:702, 1996.

44. Ettl A, Zonneveld F, Daxer A, Koornneef L: Is Whitnall's ligament responsible for the curved course of the levator palpebrae superioris muscle? *Ophthalmic Res* 30:321, 1998.

45. Frueh BR: Graves' eye disease: Orbital compliance and other physical measurements. *Trans Am Ophthalmol Soc* 84:492, 1984.

46. Furnas DW: The retaining ligaments of the cheek. *Plast Reconstr Surg* 83:11, 1989.

47. Futumura R: Über die Entwicklung der facialismuskulatur des Menschen. *Anat Hefte* 30:433, 1906.

48. Gamboa GM, de La Torre JI, Vasconez LO: Surgical anatomy of the midface as applied to facial rejuvenation. *Ann Plast Surg* 52:240, 2004.

49. Gasser RF: The development of facial muscles in man. *Am J Anat* 120:357, 1967.

50. Ghassemi A, Prescher A, Riediger D, Axer H: Anatomy of the SMAS revisited. *Aesthet Plast Surg* 27:258, 2003.

51. Ghavami A, Pessa JE, Janis J, et al: The orbicularis retaining ligament of the medial orbit: Closing the circle. *Plast Reconstr Surg* 121:994, 2008.

52. Gioia VM, Linberg JV, McCormick SA: The anatomy of the lateral canthal tendon. *Arch Ophthalmol* 105:529, 1987.

53. Goold L, Kakizaki H, Malhotra R, Selva D: Absence of lateral palpebral raphe in Caucasians. *Clin Ophthalmol* 3:391, 2009.

54. Goold LA, Casson RJ, Selva D, Kakizaki H: Tarsal height. Letter to the editor. *Ophthalmology* 116:1831, 2009.

55. Gosain AK, Madiedo G, Matloub HS, Sanger JR: Surgical anatomy of the SMAS: A reinvestigation. *Plast Reconstr Surg* 92:1254, 1993.

56. Gutgesell VJ, Stern GA, Hood CI: Histopathology of Meibomian gland dysfunction. *Am J Ophthalmol* 94:383, 1982.

57. Haramoto U, Kubo T, Tamatani M, Hosokawa K: Anatomic study of the insertions of the levator aponeurosis and Müller's muscle in Oriental eyelids. *Ann Plast Surg* 47:528, 2001.

58. Harvey JT, Anderson RL: The aponeurotic approach to eyelid retraction. *Ophthalmology* 88:513, 1981.

59. Hawes MJ, Dortzbach RK: The microscopic anatomy of the lower eyelid retractors. *Arch Ophthalmol* 100:1313, 1982.

60. Hreczko T, Farkas LG, Katic M: Clinical significance of age-related changes of the palpebral fissures between 2 and 18 years in healthy Caucasians. *Acta Chir Plast* 32:194, 1990.

61. Humphrey GM: *A Treatise on the Human Skeleton.* Cambridge, England, MacMillan, 1858.

62. Hwang K, Cho HJ, Chung IH: Pattern of temporal branch of the facial nerve in the upper orbicularis oculi muscle. *J Craniofac Surg* 15:373, 2004.

63. Hwang K, Chung RS, Lee SI, Hiraga Y: An anatomical study of the junction of the orbital septum and the levator aponeurosis in Orientals. *Br J Plast Surg* 51:594, 1998.

64. Hwang SH, Hwang K, Jin S, Kim DJ: Location and nature of retro-orbicularis oculus fat and suborbicularis oculi fat. *J Craniofac Surg* 18:387, 2007.

65. Hwang K, Jin S, Park JH, Chung IH: Innervation of the procerus muscle. *J Craniofac Surg* 17:484, 2006.

66. Hwang K, Kim DJ, Chung IH: Innervation of the corrugator supercilii muscle. *Ann Plast Surg* 52:140, 2004.

67. Hwang K, Kim DJ, Hwang SH, Chung IH: The relationship of capsulopalpebral fascia with orbital septum of the lower eyelid: An anatomic study under magnification. *J Craniofac Surg* 17:1118, 2006.

68. Hwang K, Nam YS, Kim DJ, et al: Anatomic study of the lateral palpebral raphé and lateral palpebral ligament. *Ann Plast Surg* 62:232, 2009.

69. Hwang K, Shin YH, Kim DJ: Conjoint fascial sheath of the levator and superior rectus attached to the conjunctival fornix. *J Craniofac Surg* 19:241, 2008.

70. Issue NG: Endoscopic facial rejuvenation: Endoforehead, the functional lift. *Aesthet Plast Surg* 18:21, 1994.

71. Janis JE, Ghavami A, Lemmon JA, et al: Anatomy of the corrugator supercilii muscle: Part I. Corrugator topography. *Plast Reconstr Surg* 120:1647, 2007.

72. Johnson CC: Epiblepharon. *Arch Ophthalmol* 66:1172, 1968.

73. Jones LT: The anatomy of the lower eyelid and its relation to the cause and cure of entropion. *Am J Ophthalmol* 49:29, 1960.

74. Jones LT, Quickert MH, Wobig JL: The cure of ptosis by aponeurotic repair. *Arch Ophthalmol* 93:629, 1975.

75. Jordan DR, Gupta S, Hwang I: The superior and inferior components of Whitnall's ligament. *Ophthal Surg Lasers* 32:173, 2001.

76. Kakizaki H, Madge SN, Malhotra R, Selva D: The levator aponeurosis contains smooth muscle fibers: New findings in Caucasians. *Ophthal Plast Reconstr Surg* 25:267, 2009.

77. Kakizaki H, Malhotra R, Madge SM, Selva D: Lower eyelid anatomy. An update. *Ann Plast Surg* 63:344, 2009.

78. Kakizaki H, Prabhakaran V, et al: Peripheral branching of levator superioris muscle and Müller muscle origin. *Am J Ophthalmol* 148:800, 2009.

79. Kakizaki H, Zako M, Miyaishi O, et al: Posterior aspect of the orbital septum is reinforced by ligaments anchored to the septum by bundles of fibrous tissue. *Jpn J Ophthalmol* 49:477, 2005.

80. Kakizaki H, Zako M, Nakano T, et al: No raphé identified in the orbicularis muscle. *Okajimas Folia Anat Jpn* 81:93, 2004.

81. Kakizaki H, Zako M, Nakano T, et al: The levator aponeurosis consists of two layers that include smooth muscle. *Ophthal Plast Reconstr Surg* 21:379, 2005.

82. Kakizaki H, Zako M, Nakano T, et al: The medial horn and capsulopalpebral fascia in the medial canthus are significant antagonists of the orbicularis oculi muscle for lacrimal drainage. *Ophthalmologica* 218:419, 2004.

83. Kakizaki H, Zako M, Nakano T, et al: Microscopic findings of lateral tarsal fixation in Asians. *Ophthal Plast Reconstr Surg* 24:131, 2008.

84. Kawai K, Imanishi N, Nakajima H, et al: Arterial anatomical features of the upper palpebra. *Plast Reconstr Surg* 113:479, 2004.

85. Kestinbaum A: *Applied Anatomy of the Eye.* New York, Grune and Stratton, 1963, p 264.

86. Khazanchi R, Aggarawal A, Johar M: Anatomy of the aging face. *Indian J Plast Surg* 40:223, 2007.

87. Kikkawa DO, Lemke BN, Dortzback RK: Relationships of the superficial musculoaponeurotic system to the orbit and characterization of the orbitomalar ligament. *Ophthal Plast Reconstr Surg* 12:77, 1996.

87A. Klodt J: Zur vergleichenden anatomie der lidmusculatur. *Arch fur Mikos Anat*, xli:1, 1893.

88. Knize DM: An anatomically based study of the mechanism of eyebrow ptosis. *Plast Reconstr Surg* 97:1321, 1996.

89. Knize DM: Muscles that act on glabellar skin: A closer look. *Plast Reconstr Surg* 105:350, 2000.

90. Knize DM: *The Forehead and Temporal Fossa. Anatomy and Technique.* Philadelphia, Lippincott Williams & Wilkins, 2001.

91. Knop N, Knop E: Meibomian glands. Part I: Anatomy, embryology and histology of the Meibomian glands. *Ophthalmologe* 106:827, 2009.

92. Kuwabara T, Cogan DG, Johnson CC: Structure of the muscles of the upper eyelid. *Arch Ophthalmol* 93:1189, 1975.

93. Lemke BN: Anatomic considerations in upper eyelid retraction. *Ophthal Plast Reconstr Surg* 7:158, 1991.

94. Lemke BN, Stasior OG: The anatomy of eyebrow ptosis. *Arch Ophthalmol* 100:981, 1982.

95. Lemke BN, Stasior OG, Rosenberg PN: The surgical relations of the levator palpebrae superioris muscle. *Ophthal Plast Reconstr Surg* 4:25, 1988.

96. Letourmeau A, Daniel RK: The superficial musculoaponeurotic system of the nose. *Plast Reconstr Surg* 82:48, 1988.

97. Likas JR, Priglinger S, Denk M, Mayr R: Two fibromuscular transverse ligaments related to the levator palpebrae superioris: Whitnall's ligament and an intermuscular transverse ligament. *Anat Rec* 246:415, 1996.

98. Lim HW, Paik DJ, Lee YJ: A cadaveric anatomic study of the levator aponeurosis and Whitnall's ligament. *Korean J Ophthalmol* 23:183, 2009.

99. Linberg JV, McDonald MB, Safir A, et al: Ptosis following radial keratotomy: Performed using a rigid eyelid speculum. *Ophthalmology* 93: 1509, 1986.

100. Lipham WJ, Tawfik HA, Dutton JJ: A histologic analysis and three-dimensional reconstruction of the muscle of Riolan. *Ophthal Plast Reconstr Surg* 18:93, 2002.

101. Loeffler M, Solomon LD, Renaud M: Postcataract extraction ptosis: Effect of the bridle suture. *J Cataract Refract Surg* 16:501, 1990.

102. Makino K: On the distribution and growth of nerves in the eyelid of human embryo. *Igaku Kenkyo* 30:124, 1960.

103. Manson PN, Lazarus RB, Morgan R, Iliff N: Pathways of sympathetic innervation to the superior and inferior (Müller's) tarsal muscles. *Plast Reconstr Surg* 78:33, 1986.

104. Matsuo K: Stretching of the Muller muscle results in involuntary contraction of the levator muscle. *Ophthal Plast Reconstr Surg* 18:5, 2002.

105. Matsuo K: Restoration of involuntary tonic contraction of the levator muscle in patients with aponeurotic blephroptosis or Horner's syndrome by aponeurotic advancement using the orbital septum. *Scand J Plast Reconstr Surg Hand Surg* 37:81, 2003.

106. Mendelson BC: Surgery of the superficial musculoaponeurotic system: Principles of release, vectors, and fixation. *Plast Reconstr Surg* 107:1545, 2001.

107. Mendelson BC, Jacobson SR: Surgical anatomy of the mid cheek: Facial layers, spaces, and the mid cheek segments. *Clin Plastic Surg* 35:385, 2008.

108. Meyer DR, Linberg JV, Wobig JL, McCormick SA: Anatomy of the orbital septum and associated eyelid connective tissue. *Ophthal Plast Reconstr Surg* 7:104, 1991.

109. Morton AD, Elner VM, Lemke BN, White VA: Lateral extensions of the Müller muscle. *Arch Ophthalmol* 114:1486, 1996.

110. Moss CJ, Mendelson BC, Taylor GI: Surgical anatomy of the ligamentous attachments I: The temple and periorbital regions. *Plast Reconstr Surg* 105:1475, 2000.

111. Most SP, Mobley SR, Larrabee WF: Anatomy of the eyelids. *Fac Plast Surg Clin NA* 13:487, 2005.

112. Muzaffar AR, Mendelson BC, Adams WP: Surgical anatomy of the ligamentous attachments of the lower lid and lateral canthus. *Plast Reconstr Surg* 110:873, 2002.

113. Nemato Y, Sekino Y, Kaneko H: Facial nerve anatomy in eyelids and periorbit. *Jpn J Ophthalmol* 45:445, 2001.

114. Oh CS, Chung IH, Kim YS, et al: Anatomic variations of the infraorbital fat compartment. *J Plast Reconstr Aesthet Surg* 59:376, 2006.

115. Ozanics V, Jakobiec FA: Prenatal development of the eye and its adnexa. In: Duane TD, Jaeger EA (eds): *Biomedical Foundations of Ophthalmology*, Vol. I. Philadelphia, JB Lippincott, 1988, pp 1–86.

116. Özdemir R, Kilinç H, Ünlü RE, et al: Anatomicohistologic study of the retaining ligaments of the face and use in face lift: Retaining ligament correction and SMAS plication. *Plast Reconstr Surg* 110:1134, 2002.

117. Paris GL, Quickert MH: Disinsertion of the aponeurosis of the levator palpebrae superioris muscle after cataract extraction. *Am J Ophthalmol* 81:337, 1976.

118. Park JI, Hoagland TM, Park MS: Anatomy of the corrugator supercilii muscle. *Arch Facial Plast Surg* 5:412, 2003.

119. Persichetti P, Di Lella F, Delfino S, et al: Adipose compartments of the upper eyelid: Anatomy applied to blepharoplasty. *Plast Reconstr Surg* 113:373, 2004.

120. Pessa JE: An algorithm of facial aging: Verification of Lambro's theory by three- dimensional stereolithography, with reference to the pathogenesis of midfacial aging, scleral show, and the lateral suborbital trough deformity. *Plast Reconstr Surg* 106:479, 2000.

121. Pessa JE, Zadoo VP, Matimer KL, et al: Relative maxillary retrusion as a natural consequence of aging: Combining skeletal and soft-tissue changes into an integrated model of midfacial aging. *Plast Reconstr Surg* 102:205, 1998.

122. Putterman AM: *Cosmetic Blepharoplasty.* New York, Grune and Stratton, 1982.

123. Putterman AM, Urist MJ: Surgical anatomy of the orbital septum. *Ann Ophthalmol* 6:290, 1974.

124. Rein RR, Said HK, Yu M, et al: Revisiting upper eyelid anatomy: Introduction of the septal extension. *Plast Reconstr Surg* 117:65, 2006.

125. Richard MJ, Morris C, Deen BF, et al: Analysis of the anatomic changes of the aging facial skeleton using computer-assisted tomography. *Ophthal Plast Reconstr Surg* 25:382, 2009.

126. Riolan J: Anthropography et nostalgia. Paris, Moreau, 1626.

127. Rohrich RJ, Ahmad J, Hammawy AH, Pessa JE: Is intraorbital fat extraorbital? Results of cross-sectional anatomy of the lower eyelid fat pads. *Aesthet Surg J* 29:189, 2009.

128. Rohrich RJ, Arbique GM, Wong C, et al: The anatomy of suborbicularis fat: Implications for periorbital rejuvenation. *Plast Reconstr Surg* 124:946, 2009.

129. Rohrich RJ, Pessa JE: The fat compartments of the face: Anatomy and clinical implications for cosmetic surgery. *Plast Reconstr Surg* 119:2219, 2007.

130. Schrom T, Bloching W, Wernecke K, et al: Measurement of upper eyelid implants curvature by ultrasound. *Laryngoscope* 115:884, 2005.

131. Sevel D: A reappraisal of the development of the eyelids. *Eye* 2:123, 1988.

132. Shaw JA, Katzel EB, Koltz PF, et al: Aging of the facial skeleton: Aesthetic implications and rejuvenation strategies. *Plast Reconstr Surg* 125:332, 2010.

133. Shinohara H, Kominami R, Yasutaka S, Taniguchi Y: The anatomy of the lacrimal portion of the orbicularis oculi muscle (tensor tarsi or Horner's muscle). *Okijimas Folia Anat Jpn* 77:225, 2001.

134. Sires BS, Lemke BN, Dortzbach RK, Gonnering RS: Characterization of human orbital fat and connective tissue. *Ophthal Plast Reconstr Surg* 14:403, 1998.

135. Soll DB: Evolution and current concepts in the surgical management of the anophthalmic orbit. *Ophthal Plast Reconstr Surg* 2:163, 1986.

136. Standring S (ed): *Gray's Anatomy*. 40th ed. London, Churchill Livingstone, 2009.

137. Stasior GO, Lemke BN, Wallow IH, Dortzbach RK: Levator aponeurosis elastic fiber network. *Ophthal Plast Reconstr Surg* 9:1, 1993.

138. Stuzin JM, Baker TJ, Gordon HL: The relationship of the superficial and deep facial fascias: Relevance to rhytidectomy and aging. *Plast Reconstr Surg* 89:441, 1992.

139. Tse D, Anderson RL: Aponeurosis disinsertion in congenital entropion. *Arch Ophthalmol* 101:436, 1983.

140. Virchow H: Mikroscopiche anatomie der ausseren augenhaut und des lidapparatus. *Handbuch der Augenheilkunde*, 2nd ed. Paris, Graefe-Saemisch, 1908.

141. Waller RR: Eyelid malpositions in Graves' ophthalmopathy. *Trans Am Ophthalmol Soc* 80:855, 1982.

142. Washio H: Rhytidoplasty of the forehead: An anatomical approach. In: Marcha D, Hueston JT (eds): *Transactions of the Sixth International Congress of Plastic and Reconstructive Surgery*. Paris, Masson, 1976, pp 430–433.

143. Wolfram-Gabel R, Kahn JL: Adipose body of the orbit. *Clin Anat* 15:186, 2002.

144. Wulc AE, Popp JC, Bartlett SP: Lateral wall advancement in orbital decompression. *Ophthalmology* 97:1358, 1990.

145. Yamamoto H, Morikawa K, Uchinuma E, Yamashina S: An anatomical study of the medial canthus using a three-dimensional model. *Aesth Plast Surg* 25:189, 2001.

146. Yousif NJ, Matloub H, Summers AN: The midface sling: A new technique to rejuvenate the midface. *Plast Reconstr Surg* 110:1541, 2992.

CHAPTER 9

The Lacrimal Systems

The lacrimal secretory and drainage systems provide for the production and maintenance of the precorneal tear film, and the drainage of tears from the eye. Their normal functions are essential for proper optical refraction, preservation of corneal integrity, and ocular comfort. Physiology of tear production and distribution requires normal eyelid anatomy and mobility. Blinking spreads the tears vertically over the ocular surface. It also adds essential components of lipid from the meibomian glands and mucin from the conjunctival goblet cells. Horizontal flow of tears to the medial canthus is along the tear meniscus at the eyelid margin. This requires normal contour and eyelid apposition to the globe, and an adequately functioning orbicularis pump mechanism. Both of these functions may be compromised by eyelid laxity or marginal deformities.

Tear production typically declines with advancing age, often correlated with clinical dry eye problems seen so commonly in older patients. Obata[37] noted age-related histopathologic changes in the lacrimal gland including acinar atrophy, periacinar and periductal fibrosis, lymphocytic and fatty infiltration, interlobular ductal dilatation, and stensosis of the excretory ducts in the conjunctival fornix. The mechanisms governing these changes are not yet clear.

The lacrimal gland

Embryology

The lacrimal gland is first seen in the 17 mm (6-week) embryonic stage as solid buds of epithelium arising from ectoderm of the superolateral conjunctival fornix.[11,40,41] Mesenchyme derived from neural crest condenses around these buds. By the 19–21 mm (7-week) stage the primordial gland become well-defined as an ovoid condensation of epithelial buds with surrounding mesenchymal cells. The lacrimal artery enters the gland in the 26 mm (7.5-week) stage, and central lumina appear in the epithelial buds by the 27–28 mm (8-week) stage. Secondary development during the 40–60 mm (11–12-week) fetal period forms the palpebral lobe. The levator aponeurosis differentiates between the 38 and 60 mm (9–11-week) stages, separating the orbital and palpebral lobes of the lacrimal gland. Glandular acini develop in the 90 mm (13-week) stage, as arborization of glandular parenchyma proceeds. Anastomosis of the sensory lacrimal nerve and the motor component of the zygomatic nerve occurs within the gland at this time. Canalization of the glandular tissue to form ducts begins at about the 60 mm (12-week) stage, but full development of the gland does not occur until 3 to 4 years postnatally.[41]

The adult lacrimal gland

The main lacrimal gland provides the principal aqueous secretory component to the tear film. The gland lies in the anterior orbit under the superolateral orbital rim. It is situated within a shallow concavity in the frontal bone, the fossa glandulae lacrimalis. The gland is anatomically divided into two portions by the lateral horn of the levator aponeurosis. Anteriorly, the orbital lobe lies behind the orbital septum and above the lateral horn of the levator aponeurosis. It measures approximately 20 mm long, by 12 mm wide, by 5 mm thick. The secretory acini are composed of an inner layer of columnar epithelium surrounded by a basal layer of myoepithelial cells that aid in secretion.[30] Two to six ductules collect secretions from the orbital lobe and pass through the palpebral lobe.

The smaller palpebral lobe lies more inferiorly and extends behind the levator aponeurosis where it project into the lateral portion of the upper eyelid. It may be visible on the palpebral surface of the lid just behind the superotemporal conjunctiva when the lid is everted. The palpebral and orbital lobes are continuous posteriorly where the gland bends around the free edge of the aponeurosis. The secretory ductules of the orbital lobe pass around the posterior edge of the lateral horn of the levator aponeurosis and through the substance of the palpebral lobe where they are joined by the ductules of the palpebral lobe. They exit as 6–12 openings on the lateral superior conjunctival surface, approximately 4–5 mm above the tarsus. Resection of conjunctiva in the superolateral eyelid, or excision of a prolapsed palpebral lobe may result in loss of secretory function.[50]

The lacrimal gland is a pinkish-gray, serous gland with a lobulated surface. It is composed of acini arranged into numerous lobules, and drained by tubules. Although histochemical evidence demonstrates that some of these cells have both serous and mucous secretory functions,[13] more recent observations suggest that the gland is primarily serous in nature.[15,39] The acini are surrounded by myoepithelial cells, which, on contraction, help force secretions into the tubular drainage system. The spaces surrounding the acini are filled with firboadipose tissue. Although the gland lacks a true capsule, portions of it are covered by a connective tissue layer continuous with periorbita. This layer can be seen to divide into septae that pass into the gland between lobulae. The lacrimal acini drain into approximately 2 to 6 ductules that pass from the orbital portion, through the palpebral portion, to open into the superior conjunctival fornix. Additional ductules originating in the palpebral part of the gland open independently into the superior fornix.

The lacrimal nerve transmits sensory stimuli for pain and temperature via the trigeminal nerve. Sensory fibers exit the gland posteriorly adjacent to the entrance of the lacrimal artery. They travel in the lacrimal nerve to the ophthalmic division of the trigeminal nerve, and on to the gasserian (semilunar) ganglion. Here they synapse with neurons that continue posteriorly through the tegmentum of the pons to the spinal nucleus of the trigeminal nerve. Additional fibers project to the thalamus, as well as to various motor nuclei in the pons and medulla.

Parasympathetic secretomotor fibers have a more complex course. They originate in the lacrimal nucleus of the pons, adjacent to the superior salivatory nucleus.[10] The fibers travel in the pons and exit from the ventrolateral portion of the brainstem at the cerebellopontine angle as the nervus intermedius in company with the motor division of the facial nerve. The nervus intermedius enters the auditory canal and runs to the geniculate ganglion. Here, parasympathetic fibers join with sensory neurons to form the greater superficial petrosal nerve. This nerve emerges in the middle cranial fossa through a hiatus in the facial canal. It continues forward beneath dura, and crosses lateral to the internal carotid artery. At this point it unites with the deep petrosal nerve carrying postganglionic sympathetic fibers from the superior cervical ganglion, and together they form the nerve of the pterygoid canal (vidian nerve). The latter passes through the pterygoid canal and traverses the pterygopalatine fossa where the parasympathetic fibers synapse in the pterygopalatine ganglion.

Postganglionic parasympathetic fibers leave the pterygopalatine ganglion via the small pterygopalatine nerves, some of which run along the numerous fascicles of the maxillary division of the trigeminal nerve. These fibers enter the orbit through the inferior orbital fissure via several distinct pathways. Some may join a branch from the maxillary division, the zygomatic nerve, which passes through the inferior orbital fissure. This further divides into several branches (zygomaticotemporal and zygomaticofacial nerves) that gradually ascend along the lateral orbital wall, within a split in periorbita. One or more small branches continue upward from the zygomatic nerve, penetrate the lateral horn of the levator aponeurosis, and often join the lacrimal nerve prior to penetrating the lacrimal gland. However, this association between the zygomatic and lacrimal nerves is inconsistent,[52] and branches from the zygomatic nerve can be observed to ramify and enter the lacrimal gland directly.

Although the zygomatic nerve has been thought to carry the sole parasympathetic secretomotor innervation to the lacrimal gland, disruption of this nerve during lateral orbitotomy procedures does not usually result in dry eyes. Ruskell[44,45] demonstrated, both anatomically and physiologically, the direct passage of parasympathetic fibers from the pterygopalatine ganglion to the lacrimal gland in monkeys. These pass through a fine network of orbital nerve fibers, the rami orbitales, or via the retro-orbital autonomic plexus. In humans, fine nerve fibers, presumably from the retro-orbital plexus, can be traced along the lacrimal artery and into the substance of the lacrimal gland, independent of the lacrimal nerve. There is also experimental evidence that secretomotor fibers may also run within the lacrimal nerve of the cat. Thus, there may be at least three potential pathways for parasympathetic innervation of the gland: along branches from the retro-orbital plexus, either independently or with the lacrimal nerve; along the rami orbitale direct from the pterygopalatine ganglion; or via the zygomatic nerve. The relative contributions of these three pathways in humans remain unclear. Along with the afferent arc supplied by the trigeminal nerve, these parasympathetic efferent pathways are responsible for reflex tearing.

The lacrimal gland is invested in a thin pseuodcapsule of connective tissue that is continuous with the interlobular septa. This layer is surgically distinct and is important in the management of lacrimal gland tumors.[22] The fibrous interlobular septa within the gland continue beyond the capsule superiorly as loose connective tissue strands that attach the gland to periorbita of the frontal bone. These are sometimes referred to as Sommering's ligaments.[16] Major support of the gland, however, is from Whitnall's ligament and from the lateral horn of the levator aponeurosis, which lies between the two lobes. Fibers from Whitnall's ligament pass through the orbital lobe where they intermingle with the connective tissue of the gland before inserting onto the lateral orbital wall.[1] Some septa from the lateral orbital suspensory system, associated with the lacrimal artery and nerve, support the posterior portion of the gland as the inferior ligament of Schwalbe.[31] Disruption of Whitnall's ligament or other suspensory structures during ptosis or anterior orbital surgery may result in prolapse of the lacrimal gland. Although some authorities have suggested resection of this for cosmetic purposes, refixation of the gland is preferred, and avoids the risk of postoperative dry eyes.[50] During any eyelid surgery the lacrimal gland usually can be distinguished from orbital fat, but sometimes it can be mistaken for a preaponeurotic extraconal fat pocket, and inadvertently excised during blepharoplasty operations. Although there is no lateral fat pocket in the upper eyelid, as discussed in Chapter 8 there is sometimes a thin lateral extension of fat covering the anterior pole of the lacrimal gland.

In addition to the main lacrimal gland there are accessory glands in the substantia propria of the palpebral conjunctiva. Although these have been widely believed to be responsible for basic tear secretion,[23] more recent evidence suggests these also respond to reflex stimulation.[25,47] These consist of approximately 20–40 glands of Krause in the superior conjunctival fornix. Although 6–8 accessory glands are believed to be present in the inferior fornix,[21,24,25] Hawes and Dortzbach[18] failed to identify any such glands in the lower eyelid. Three to four accessory glands of Wolfring are found along the superior tarsal border in the upper eyelid and are easy to identify during recession procedures on the upper eyelid. The mucin layer of the tear film is provided by goblet cells concentrated in the conjunctival fornices. During eyelid surgery, every attempt should be made to avoid injury to these accessory glands. Some operations, such as the Fasanella-Servat procedure or the posterior tarsoconjunctival resection for ptosis repair, are particularly liable to destroy these structures.[26]

A superficial lipid layer is added to the tear film by the meibomian glands, and to a lesser extent by the glands of Zeiss and Moll. The meibomian glands are sebaceous glands located within the tarsal plates. There are about 25–30 glands in the upper eyelid and about 15–20 in the lower eyelid. Under inflammatory conditions, they are capable of atavistic metaplasia that can result in the production of hair shafts clinically manifest as acquired distichiasis.[2] The glands of Zeiss are also sebaceous glands. They are associated with each eyelash follicle. The glands of Moll are eccrine sweat glands. A single gland is found along each lash follicle. Like the Zeiss glands, Moll's glands discharge their secretions around the eyelash shaft.

The lacrimal drainage system

Embryology

The lacrimal drainage system begins its development in the 7 mm embryonic stage as the nasooptic fissure or groove is formed, bordered above by the lateral nasal process and below by the incipient maxillary process.[8] During the 8–9 mm (32–34-day) stage the frontonasal and maxillary processes develop as mesenchymal folds extending from the eyes forward to the nasal pit. The nasooptic fissure contains a thickened cord of ectoderm which becomes buried as the maxillary process grows upward and fuses with the frontonasal process.[41] As the fissure is slowly obliterated by growth of adjacent tissues the cord becomes buried, connected to surface epithelium only at its two ends by the 13–14 mm (6-week) embryonic period.[46] The upper end of the cord slowly enlarges to form the lacrimal sac, and two buds of cells grow toward the eyelid margins to form the canaliculi.[19] Occasionally, additional buds arise that may develop into additional canaliculi, fistulae or diverticulae. Differential lateral growth of the canaliculi occurs along with formation of the medial canthus and caruncle.[48]

Canalization of the solid epithelial cord begins in the lacrimal sac during the 60 mm (12-week) fetal stage, but may begin as early as the 28 mm (8-week) stage.[11,41] The process occurs by disintegration of the central cord cells.[4] It proceeds proximally to the canaliculi, and distally to the lower nasolacrimal duct. Remnants of the epithelial cord remain within the lumen as valve-like folds. Columnar epithelium develops in the sac and duct, but the substantia propria and goblet cells are not seen until after term.[48] Because of the rapid growth of the maxillae compared to that of the frontal bone there is greater lateral migration of the lower eyelid. This causes the inferior canaliculus to be pulled laterally so that in the adult the inferior punctum lies about 1–2 mm more lateral than the upper.[20] The canaliculi gradually become surrounded by a dense layer of connective tissue and are invested by striated muscle fibers that eventually become Horner's muscle and the muscle of Riolan (see Chapter 8).

The proximal and distal ends of the lacrimal drainage system remain occluded by membranes. At the puncta, this membrane is formed by an inner layer of canalicular epithelium and an outer layer of conjunctival epithelium. This usually perforates just before or at term. The inferior extent of the lacrimal duct extends to the nasal cavity from which it is separated by the thin membrane of Hasner. This is formed by an inner layer of lacrimal epithelium and an outer layer of nasal mucosa. At birth, this membrane is imperforate in 60–70% of newborns,[48] but generally opens within the first postpartum month.[58] In a small number of children it may remain imperforate, requiring probing for relief of epiphora.[6,55] In at least 60% of young children the lacrimal apparatus shows a marked angulation at the sac/duct junction. This bend may be directed laterally, anteriorly or posteriorly and may explain the significant incidence of false passages and failed probings in this age group.[35] In many cases of congenital NLD obstruction, mechanical probing may be unnecessary, and forced irrigation alone will often perforate Hasner's membrane.

The adult lacrimal drainage system

In the adult the lacrimal drainage system is situated in the anterior inferomedial orbit. The lacrimal sac sits in a depression, the lacrimal sac fossa. It is bounded anteriorly by the anterior lacrimal crest on the frontal process of the maxillary bone, and posteriorly by the posterior lacrimal crest on the lacrimal bone. The fossa is variable in size, but generally measures 14–16 mm vertically, 4–8 mm anteroposteriorly, and 2–4 mm deep.[20] The lower end of the fossa opens into the bony nasolacrimal duct. This duct is bounded by the maxillary bone anteriorly, posteriorly, and laterally. On the medial side it is usually bordered by the lacrimal bone above and by the inferior turbinate below. The diameter is variable, averaging 5.6 mm anteroposteriorly and 5.0 mm in the transverse diameter, but ranges from 2–10 mm,[49] and is slightly smaller in females.[33] The canal is directed inferiorly and slightly posteriorly at an angle of about 15–30° to the frontal plane, and is approximately 11–15 mm in length. It enters the nose about 25–30 mm behind the lateral margin of the anterior nares, at an angle averaging 78° to the plane of the nasal floor.

The lacrimal puncta and canaliculi

The lacrimal excretory system consists of the puncta, canaliculi, lacrimal sac, and nasolacrimal duct. Tears collect in the medial canthal angle where they drain into the puncta of upper and lower eyelids. The upper and lower puncta are tiny openings about 0.3 mm in diameter. The superior punctum lies about 4.5–6.0 mm, and the inferior punctum about 5.5–6.5 mm from the medial canthal angle. Each is situated on the summit of a small elevated papilla. From each punctum, the canaliculus initially passes vertically for about 2 mm to a dilated receptacle called the ampulla. The horizontal portions of the canaliculi measure about 0.5–1.0 mm in diameter, and extend medially from the ampullae toward the medial canthal angle. The canaliculi measure about 8 mm in length in the upper eyelid and 9 mm in the lower eyelid. They run just below the eyelid margins and initially lie anterior to the crura of the medial canthal ligament. As they course medially, the canaliculi pass either through the substance of their respective crura, or around them (over in the upper lid and under in the lower lid) to a position posterior to the canthal ligament. The canaliculi continue toward the lacrimal sac within the fascial tissue of the posterior arm of the canthal ligament. The canaliculi are invested with fibrous tissue.

In 90–94% of individuals the two canaliculi join at an angle of about 57–65° to form a common canaliculus.[9] Tucker et al., noted that the common canaliculus abruptly turns anteriorly at an angle of about 118°, passing through the posterior arm of the medial canthal ligament, before entering the lacrimal sac at an acute angle of about 58°.[54] They suggested that this could help form a functional valve-like mechanism. Contrary to this observation, Kakizaki et al.[27]

stated that the common canaliculus enters the sac almost perpendicularly. The common canaliculus has an average length of about 1–2 mm and its internal lining shows fine corrugations in the wall. In another report, Kakizaki et al.[28] reported that in Japanese cadavers more than half of the common canaliculus length was located within the lacrimal sac wall, and that no true structural valve was present around the internal ostium. They suggested that this relationship, along with changes in the thickness of the lacrimal sac induced by sympathetic and parasympathetic stimulations,[36] might provide a functional valve-like mechanism.

Throughout their length, the canaliculi are covered by a layer of connective tissue to help prevent collapse. During contraction of the orbicularis muscles and eyelid closure they become tortuous and convoluted, so that the folded structure helps occlude the canalicular channels. During any probing procedure, the eyelid must be pulled laterally to straighten these canals in order to prevent injury to their folded walls. Along their course, the canaliculi are surrounded posteriorly and inferiorly by the delicate fibers of the muscles of Riolan. Anteriorly and superiorly, the canaliculi of both lids are covered by thickened portions of the pretarsal orbicularis muscles. These fibers maintain an intimate relationship with the canaliculi as the latter pass around the canthal crura. The pretarsal fibers gradually roll around the canaliculi and come to lie along their posterior surface where they merge with the muscles of Riolan. These united bundles fuse at the level of the common canaliculus to form Horner's muscle, which passes backward to the posterior lacrimal crest.

Just prior to reaching the lacrimal sac the common canaliculus dilates slightly to form the sinus of Maier. It then enters the posterolateral wall of the lacrimal sac at the common internal punctum. In about 4% of individuals, the two canaliculi meet at the internal punctum without forming a common channel, and in about 2% they enter the sac completely independently.[57] At the internal punctum the canaliculus opens at an angle to form an inconsistent fold, often referred to as the valve of Rosenmüller. The existence of this valve has been controversial and retrograde reflux through this junction point has been documented.[54] Nevertheless, at least a functional barrier to reflux from the lacrimal sac to the conjunctival fornix is commonly observed clinically in many cases of dacryocystitis and congenital dacryocele where the lacrimal sac does not spontaneously decompress. This barrier also prevents retrograde reflux of tears from the sac, and is relatively more competent in children than in adults. In the presence of nasolacrimal duct obstruction, competency of this barrier, either from edema or from inflammation, will prevent reflux of mucopurulent material, and the clinical condition of dacryocystitis with abscess. As mentioned above, the angulation of entrance of the common canaliculus may contribute to this phenomenon. Using subtraction dacryocystography, Yazici et al.[56] showed that in 83% of cases of dacryocystitis with a dilated palpable sac there was increased angulation between the common canaliculus and lacrimal sac. In contrast, in cases with a non-dilated lacrimal sac the common canaliculus entered the sac in a more direct horizontal orientation. Not only does this finding confirm the earlier proposal of Tucker et al.[54] but also it should be kept in mind during probing in patients with dacryocystitis.

The lacrimal sac

The lacrimal sac is a membranous conduit lined by modified, nonciliated respiratory epithelium. It lies in a depression, the lacrimal sac fossa, formed by the frontal process of the maxillary bone and the lacrimal bone. The fossa is bounded anteriomedially by the anterior lacrimal crest on the maxillary bone, and posteromedially by the posterior lacrimal crest, which is a vertical ridge on the lacrimal bone. The bony fossa is relatively thick anteriorly where it is formed by the maxillary bone, but paper-thin posteriorly at the lacrimal bone where it may be only 0.1 mm in thickness. During dacryocystorhinostomy procedures entrance into the nose with a hemostat is easily achieved through this thin posterior region. However, the maxillary-lacrimal suture may be positioned more posteriorly in some individuals, most notably in Asians, so that the fossa is underlain by the thicker maxillary bone. In these cases entrance into the nose may require thinning the bone with a burr.

An anterior extension of the ethmoid sinus air cells, the agger nasi cells, is often located medial to the lacrimal sac fossa, and may continue to, or even lie anterior to the anterior lacrimal crest. Blaylock[7] found that theses cells extend anterior to the posterior lacrimal crest in 93% of cases, and anterior to the maxillary-lacrimal suture line in 40% of orbits. Here, these air cells lay adjacent to the upper portion of the lacrimal sac. These may be entered during lacrimal bypass surgery, and if not recognized, the lacrimal sac may be opened into the ethmoid sinus instead of the nose. Passing a cotton-tipped applicator or Freer elevator into the nose and applying pressure against the lateral wall in the region of the lacrimal sac will distinguish between bare nasal mucosa and intervening ethmoid bone. In the latter case, the medial wall of the ethmoid labyrinth must be removed, and the lacrimal sac flaps bridged across the sinus where they are anastomosed to nasal mucosa. The position of the floor of the anterior cranial fossa is quite variable, and is located 1–30 mm above the medial canthal ligament.[29] In 21% of cases this distance is 3 mm or less. Therefore, during dacryocystorhinostomy procedures, the medial canthal ligament should be disinserted only with extreme caution, if at all, since this serves as a useful anatomic landmark for placing the uppermost border of the DCR osteum.

Except for the bony lacrimal sac fossa medially, the lacrimal sac is surrounded by a complex soft-tissue system bounded in front and behind by the anterior and posterior arms of the medial canthal ligament, and closed above by the superior arm. The orbital septum from each eyelid splits into several wings that insert onto the bony crests and along the arms of the medial canthal ligament. Thus, the lacrimal sac is almost completely enclosed within its own septal compartment, isolated from both the eyelids and the orbit. Dense fibroconnective tissue joins the membranous sac to its enclosing walls. A deep head of the preseptal orbicularis muscle in the upper eyelid inserts onto the superior arm of the canthal ligament, and through this it may influence fluid dynamics in the lacrimal sac. In addition, Horner's muscle inserts along the posterior arm of the ligament and onto the posterior lacrimal crest, passing immediately posterolateral to the sac. It also has some attachments to the posterolateral sac wall. Contraction of the orbicularis muscle may alter the volume of the lacrimal sac. The inferior edge of the medial canthal ligament does not continue to the nasolacrimal canal so that the inferior-most segment of the lacrimal sac is covered only by orbital septum.[32,34] This is the weakest portion of the sac mechanically, and therefore is vulnerable to development of fistulas associated with dacryocystitis.

The lacrimal sac measures 4–6 mm in diameter and is approximately 12–15 mm in vertical length. It extends 3–5 mm above the medial canthal ligament, and 9–10 mm below the ligament to the opening of the nasolacrimal canal. The sac is separated from the investing lacrimal fascia by a thin layer of loose connective tissue containing a plexus of venules. It is lined with a double layer of columnar epithelial cells. The sac is usually in a semi-collapsed state, but with partial or complete nasolacrimal duct obstruction it may be dilated to many times its normal size. At the entrance of the nasolacrimal canal the sac narrows to form an isthmus at the junction of the sac and nasolacrimal duct.

The nasolacrimal duct

The nasolacrimal duct begins at the entrance of the bony canal. It continues within the maxillary bone, along the medial wall of the maxillary sinus to its opening in the nose, beneath the inferior nasal turbinate. It measures about 3.5–4 mm in diameter, and 16–22 mm in overall length from its junction with the lacrimal sac. About 11–15 mm of the duct lie within the bony nasolacrimal canal and another 3–5 mm are situated within a membranous papilla in the inferior nasal meatus. The duct is lined by a double layer of columnar epithelium similar to that of the lacrimal sac. A venous plexus surrounds the lacrimal sac and duct, interconnected to the veins of the inferior turbinate. Groessl et al.[17] confirmed a smaller dimension of the nasolacrimal drainage system in females and suggested that this might predispose females to NLD obstruction. This is in keeping with clinical observations. Mucosal folds within the lacrimal duct have been described, but their presence is variable and inconsistent.

The normal orientation of the duct as it descends to the nose is backward at about 15–30° to the frontal plane, and slightly lateral. This angulation is important to keep in mind during nasolacrimal duct probings in order to avoid a traumatic submucosal pass of the probe and possible scarring. However, this orientation may be vertical or even slightly more medial or lateral, depending upon the intercanthal distance. Young children may have an angulation at the sac-duct junction, potentially making probing in neonates more difficult. The nasal opening of the nasolacrimal duct is situated beneath the inferior turbinate, about 25 mm posterior to the anterior nasal spine, 30–35 mm from the external nares, and 4–18 mm above the nasal floor.[38,51] Prior to penetrating the nasal mucosa the lacrimal duct continues as a variably developed papilla. A fold of mucosa at the meatal termination of the duct forms what has been termed the lacrimal fold or valve of Hasner. This is present in 80% of normal individuals.[31] The duct is vulnerable to injury during transnasal polypectomy procedures, or the creation of a naso-antral window for maxillary sinus drainage.

The lacrimal pump mechanism

The lacrimal excretory pump functions to propel tears through the drainage system into the nose. Its exact physiologic properties remain a matter of dispute. Jones and Wobig[24] postulated that during eyelid blinking, with contraction of the orbicularis muscle, the ampulae become occluded and the canaliculi compressed. This pushes tears toward the lacrimal

sac. At the same time, they suggested that the lacrimal sac is expanded by contraction of the preseptal orbicularis muscle attached to its lateral wall, thus creating a negative pressure. The net flow of tears is thus into the sac and down the duct to the nose. Using high-speed photography, Doane[12] suggested a different mechanism of tear propulsion. He noted mechanical occlusion of the puncta during the early phases of eyelid closure, followed by compression of both the canaliculi and lacrimal sac by the contracting orbicularis muscle. Thus, the collapsing lacrimal drainage conduit pushed the tears through the system into the nose without the suction phase postulated by Jones and Wobig.

Using endoscopic observation of the lacrimal sac walls and an air bubble at the nasolacrimal opening, Becker[6] demonstrated a more complex process of pressure variations within the lacrimal drainage system. He showed that on eyelid closure and orbicularis muscle contraction, the canaliculi close and the upper lacrimal sac widens by movement of the lateral wall laterally, causing a negative pressure within the sac. At the same time, the lower sac compresses. The resulting negative pressure in the upper sac draws tears in from the canaliculi. During eyelid opening and orbicularis muscle relaxation the canaliculi open, the upper sac compresses, the valve of Rosemüller closes, and the lower sac widens. The resulting positive pressure in the upper sac and negative pressure in the lower sac propels the tears down the system into the nose.

A contrary view holds that the pump mechanism uses a positive pressure mechanism in the sac. Based on histologic, immunohistochemical, and electron microscopic studies of the lacrimal drainage system, Thale et al.[53] found that the sac walls are made up of collagen bundles with elastic and reticular fibers arranged in a helical pattern. Wide luminal vascular plexuses were found embedded within the helical system and connected to the cavernous tissue of the inferior turbinate in the region of the inferior lacrimal duct and Hasner's valve. These authors proposed that with eyelid closure and orbicularis muscle contraction, the fornix of the lacrimal sac moves superiorly and laterally thus distending. They further suggested that this, coupled with the medial attachments of the sac and the helically arranged fibrillar structure of its walls might "wring-out" the sac thus propelling tears into the nasolacrimal duct. In addition, the vascular plexus might play a role in tear fluid dynamics and absorption within the nasolacrimal system, a concept also supported by the epithelial lining with microvilli and seromucous glands.[42,43] Paulsen[43] proposed a more active mechanism of tear drainage through autonomic control of embedded blood vessels (cavernous body of the lacrimal sac) that could regulate lacrimal passage lumen size, and therefore mediate tear outflow. Inflammatory stimuli from the eye or nose could initiate mucous membrane swelling with reactive hyperemia and temporary occlusion of the lacrimal passages. There appears to be a complex feedback mechanism starting with sensory nerves in the cornea and ending with innervation of the lacrimal cavernous body. This could provide an important protective reflex controlling tear drainage.[3]

Based on the fine muscular anatomy of the medial canthal region it seems almost certain that the muscle of Riolan, in conjunction with the pretarsal and preseptal orbicularis and Horner's muscles can exert considerable influence of fluid dynamics within the lacrimal drainage system. During blinking, there is compression of the ampullae and canaliculi, and concomitant expansion of the lacrimal sac fundus. Compression and folding of the proximal canaliculi alone would appear sufficient to prevent regurgitation. Since the two canaliculi on each side can hold approximately 0.3 mL of tears, this pump mechanism is potentially capable of moving 1 mL with every 3–4 blinks.

Clinical correlations

Adult acquired nasolacrimal duct obstruction is most commonly the result of inflammatory fibrosis of the duct walls.[1] Clinically it causes intermittent or complete epiphora, and occasionally dacryocystitis. Commonly, this may be associated with canalicular obstruction, although the latter may be seen as an isolated disorder. Preoperative evaluation is essential to determine the exact site of obstruction, and the most appropriate surgical approach.[8] Radiographic imaging and ultrasound have both been shown to be useful in the evaluation of nasolacrimal pathology.[14] In most cases a dacryocystorhinostomy bypass procedure will result in a cure when the defect is located in the lower lacrimal sac or duct. When the canaliculi are obstructed, canalicular reconstruction may be attempted, but in many patients a conjunctivodacryocystorhinostomy with placement of a Jones tube will be necessary for relief of epiphora.

In congenital nasolacrimal duct obstruction the pathology is usually an imperforate Hasner's membrane at the nasal aperture of the lacrimal duct. Spontaneous opening of this membrane will occur in most affected children by about 6 months of age. If persistent, nasolacrimal duct probing between 6 and 12 months of age is usually curative. However, to avoid failure from false passage, the probe must be visualized in the inferior meatus. Infracturing of the inferior turbinate may improve the success rate.

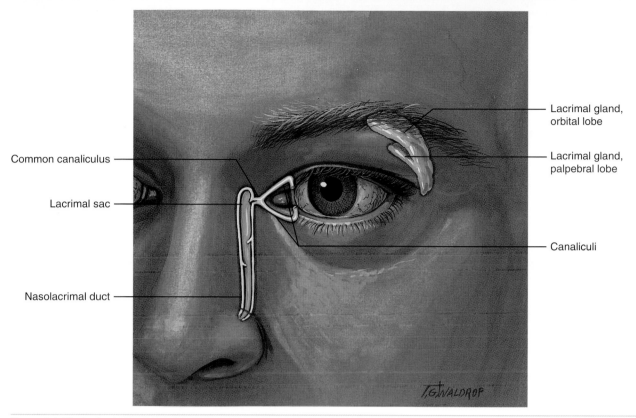

Lacrimal gland, orbital lobe

Lacrimal gland, palpebral lobe

Common canaliculus

Lacrimal sac

Canaliculi

Nasolacrimal duct

Figure 9-1 The lacrimal secretory and drainage systems.

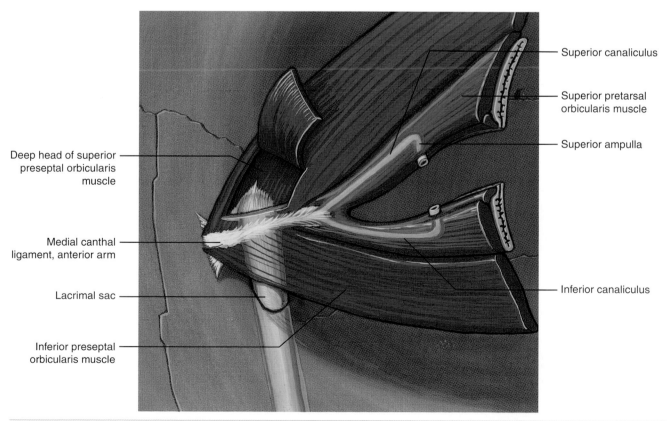

Superior canaliculus

Superior pretarsal orbicularis muscle

Superior ampulla

Deep head of superior preseptal orbicularis muscle

Medial canthal ligament, anterior arm

Lacrimal sac

Inferior canaliculus

Inferior preseptal orbicularis muscle

Figure 9-2 Lacrimal drainage system, medial canthal ligament, and orbicularis muscle.

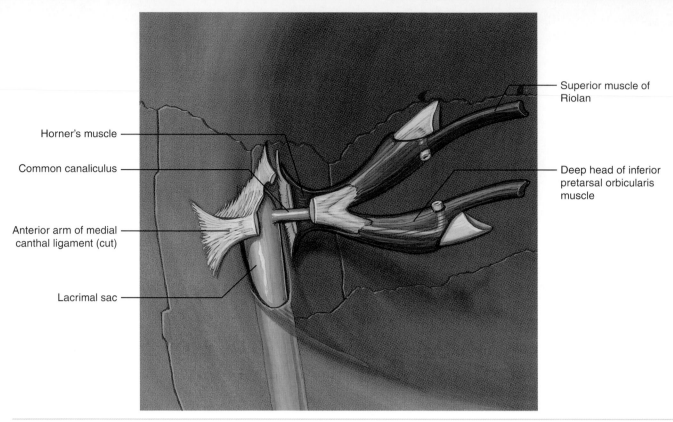

Superior muscle of
Riolan

Horner's muscle

Common canaliculus

Deep head of inferior
pretarsal orbicularis
muscle

Anterior arm of medial
canthal ligament (cut)

Lacrimal sac

Figure 9-3 Nasolacrimal sac and duct, and deep heads of the orbicularis muscle.

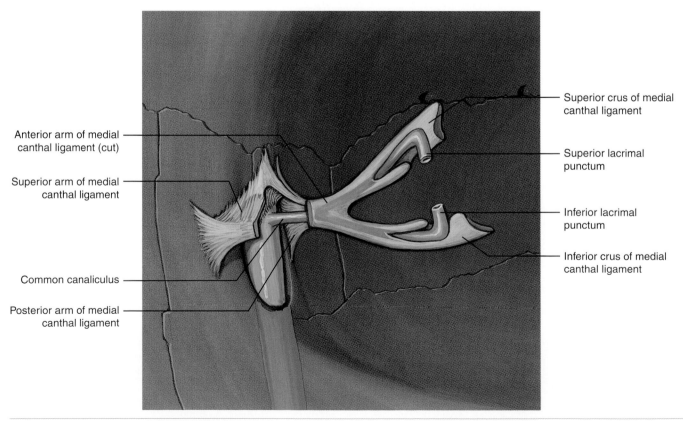

Anterior arm of medial
canthal ligament (cut)

Superior arm of medial
canthal ligament

Common canaliculus

Posterior arm of medial
canthal ligament

Superior crus of medial
canthal ligament

Superior lacrimal
punctum

Inferior lacrimal
punctum

Inferior crus of medial
canthal ligament

Figure 9-4 Nasolacrimal system with the medial canthal ligament.

References

1. Anderson RL, Dixon RS: Role of Whitnall's ligament in ptosis surgery. *Arch Ophthalmol* 97:705, 1979.

2. Anderson RL, Harvey JT: Lid splitting and posterior lamellar cryosurgery for congenital and acquired distichiasis. *Arch Ophthalmol* 99:631, 1981.

3. Ayub M, Thale AB, Hedderich J, et al: The cavernous body of the human efferent tear ducts contributes to regulation of tear outflow. *Invest Ophthalmol Vis Sci* 44:4900, 2003.

4. Barber AN: *Embryology of the Human Eye*. St. Louis, CV Mosby Co, 1955.

5. Becker BB: Tricompartment model of the lacrimal pump mechanism. *Ophthalmology* 99:1139, 1992.

6. Becker BB: The treatment of congenital dacryocystocele. *Am J Ophthalmol* 142:835, 2006.

7. Blaylock WK, Moore CA, Linberg JV: Anterior ethmoid anatomy facilitates dacryocystorhinostomy. *Arch Ophthalmol* 108:1774, 1990.

8. Burkat CN, Lucarelli MJ: Anatomy of the lacrimal system. In: Cohen AJ, Mercandetti M, Brazzo BG (eds): *The Lacrimal System, Diagnosis, Management, and Surgery*. New York, Springer, 2006, pp 3–19.

9. Corin SM, Hurwitz JJ, Jaffer N, Boota EP: The true canalicular angle: A mathematical model. *Ophthalm Plast Reconstr Surg* 6:42, 1990.

10. Crosby DG, Humphrey T, Lauer EW: *Correlative Anatomy of the Nervous System*. New York; Macmillan, 1962.

11. de la Cuadra-Blanco C, Peces-Pena MD, Merida-Velasco JR: Morphogenesis of the human lacrimal gland. *J Anat* 203:531, 2003.

12. Doane MG: Blinking and the mechanics of the lacrimal drainage system. *Ophthalmology* 88:844, 1981.

13. Duke-Elder S, Wybar KC. The anatomy of the visual system. In: Duke-Elder S (ed): *System of Ophthalmology*, Vol. 2. St. Louis, CV Mosby, 1961.

14. Dutton JJ: Diagnostic and imaging techniques. In: Linberg JV (ed): *Lacrimal Surgery*. New York, Churchill Livingstone, 1988.

15. Egeberg J, Jensen OA: The ultrastructure of the acini of the human lacrimal gland. *Acta Ophthalmol* 47:400, 1969.

16. Friedhofer H, Orel M, Saito FL, et al: Lacrimal gland prolapse: Management during aesthetic blepharoplasty: Review of the literature and case report. *Aesth Plast Surg* 33:647, 2009.

17. Groessl SA, Sires BS, Lemke BN: An anatomic basis for primary acquired nasolacrimal duct obstruction. *Arch Ophthalmol* 115:71, 1997.

18. Hawes MJ, Dortzbach RK: The microscopic anatomy of the lower eyelid retractors. *Arch Ophthalmol* 100:1313, 1982.

19. Hurwitz JJ: Embryology of the lacrimal drainage system. In: Hurwitz JJ (ed): *The Lacrimal System*. Philadelphia, Lippincott-Raven, 1996, pp 9–13.

20. Hurwitz JJ: *The Lacrimal System*. Philadelphia, Lippincott-Raven, 1996, pp 15–21.

21. Iwamoto T, Jakobiec FA: Lacrimal glands. In: Duane TD, Jaeger FA (eds): *Biomedical Foundations of Ophthalmology*, Vol. 1. Philadelphia, Harper and Row, 1982, Chapter 30.

22. Jakobiec FA, Yeo JH, Trokel SL: Combined clinical and computed tomographic diagnosis of primary lacrimal fossa lesions. *Am J Ophthalmol* 94:785, 1982.

23. Jones LT: The lacrimal secretory system and its treatment. *Am J Ophthalmol* 62:47, 1966.

24. Jones LT, Wobig JL: *Surgery of the Eyelids and Lacrimal System*. Birmingham; Aesculapius, 1976.

25. Jordan A, Baum J: Basic tear flow. Does it exist? *Ophthalmology* 87:920, 1980.

26. Jordan DR, Anderson RL, Mamalis N: Accessory lacrimal glands (Letter to the editor). *Ophthalm Surg* 21:146, 1990.

27. Kakizaki H, Masahiro Z, Osamu M, et al: Overview of the lacrimal canaliculus in microscopic cross-section. *Orbit* 26:237, 2007.

28. Kakizaki H, Selva D, Leibovitch I: Lacrimal canaliculus. Letter to the editor. *Ophthalmology* 117:644, 2010.

29. Kurihashi K, Yamashita A: Anatomical considerations for dacryocystorhinostomy. *Ophthalmologica* 203:1, 1991.

30. Lemke BN, Lucarelli MJ: Anatomy of the ocular adnexa, orbit, and related facial structures. In: Nesi FA, Lisman RD, Levine MR, Brazzo BG, Glastone GJ (eds): *Smith's Ophthalmic Plastic and Reconstructive Surgery*. 2nd ed. St Louis; Mosby, 1998, pp. 3-78.

31. Linberg JV: Surgical anatomy of the lacrimal system. In: Linberg JV (ed): *Lacrimal Surgery*. New York, Churchill Livingston, 1988.

32. Linberg JV, McCormick SA: Primary acquired nasolacrimal duct obstruction: A clinicopathologic report and biopsy technique. *Ophthalmology* 93:1055, 1986.

33. McCormick A, Sloan B: The diameter of the nasolacrimal canal measured by computed tomography: Gender and racial differences. *Clin Exp Ophthalmol* 37:357, 2009.

34. Meyer DR, Linberg JV, Wobig JL, McCormick SA: Anatomy of the orbital septum and associated eyelid connective tissues. Implications for ptosis surgery. *Ophthal Plast Reconstr Surg* 7:104, 1991.

35. Müller K-M, Busse H, Osmers F: Anatomy of the nasolacrimal duct in new-borns. *Eur J Pediatr* 129:83, 1978.

36. Narioka J, Ohiashi Y: Changes in lumen width of nasolacrimal drainage system after adrenergic and cholinergic stimulation. *Am J Ophthalmol* 141:689, 2006.

37. Obata H: Anatomy and histopathology of the human lacrimal gland. *Cornea* 25(Suppl.):S82, 2006.

38. Orhan M, Ikiz ZAA, Saylam CY: Anatomical features of the opening of the nasolacrimal duct and the lacrimal fold (Hasner's valve) fort intranasal surgery: A cadaveric study. *Clin Anat* 22:925, 2009.

39. Orzales N, Riva A, Testa F: Fine structure of the human lacrimal gland. I. The normal gland. *J Submicro Cytol* 3:283, 1971.

40. Older JJ: Congenital lacrimal disorders. In: Linberg JV (ed): *Lacrimal Surgery*. New York, Churchill Livingstone, 1988, pp 91–95.

41. Ozanics V, Jakobiec FA: Prenatal development of the eye and its adnexa. In: Jakobiec FA (ed): *Ocular Anatomy, Embryology and Teratology*. Philadelphia, Harper and Row, 1982, pp 11–96.

42. Paulsen F: The human nasolacrimal ducts. *Adv Anat Embryol Cell Biol* 170:III–IX, 1, 2003.

43. Paulsen F, Thale A, Kohla G, et al: Functional anatomy of human lacrimal duct epithelium. *Anat Embryol (Berl)* 198:1, 1998.

44. Ruskell GL: The orbital branches of the pterygopalatine ganglion and their relationship with internal carotid nerve branches in primates. *J Anat* 106:323, 1970.

45. Ruskell GL: The distribution of autonomic post-ganglionic nerve fibers to the lacrimal gland in monkeys. *J Anat* 109:229, 1971.

46. Schaeffer JP: The genesis and development of the nasolacrimal passages in man. *Am J Anat* 13:1, 1912.

47. Scherz W, Dohlman CH: Is the lacrimal gland dispensable? Keratoconjunctivitis sicca after lacrimal gland removal. *Arch Ophthalmol* 93:281, 1975.

48. Sevel D: Development and congenital abnormalities of the nasolacrimal apparatus. *J Pediatr Ophthalmol Stab* 18:13, 1981.

49. Shigeta K, Takegoshi H, Kikuchi S: Sex and age differences in the bony nasolacrimal canal. *Arch Ophthalmol* 125:1677, 2007.

50. Smith B, Petrelli R: Surgical repair of the prolapsed lacrimal glands. *Arch Ophthalmol* 96:113, 1978.

51. Tatisumak E, Aslan A, Cömert A, et al: Surgical anatomy of the nasolacrimal duct on the lateral nasal wall as revealed by serial dissections. *Anat Sci Int* 85:8, 2010.

52. Testut L: *Système Nerveux Périphérique—Organs des Sens. Traité d'Anatomie Humaine*, 4th ed., pt 3, Paris, Octave Doin, p 58.

53. Thale A, Paulsen TA, Rochels R, Tillmann B: Functional anatomy of the human efferent tear ducts: A new theory of tear outflow mechanism. *Graefes Arch Clin Exp Ophthalmol* 236:674, 1998.

54. Tucker NA, Tucker SM, Linberg JV: The anatomy of the common canaliculus. *Arch Ophthalmol* 114:1231, 1996.

55. Wong RK, VanderVeen DK: Presentation and management of congenital dacryocystocele. *Pediatrics* 122:e1108, 2008.

56. Yazici B, Yazici Z: Frequency of the common canaliculus: A radiological study. *Arch Ophthalmol* 118:1381, 2000.

57. Yazici B, Yazici Z: Anatomic position of the common canaliculus in patients with a large lacrimal sac. *Ophthal Plast Reconstr Surg* 24:90, 2008.

58. Yuen SJ, Oley C, Sullivan TJ: Lacrimal outflow dysgenesis. *Ophthalmology* 111:1782, 2004.

CHAPTER 10

Histologic Anatomy of the Orbit

As stated in the introduction, the anatomical reconstructions in this atlas were based largely on histologic sections cut through human orbits. The specimens were fixed and demineralized, and then embedded in a celoidin block for 4 months. Orbits were cut into sections at 150 microns thickness in various planes. Specimens were mounted on glass slides, and stained with hematoxylin and eosin. For the coronal orientation, sectioning was perpendicular to the longitudinal axis of the orbit, thus representing an oblique coronal view with respect to the frontal section of the skull, but a true cross-section of the orbit. Other specimens were sectioned in the sagital plane.

For each anatomical system (bones, muscles, arteries, etc) every slide was back projected at 2.5 times magnification onto a transparent mylar sheet, and details traced directly. These were then superimposed in stacks, and three-dimensional reconstructions were drawn in the coronal, sagittal, and axial orientations. It became clear, however, that the fine anatomic complexity of certain features shown so dramatically on the original histologic sections could not be reproduced adequately by tracing and artistic rendering alone. We therefore include here a series of the original histologic sections with appropriate enlargements where necessary to demonstrate specific details.

Coronal cross-sectional histological anatomy

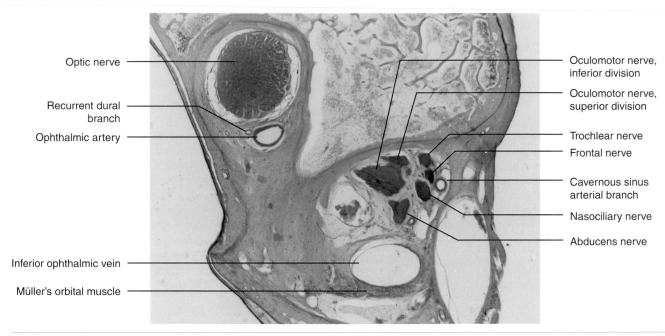

Optic nerve

Recurrent dural branch

Ophthalmic artery

Inferior ophthalmic vein

Müller's orbital muscle

Oculomotor nerve, inferior division

Oculomotor nerve, superior division

Trochlear nerve

Frontal nerve

Cavernous sinus arterial branch

Nasociliary nerve

Abducens nerve

Figure 10-1 Orbital apex at the optic strut near the confluence of the optic canal and superior orbital fissure.

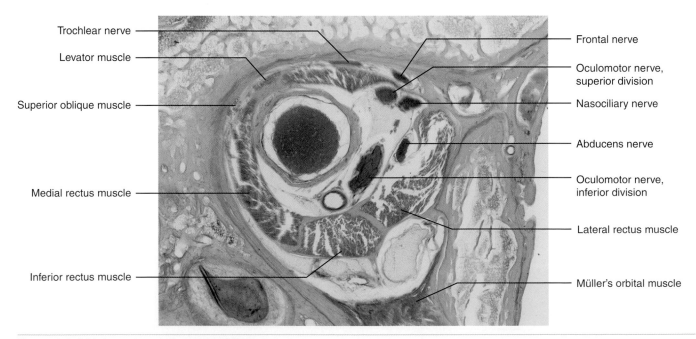

Trochlear nerve

Levator muscle

Superior oblique muscle

Medial rectus muscle

Inferior rectus muscle

Frontal nerve

Oculomotor nerve, superior division

Nasociliary nerve

Abducens nerve

Oculomotor nerve, inferior division

Lateral rectus muscle

Müller's orbital muscle

Figure 10-2 Orbital apex through the annulus of Zinn.

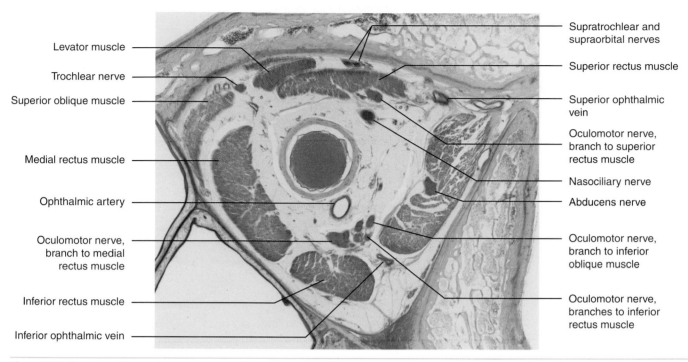

Levator muscle

Trochlear nerve

Superior oblique muscle

Medial rectus muscle

Ophthalmic artery

Oculomotor nerve, branch to medial rectus muscle

Inferior rectus muscle

Inferior ophthalmic vein

Supratrochlear and supraorbital nerves

Superior rectus muscle

Superior ophthalmic vein

Oculomotor nerve, branch to superior rectus muscle

Nasociliary nerve

Abducens nerve

Oculomotor nerve, branch to inferior oblique muscle

Oculomotor nerve, branches to inferior rectus muscle

Figure 10-3 Posterior orbit near the anterior extent of the superior orbital fissure.

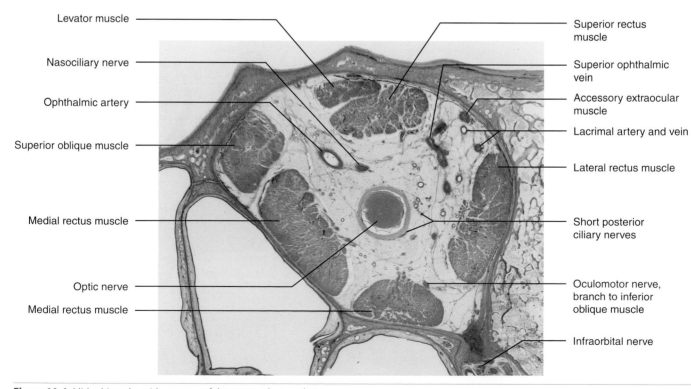

Levator muscle

Nasociliary nerve

Ophthalmic artery

Superior oblique muscle

Medial rectus muscle

Optic nerve

Medial rectus muscle

Superior rectus muscle

Superior ophthalmic vein

Accessory extraocular muscle

Lacrimal artery and vein

Lateral rectus muscle

Short posterior ciliary nerves

Oculomotor nerve, branch to inferior oblique muscle

Infraorbital nerve

Figure 10-4 Mid-orbit at the widest extent of the extraocular muscles.

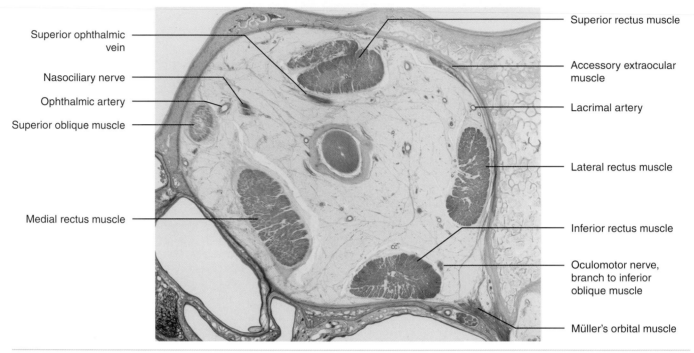

Superior ophthalmic vein

Nasociliary nerve

Ophthalmic artery

Superior oblique muscle

Medial rectus muscle

Superior rectus muscle

Accessory extraocular muscle

Lacrimal artery

Lateral rectus muscle

Inferior rectus muscle

Oculomotor nerve, branch to inferior oblique muscle

Müller's orbital muscle

Figure 10-5 Mid-orbit just behind the globe.

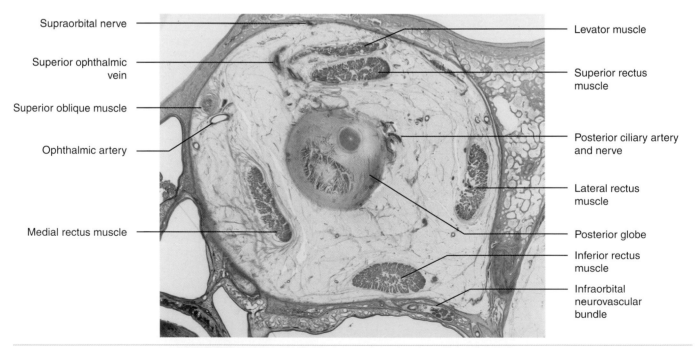

Supraorbital nerve

Superior ophthalmic vein

Superior oblique muscle

Ophthalmic artery

Medial rectus muscle

Levator muscle

Superior rectus muscle

Posterior ciliary artery and nerve

Lateral rectus muscle

Posterior globe

Inferior rectus muscle

Infraorbital neurovascular bundle

Figure 10-6 Mid-orbit cut tangentially through the posterior sclera.

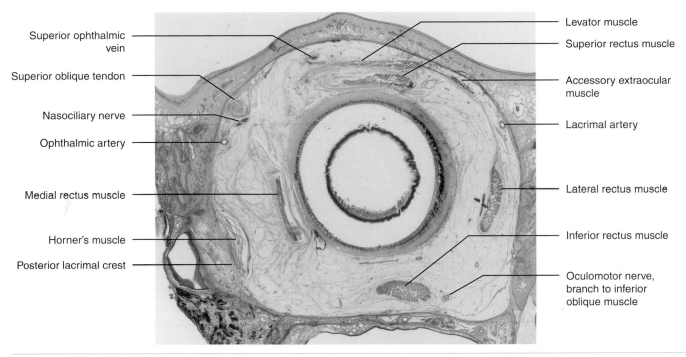

Superior ophthalmic vein

Superior oblique tendon

Nasociliary nerve

Ophthalmic artery

Medial rectus muscle

Horner's muscle

Posterior lacrimal crest

Levator muscle

Superior rectus muscle

Accessory extraocular muscle

Lacrimal artery

Lateral rectus muscle

Inferior rectus muscle

Oculomotor nerve, branch to inferior oblique muscle

Figure 10-7 Anterior orbit through the posterior globe.

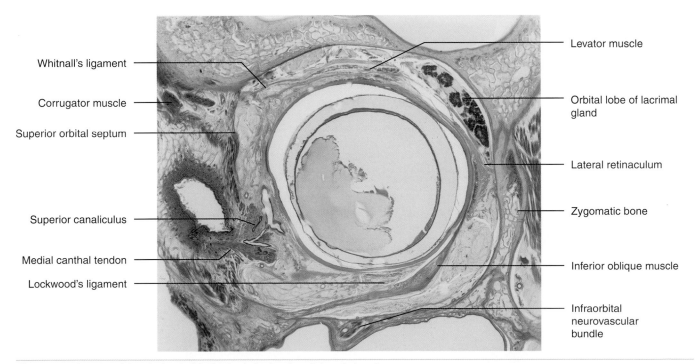

Whitnall's ligament

Corrugator muscle

Superior orbital septum

Superior canaliculus

Medial canthal tendon

Lockwood's ligament

Levator muscle

Orbital lobe of lacrimal gland

Lateral retinaculum

Zygomatic bone

Inferior oblique muscle

Infraorbital neurovascular bundle

Figure 10-8 Anterior orbit at the level of the lacrimal gland and medial canthal tendon.

Sagittal cross-sectional histological anatomy

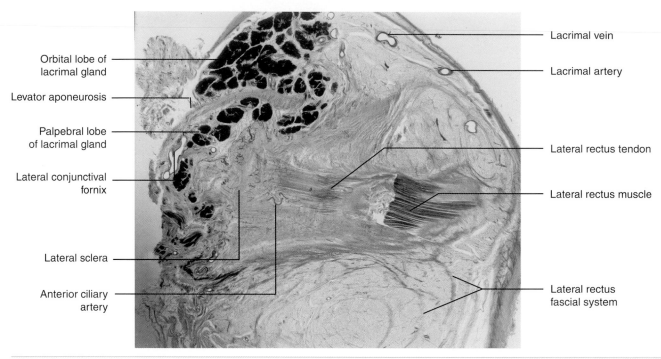

Orbital lobe of lacrimal gland

Levator aponeurosis

Palpebral lobe of lacrimal gland

Lateral conjunctival fornix

Lateral sclera

Anterior ciliary artery

Lacrimal vein

Lacrimal artery

Lateral rectus tendon

Lateral rectus muscle

Lateral rectus fascial system

Figure 10-9 Sagittal section of the lateral orbit through the insertion of the lateral rectus muscle and lacrimal gland.

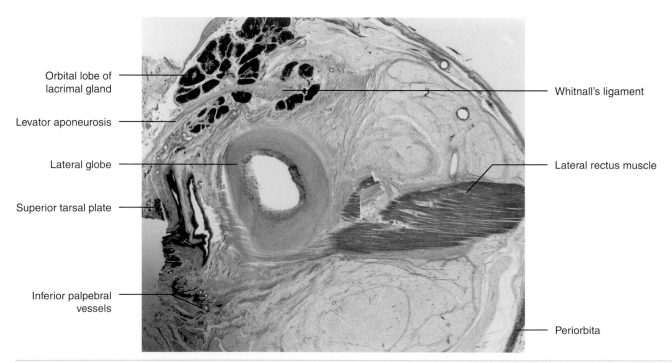

Orbital lobe of lacrimal gland

Levator aponeurosis

Lateral globe

Superior tarsal plate

Inferior palpebral vessels

Whitnall's ligament

Lateral rectus muscle

Periorbita

Figure 10-10 Sagittal section of the lateral orbit through the lateral rectus muscle and lateral sclera, at the level of the lateral conjunctival fornix.

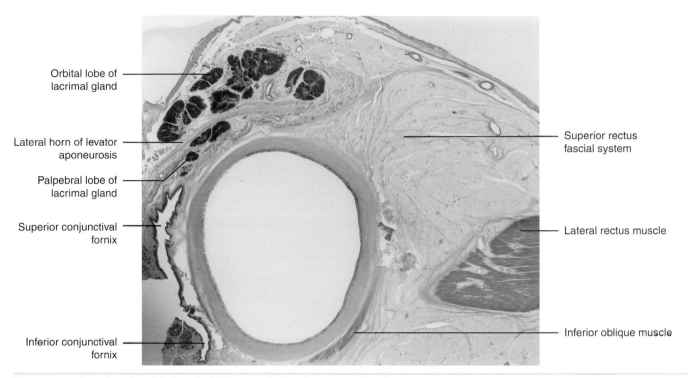

Orbital lobe of lacrimal gland

Lateral horn of levator aponeurosis

Palpebral lobe of lacrimal gland

Superior conjunctival fornix

Inferior conjunctival fornix

Superior rectus fascial system

Lateral rectus muscle

Inferior oblique muscle

Figure 10-11 Sagittal section of the lateral orbit between the lateral rectus muscle and optic nerve.

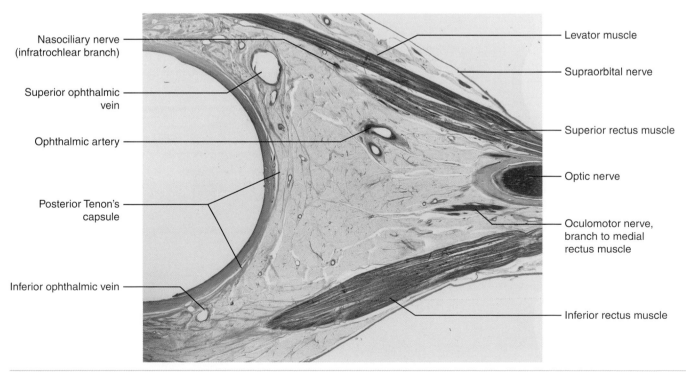

Nasociliary nerve (infratrochlear branch)

Superior ophthalmic vein

Ophthalmic artery

Posterior Tenon's capsule

Inferior ophthalmic vein

Levator muscle

Supraorbital nerve

Superior rectus muscle

Optic nerve

Oculomotor nerve, branch to medial rectus muscle

Inferior rectus muscle

Figure 10-12 Sagittal section of the mid-orbit through the inferior and superior rectus muscles.

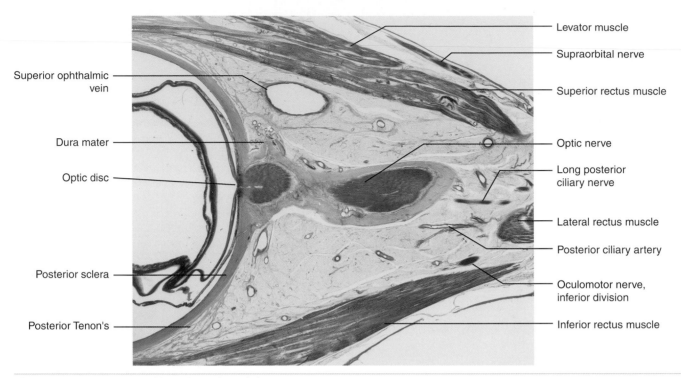

Levator muscle

Supraorbital nerve

Superior ophthalmic vein

Superior rectus muscle

Dura mater

Optic nerve

Optic disc

Long posterior ciliary nerve

Lateral rectus muscle

Posterior ciliary artery

Posterior sclera

Oculomotor nerve, inferior division

Posterior Tenon's

Inferior rectus muscle

Figure 10-13 Sagittal section of the mid-orbit through the optic nerve.

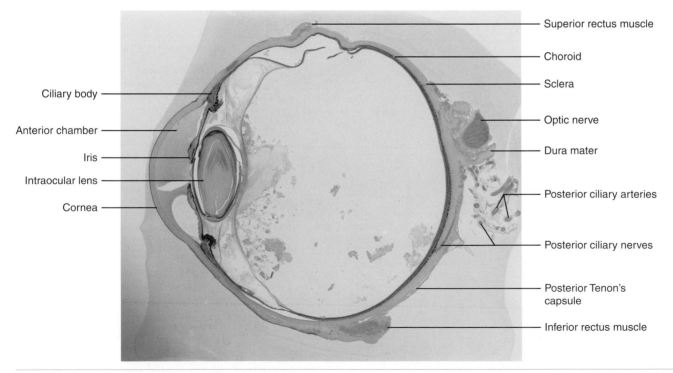

Superior rectus muscle

Choroid

Sclera

Ciliary body

Optic nerve

Anterior chamber

Dura mater

Iris

Intraocular lens

Posterior ciliary arteries

Cornea

Posterior ciliary nerves

Posterior Tenon's capsule

Inferior rectus muscle

Figure 10-14 Sagittal section through the globe at the level of the optic nerve.

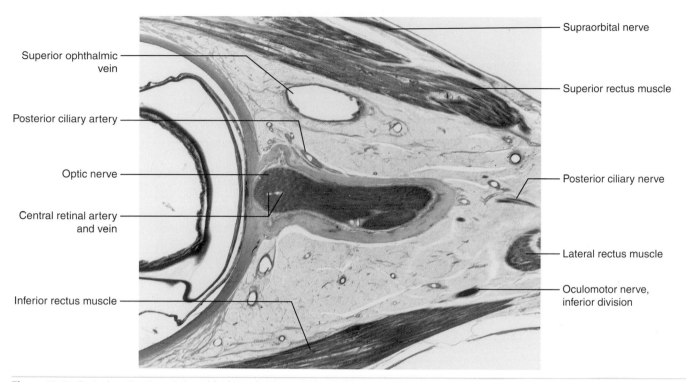

Superior ophthalmic vein

Posterior ciliary artery

Optic nerve

Central retinal artery and vein

Inferior rectus muscle

Supraorbital nerve

Superior rectus muscle

Posterior ciliary nerve

Lateral rectus muscle

Oculomotor nerve, inferior division

Figure 10-15 Sagittal section through the mid-orbit and globe at the level of the optic nerve.

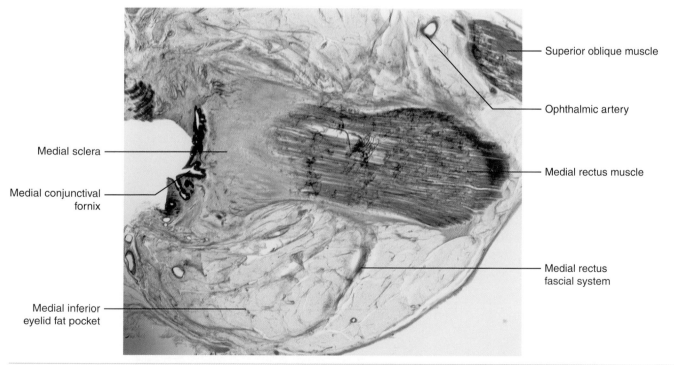

Medial sclera

Medial conjunctival fornix

Medial inferior eyelid fat pocket

Superior oblique muscle

Ophthalmic artery

Medial rectus muscle

Medial rectus fascial system

Figure 10-16 Sagittal section of the medial orbit through the insertion of the medial rectus muscle.

Annulus of Zinn

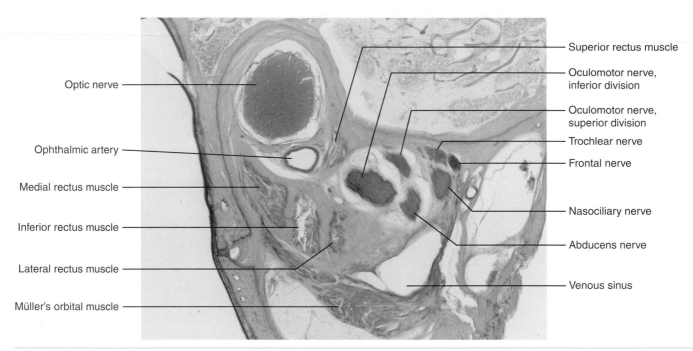

Optic nerve

Ophthalmic artery

Medial rectus muscle

Inferior rectus muscle

Lateral rectus muscle

Müller's orbital muscle

Superior rectus muscle

Oculomotor nerve, inferior division

Oculomotor nerve, superior division

Trochlear nerve

Frontal nerve

Nasociliary nerve

Abducens nerve

Venous sinus

Figure 10-17 Annulus of Zinn just anterior to the optic strut.

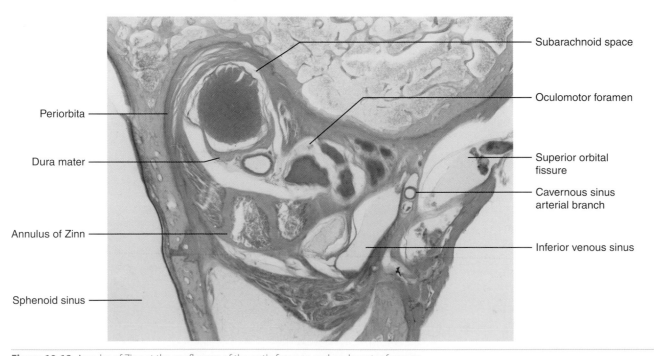

Periorbita

Dura mater

Annulus of Zinn

Sphenoid sinus

Subarachnoid space

Oculomotor foramen

Superior orbital fissure

Cavernous sinus arterial branch

Inferior venous sinus

Figure 10-18 Annulus of Zinn at the confluence of the optic foramen and oculomotor foramen.

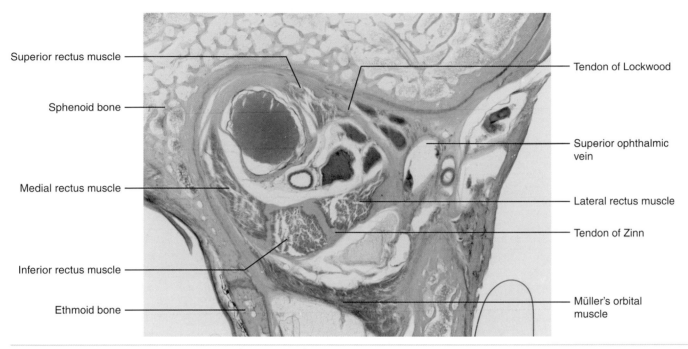

Superior rectus muscle

Sphenoid bone

Medial rectus muscle

Inferior rectus muscle

Ethmoid bone

Tendon of Lockwood

Superior ophthalmic vein

Lateral rectus muscle

Tendon of Zinn

Müller's orbital muscle

Figure 10-19 Section through the central portion of the annulus of Zinn.

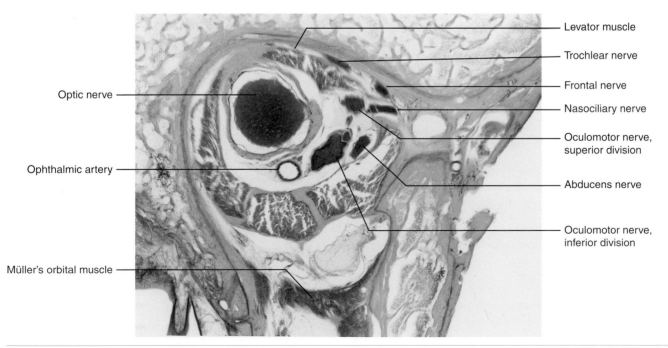

Optic nerve

Ophthalmic artery

Müller's orbital muscle

Levator muscle

Trochlear nerve

Frontal nerve

Nasociliary nerve

Oculomotor nerve, superior division

Abducens nerve

Oculomotor nerve, inferior division

Figure 10-20 Anterior annulus of Zinn.

Optic nerve

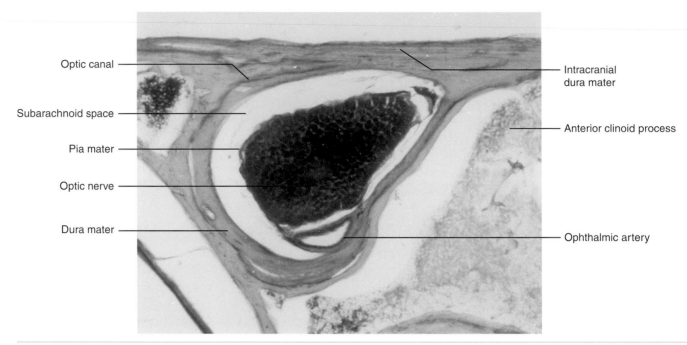

Optic canal

Subarachnoid space

Pia mater

Optic nerve

Dura mater

Intracranial
dura mater

Anterior clinoid process

Ophthalmic artery

Figure 10-21 Optic nerve and ophthalmic artery within the optic canal.

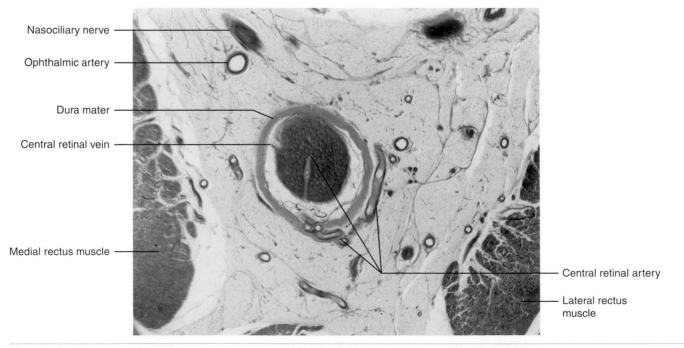

Nasociliary nerve

Ophthalmic artery

Dura mater

Central retinal vein

Medial rectus muscle

Central retinal artery

Lateral rectus
muscle

Figure 10-22 Optic nerve in the posterior orbit at the entrance of the central retinal artery.

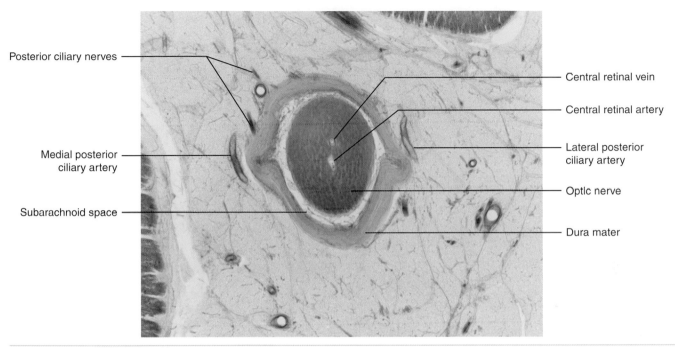

Posterior ciliary nerves

Medial posterior ciliary artery

Subarachnoid space

Central retinal vein

Central retinal artery

Lateral posterior ciliary artery

Optic nerve

Dura mater

Figure 10-23 Optic nerve in the mid-orbit just behind the globe.

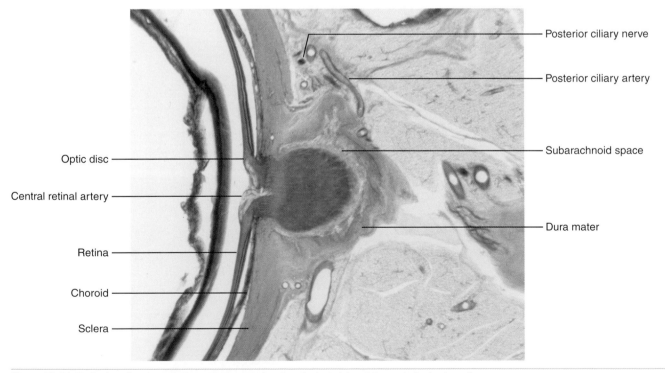

Optic disc

Central retinal artery

Retina

Choroid

Sclera

Posterior ciliary nerve

Posterior ciliary artery

Subarachnoid space

Dura mater

Figure 10-24 Sagittal section through the optic nerve and main retinal arterioles at the posterior lamina cribrosa.

Posterior globe

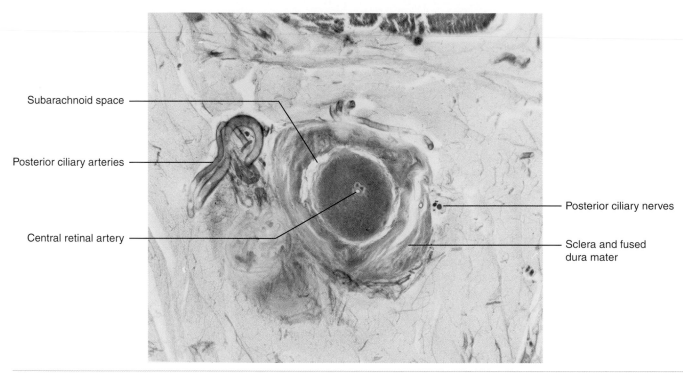

Subarachnoid space

Posterior ciliary arteries

Central retinal artery

Posterior ciliary nerves

Sclera and fused dura mater

Figure 10-25 Posterior globe at the entrance of the optic nerve and posterior ciliary arteries.

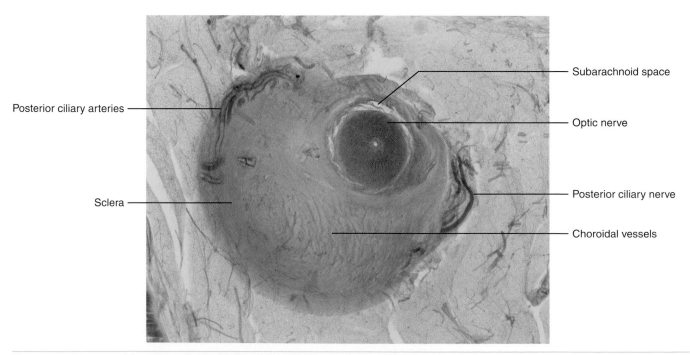

Posterior ciliary arteries

Sclera

Subarachnoid space

Optic nerve

Posterior ciliary nerve

Choroidal vessels

Figure 10-26 Posterior globe tangentially through the sclera at the entrance of the posterior ciliary nerves.

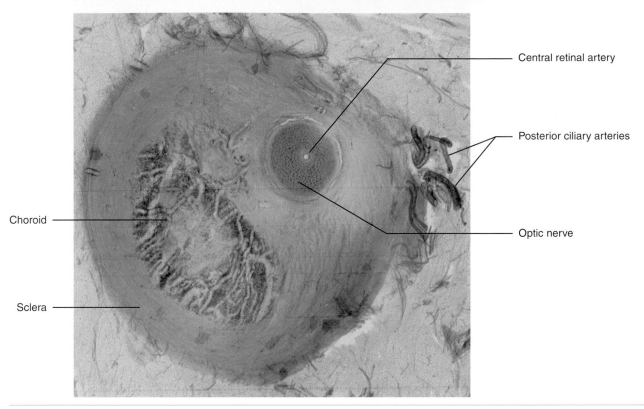

Central retinal artery

Posterior ciliary arteries

Choroid

Optic nerve

Sclera

Figure 10-27 Posterior globe tangentially through the sclera and choroid.

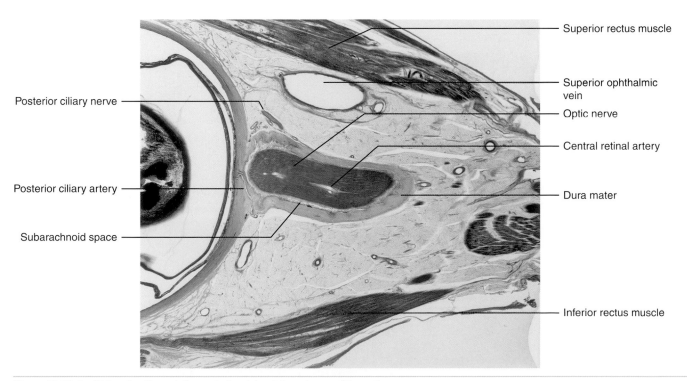

Superior rectus muscle

Posterior ciliary nerve

Superior ophthalmic vein

Optic nerve

Central retinal artery

Posterior ciliary artery

Dura mater

Subarachnoid space

Inferior rectus muscle

Figure 10-28 Sagittal section through the posterior globe at the entrance of the optic nerve.

Ciliary ganglion and nerves

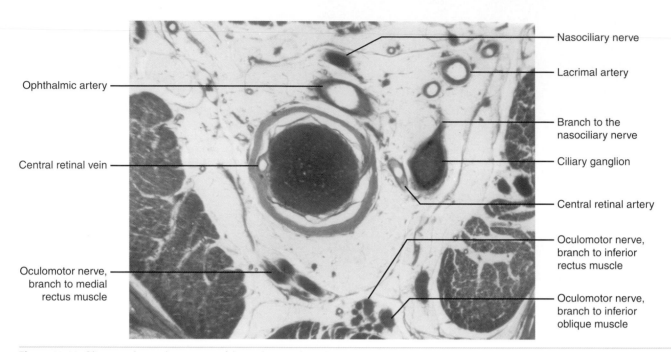

Nasociliary nerve

Lacrimal artery

Branch to the nasociliary nerve

Ciliary ganglion

Central retinal artery

Oculomotor nerve, branch to inferior rectus muscle

Oculomotor nerve, branch to inferior oblique muscle

Ophthalmic artery

Central retinal vein

Oculomotor nerve, branch to medial rectus muscle

Figure 10-29 Ciliary ganglion at the entrance of the oculomotor branch.

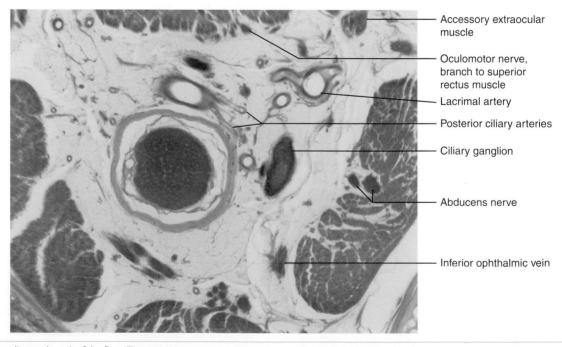

Accessory extraocular muscle

Oculomotor nerve, branch to superior rectus muscle

Lacrimal artery

Posterior ciliary arteries

Ciliary ganglion

Abducens nerve

Inferior ophthalmic vein

Figure 10-30 Ciliary ganglion at the exit of the first ciliary nerve.

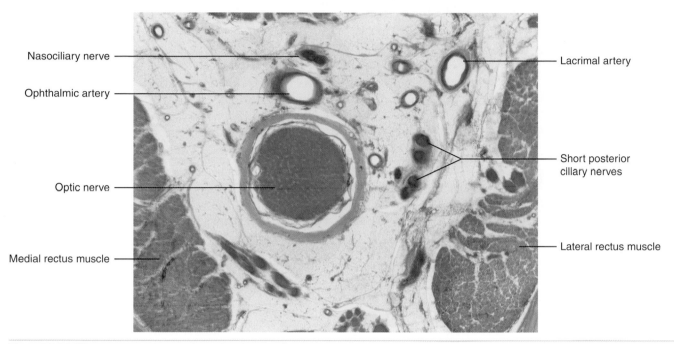

Nasociliary nerve

Ophthalmic artery

Optic nerve

Medial rectus muscle

Lacrimal artery

Short posterior ciliary nerves

Lateral rectus muscle

Figure 10-31 Ciliary nerve roots just anterior to the ciliary ganglion.

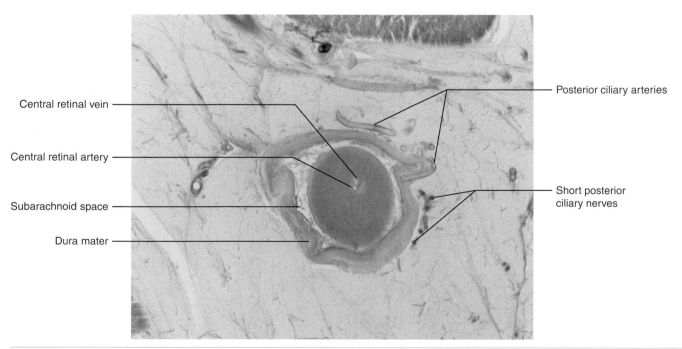

Central retinal vein

Central retinal artery

Subarachnoid space

Dura mater

Posterior ciliary arteries

Short posterior ciliary nerves

Figure 10-32 Ciliary nerves along the optic nerve just posterior to the globe.

Ophthalmic artery

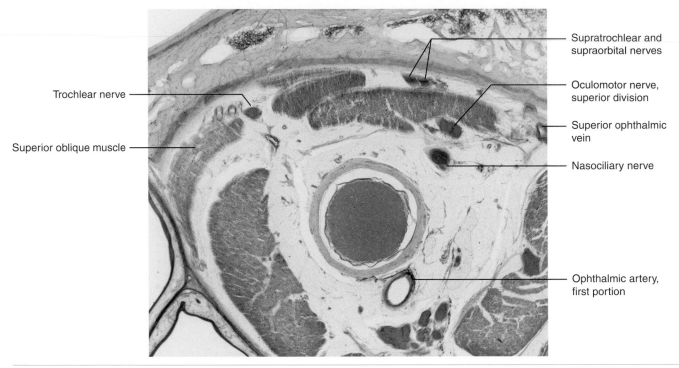

Trochlear nerve

Superior oblique muscle

Supratrochlear and supraorbital nerves

Oculomotor nerve, superior division

Superior ophthalmic vein

Nasociliary nerve

Ophthalmic artery, first portion

Figure 10-33 First portion of ophthalmic artery beneath the optic nerve in the posterior orbit.

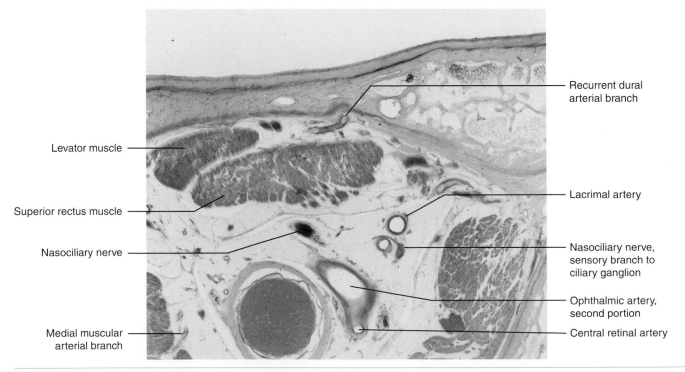

Levator muscle

Superior rectus muscle

Nasociliary nerve

Medial muscular arterial branch

Recurrent dural arterial branch

Lacrimal artery

Nasociliary nerve, sensory branch to ciliary ganglion

Ophthalmic artery, second portion

Central retinal artery

Figure 10-34 Second portion of the ophthalmic artery as it passes around the optic nerve.

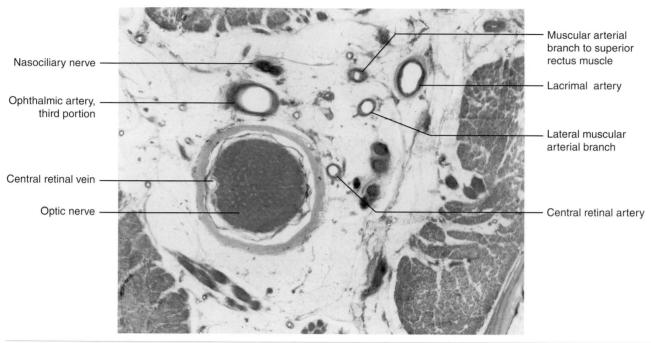

Nasociliary nerve

Ophthalmic artery, third portion

Central retinal vein

Optic nerve

Muscular arterial branch to superior rectus muscle

Lacrimal artery

Lateral muscular arterial branch

Central retinal artery

Figure 10-35 Third portion of the ophthalmic artery crossing over the optic nerve.

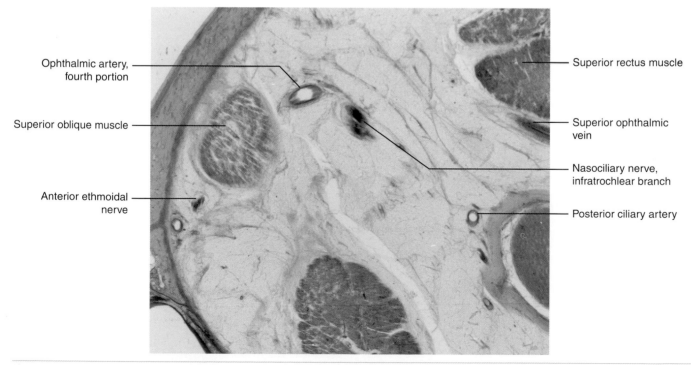

Ophthalmic artery, fourth portion

Superior oblique muscle

Anterior ethmoidal nerve

Superior rectus muscle

Superior ophthalmic vein

Nasociliary nerve, infratrochlear branch

Posterior ciliary artery

Figure 10-36 Fourth portion of the ophthalmic artery in the superomedial orbit.

Inferior rectus muscle

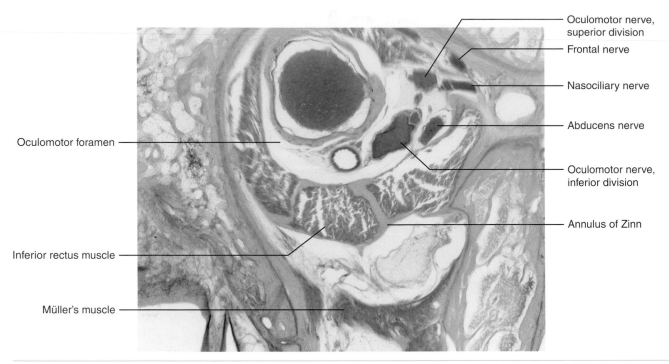

Oculomotor nerve, superior division

Frontal nerve

Nasociliary nerve

Abducens nerve

Oculomotor nerve, inferior division

Annulus of Zinn

Oculomotor foramen

Inferior rectus muscle

Müller's muscle

Figure 10-37 Inferior rectus muscle within the annulus of Zinn at the orbital apex.

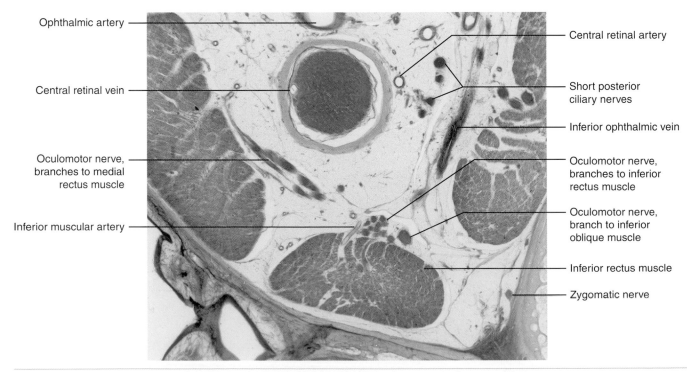

Ophthalmic artery

Central retinal vein

Oculomotor nerve, branches to medial rectus muscle

Inferior muscular artery

Central retinal artery

Short posterior ciliary nerves

Inferior ophthalmic vein

Oculomotor nerve, branches to inferior rectus muscle

Oculomotor nerve, branch to inferior oblique muscle

Inferior rectus muscle

Zygomatic nerve

Figure 10-38 Inferior rectus muscle in the posterior orbit at the entrance of the oculomotor nerve rootlets.

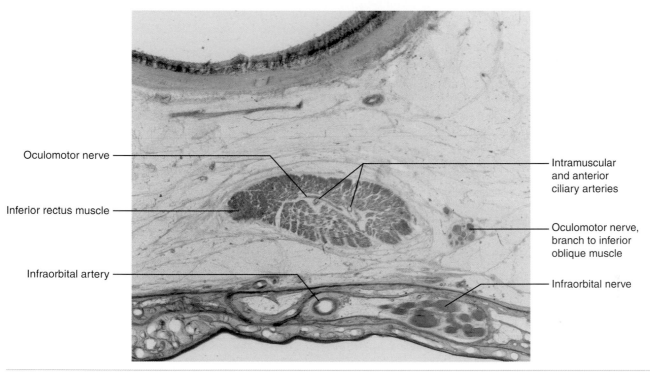

Oculomotor nerve

Inferior rectus muscle

Infraorbital artery

Intramuscular and anterior ciliary arteries

Oculomotor nerve, branch to inferior oblique muscle

Infraorbital nerve

Figure 10-39 Inferior rectus muscle in the anterior orbit at the level of the posterior globe.

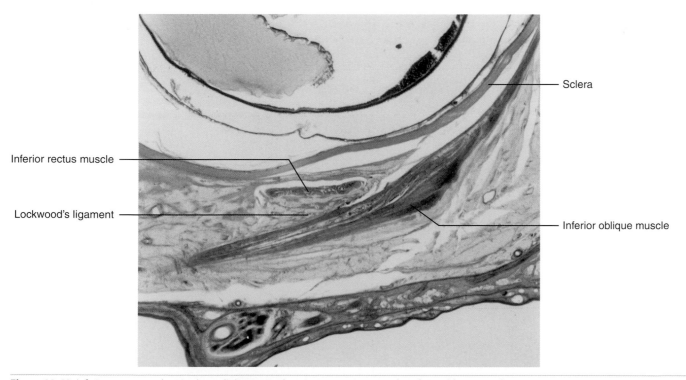

Inferior rectus muscle

Lockwood's ligament

Sclera

Inferior oblique muscle

Figure 10-40 Inferior rectus muscle at Lockwood's ligament where it crosses superior to the inferior oblique muscle.

Medial rectus muscle

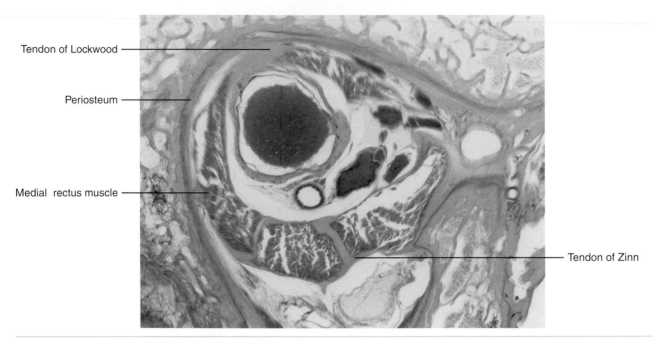

Tendon of Lockwood

Periosteum

Medial rectus muscle

Tendon of Zinn

Figure 10-41 Medial rectus muscle within the annulus of Zinn at the orbital apex.

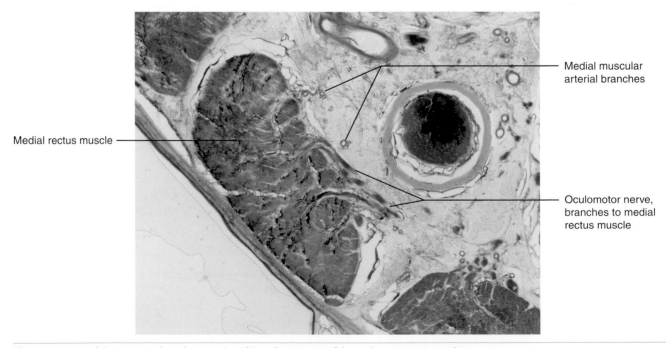

Medial rectus muscle

Medial muscular arterial branches

Oculomotor nerve, branches to medial rectus muscle

Figure 10-42 Medial rectus muscle in the posterior orbit at the entrance of the oculomotor nerve rootlets.

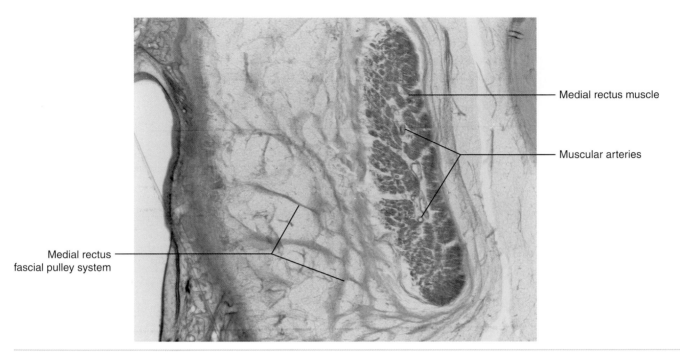

Figure 10-43 Medial rectus muscle in the anterior orbit within its fascial pulley system.

Medial rectus muscle

Muscular arteries

Medial rectus
fascial pulley system

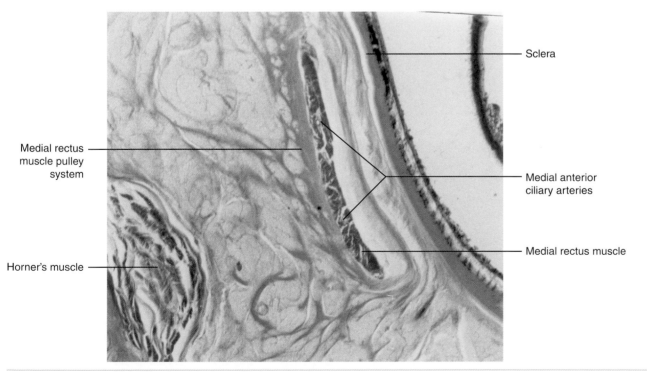

Figure 10-44 The medial rectus muscle near the transition to its tendon of insertion.

Sclera

Medial rectus
muscle pulley
system

Medial anterior
ciliary arteries

Medial rectus muscle

Horner's muscle

Superior rectus and levator palpebrae superioris muscles

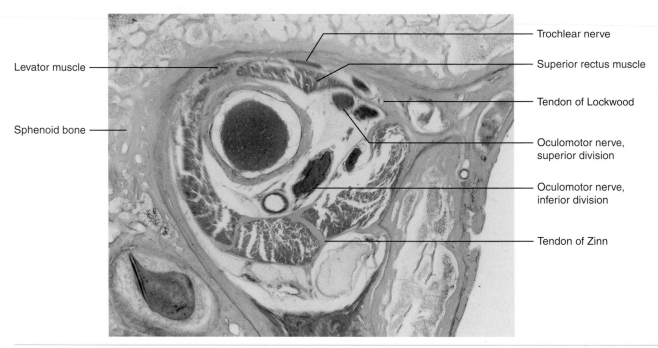

Levator muscle

Sphenoid bone

Trochlear nerve

Superior rectus muscle

Tendon of Lockwood

Oculomotor nerve, superior division

Oculomotor nerve, inferior division

Tendon of Zinn

Figure 10-45 Superior rectus and levator muscles at the annulus of Zinn in the orbital apex.

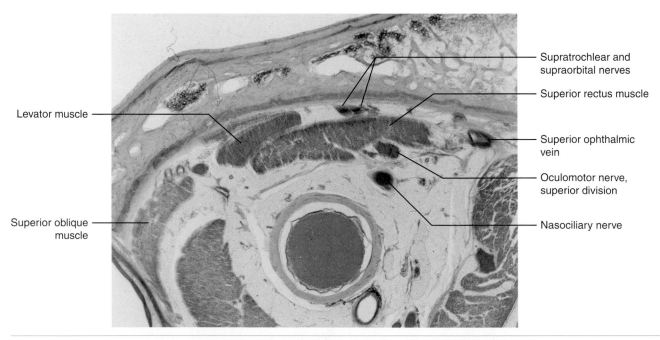

Levator muscle

Superior oblique muscle

Supratrochlear and supraorbital nerves

Superior rectus muscle

Superior ophthalmic vein

Oculomotor nerve, superior division

Nasociliary nerve

Figure 10-46 Superior rectus and levator muscles in the posterior orbit.

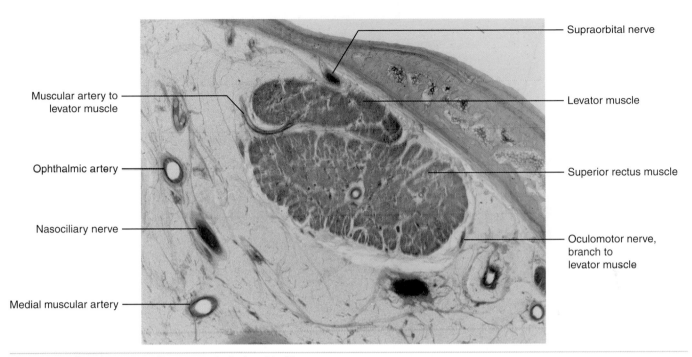

Supraorbital nerve

Muscular artery to levator muscle

Levator muscle

Ophthalmic artery

Superior rectus muscle

Nasociliary nerve

Oculomotor nerve, branch to levator muscle

Medial muscular artery

Figure 10-47 Superior rectus and levator muscles in the mid-orbit.

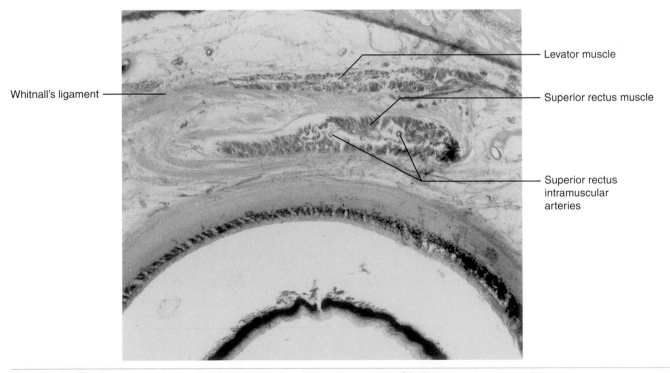

Levator muscle

Whitnall's ligament

Superior rectus muscle

Superior rectus intramuscular arteries

Figure 10-48 Superior rectus and levator muscles in the anterior orbit near the transition of the levator into its aponeurosis.

Lateral rectus muscle

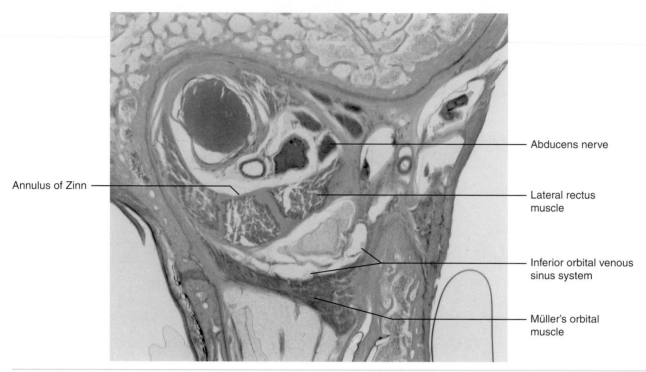

Annulus of Zinn

Abducens nerve

Lateral rectus muscle

Inferior orbital venous sinus system

Müller's orbital muscle

Figure 10-49 Lateral rectus muscle within the annulus of Zinn at the orbital apex.

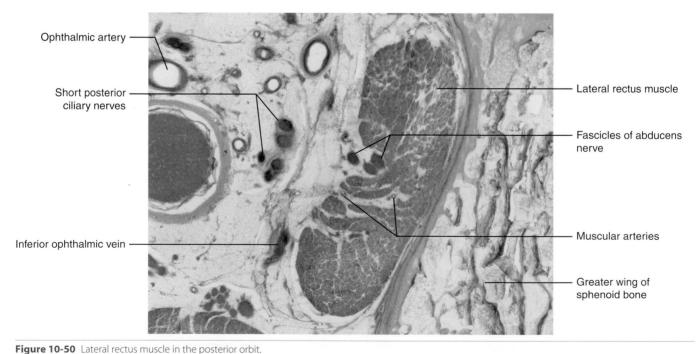

Ophthalmic artery

Short posterior ciliary nerves

Inferior ophthalmic vein

Lateral rectus muscle

Fascicles of abducens nerve

Muscular arteries

Greater wing of sphenoid bone

Figure 10-50 Lateral rectus muscle in the posterior orbit.

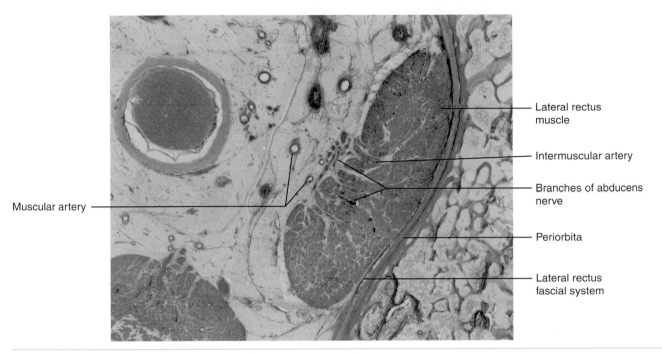

Lateral rectus muscle

Intermuscular artery

Branches of abducens nerve

Periorbita

Lateral rectus fascial system

Muscular artery

Figure 10-51 Lateral rectus muscle at the entrance of the abducens nerve rootlets.

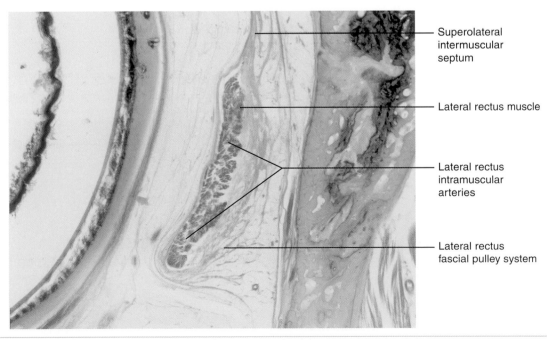

Superolateral intermuscular septum

Lateral rectus muscle

Lateral rectus intramuscular arteries

Lateral rectus fascial pulley system

Figure 10-52 Lateral rectus muscle near the transition to its tendon of insertion onto the globe.

Inferior oblique muscle

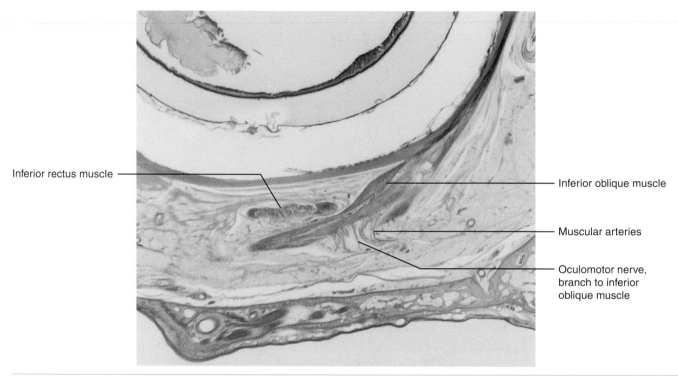

Inferior rectus muscle

Inferior oblique muscle

Muscular arteries

Oculomotor nerve, branch to inferior oblique muscle

Figure 10-53 Inferior rectus muscle at the level of its insertion onto the posterior globe.

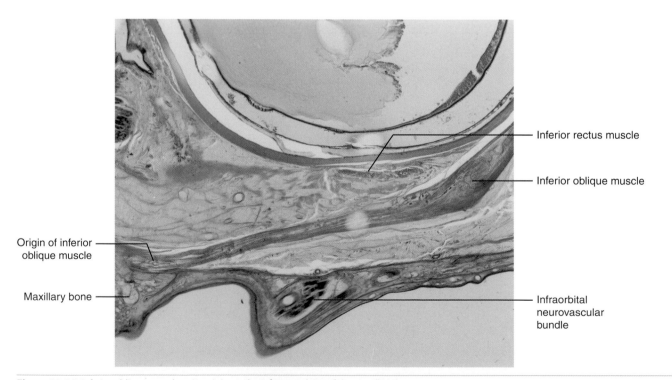

Inferior rectus muscle

Inferior oblique muscle

Origin of inferior oblique muscle

Maxillary bone

Infraorbital neurovascular bundle

Figure 10-54 Inferior oblique muscle at its origin on the inferonasal rim of the maxillary bone.

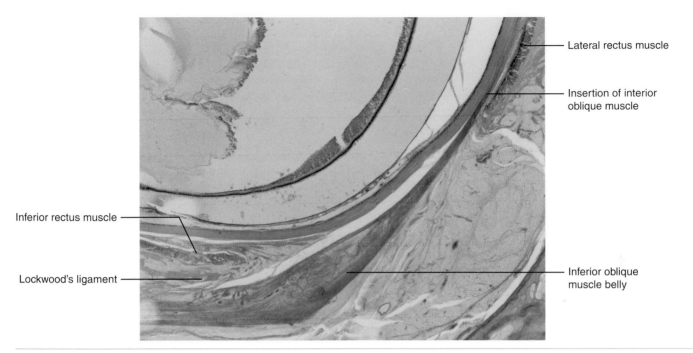

Lateral rectus muscle

Insertion of interior oblique muscle

Inferior rectus muscle

Lockwood's ligament

Inferior oblique muscle belly

Figure 10-55 Inferior oblique muscle within Lockwood's ligament as it crosses under the inferior rectus muscle.

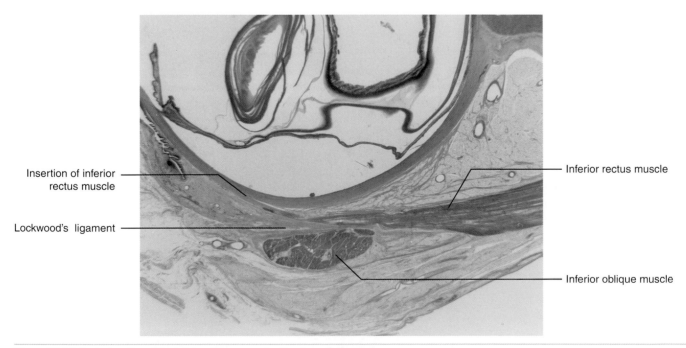

Insertion of inferior rectus muscle

Lockwood's ligament

Inferior rectus muscle

Inferior oblique muscle

Figure 10-56 Sagittal section of the inferior oblique muscle at Lockwood's ligament.

Superior oblique muscle

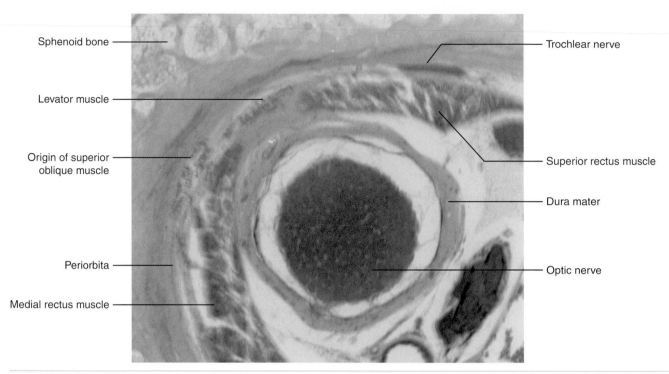

Sphenoid bone

Levator muscle

Origin of superior oblique muscle

Periorbita

Medial rectus muscle

Trochlear nerve

Superior rectus muscle

Dura mater

Optic nerve

Figure 10-57 Origin of the superior oblique muscle in the orbital apex just above the annulus of Zinn.

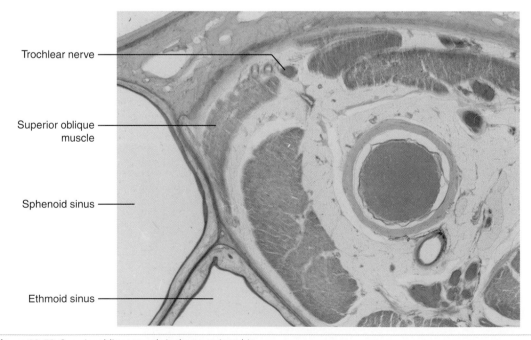

Trochlear nerve

Superior oblique muscle

Sphenoid sinus

Ethmoid sinus

Figure 10-58 Superior oblique muscle in the posterior orbit.

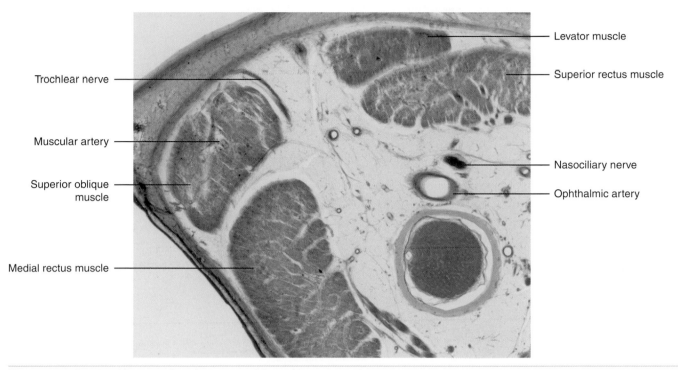

Trochlear nerve

Muscular artery

Superior oblique muscle

Medial rectus muscle

Levator muscle

Superior rectus muscle

Nasociliary nerve

Ophthalmic artery

Figure 10-59 Superior oblique muscle at the entrance of the trochlear nerve rootlets.

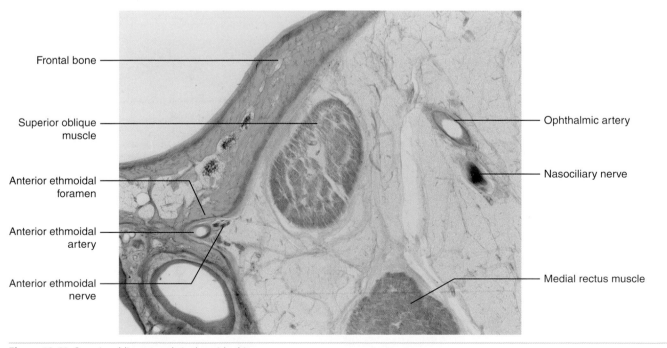

Frontal bone

Superior oblique muscle

Anterior ethmoidal foramen

Anterior ethmoidal artery

Anterior ethmoidal nerve

Ophthalmic artery

Nasociliary nerve

Medial rectus muscle

Figure 10-60 Superior oblique muscle in the mid-orbit.

Trochlea and superior oblique tendon

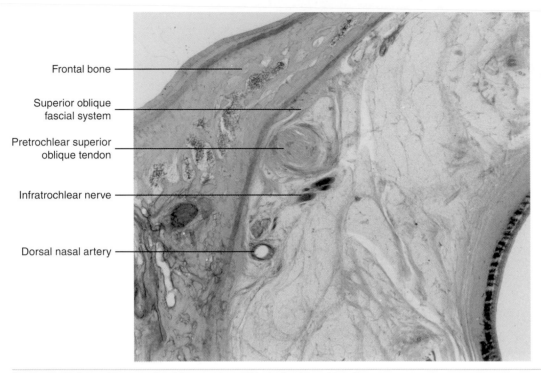

Frontal bone

Superior oblique
fascial system

Pretrochlear superior
oblique tendon

Infratrochlear nerve

Dorsal nasal artery

Figure 10-61 Pretrochlear superior oblique tendon within the fascial trochlea sling.

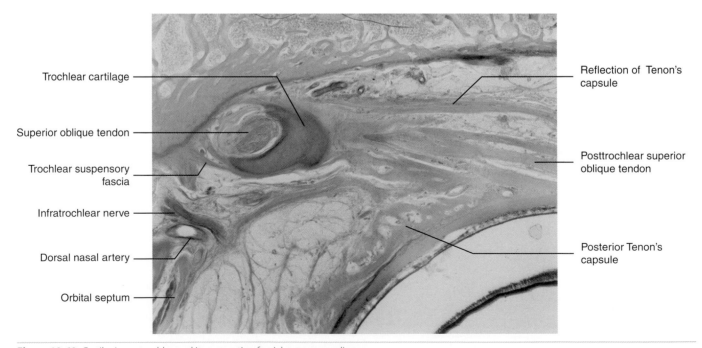

Trochlear cartilage

Superior oblique tendon

Trochlear suspensory
fascia

Infratrochlear nerve

Dorsal nasal artery

Orbital septum

Reflection of Tenon's
capsule

Posttrochlear superior
oblique tendon

Posterior Tenon's
capsule

Figure 10-62 Cartilaginous trochlea and its supporting fascial suspensory sling.

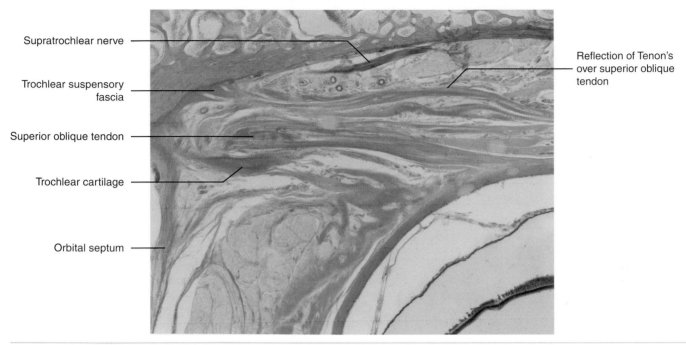

Supratrochlear nerve

Trochlear suspensory fascia

Superior oblique tendon

Trochlear cartilage

Orbital septum

Reflection of Tenon's over superior oblique tendon

Figure 10-63 Superior oblique tendon as it leaves the trochlea within its fascial sheath.

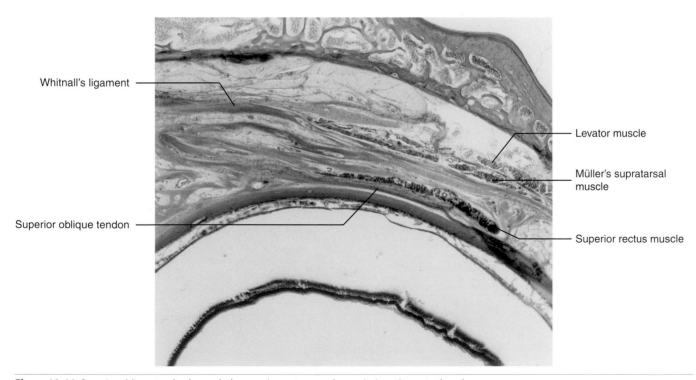

Whitnall's ligament

Superior oblique tendon

Levator muscle

Müller's supratarsal muscle

Superior rectus muscle

Figure 10-64 Superior oblique tendon beneath the superior rectus muscle near its insertion onto the sclera.

Müller's orbital muscle

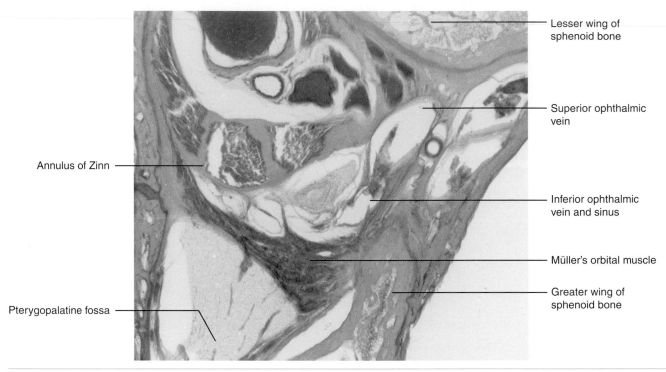

Lesser wing of
sphenoid bone

Superior ophthalmic
vein

Annulus of Zinn

Inferior ophthalmic
vein and sinus

Müller's orbital muscle

Greater wing of
sphenoid bone

Pterygopalatine fossa

Figure 10-65 Müller's orbital muscle beneath the annulus of Zinn at the orbital apex.

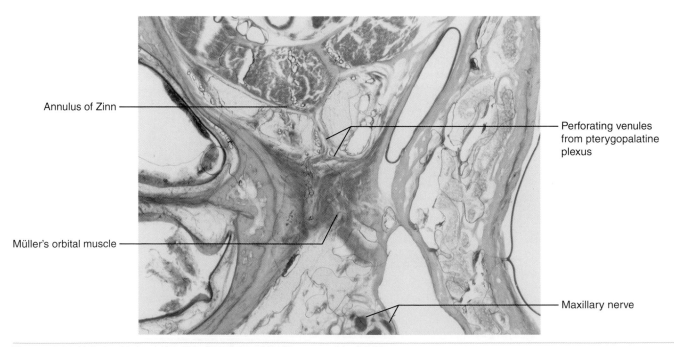

Annulus of Zinn

Perforating venules
from pterygopalatine
plexus

Müller's orbital muscle

Maxillary nerve

Figure 10-66 Müller's orbital muscle within the inferior orbital fissure near the orbital apex.

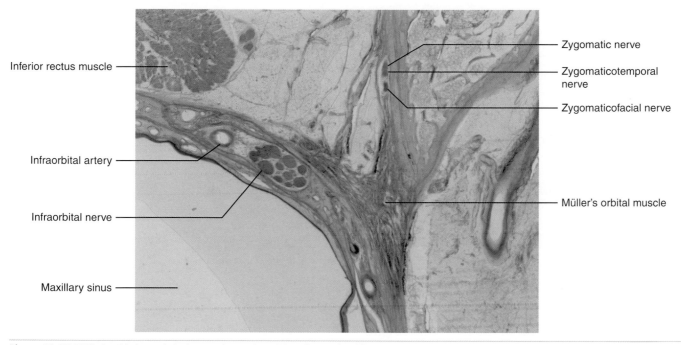

Inferior rectus muscle

Infraorbital artery

Infraorbital nerve

Maxillary sinus

Zygomatic nerve

Zygomaticotemporal nerve

Zygomaticofacial nerve

Müller's orbital muscle

Figure 10-67 Müller's orbital muscle in the anterior portion of the inferior orbital fissure.

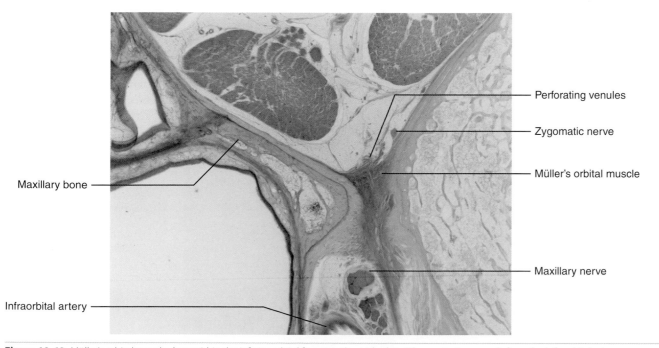

Maxillary bone

Infraorbital artery

Perforating venules

Zygomatic nerve

Müller's orbital muscle

Maxillary nerve

Figure 10-68 Müller's orbital muscle deep within the inferior orbital fissure in the mid-orbit with penetrating vessels from the infraorbital artery.

Orbital fascial connective tissue and pulley systems

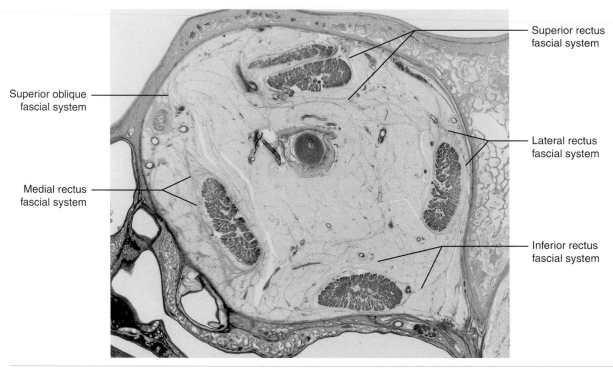

Superior oblique fascial system

Medial rectus fascial system

Superior rectus fascial system

Lateral rectus fascial system

Inferior rectus fascial system

Figure 10-69 Major orbital fascial systems in the mid-orbit.

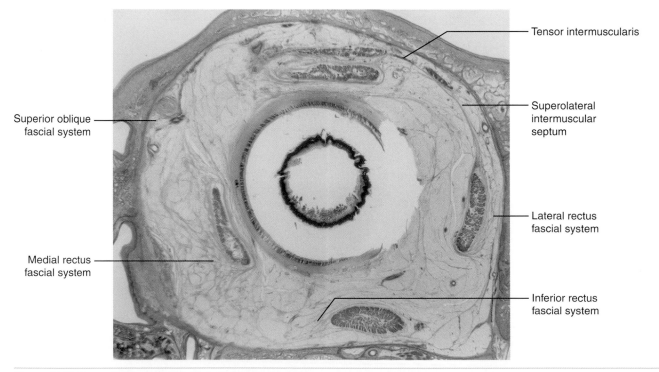

Superior oblique fascial system

Medial rectus fascial system

Tensor intermuscularis

Superolateral intermuscular septum

Lateral rectus fascial system

Inferior rectus fascial system

Figure 10-70 Connective tissue fascial systems in the anterior orbit.

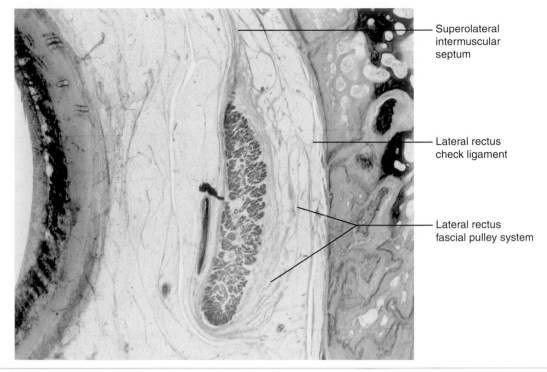

Superolateral
intermuscular
septum

Lateral rectus
check ligament

Lateral rectus
fascial pulley system

Figure 10-71 Lateral rectus suspensory and pulley system in the anterior orbit.

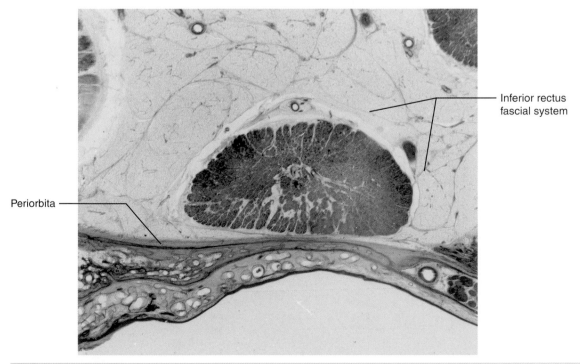

Inferior rectus
fascial system

Periorbita

Figure 10-72 Inferior rectus suspensory and pulley system in the mid-orbit.

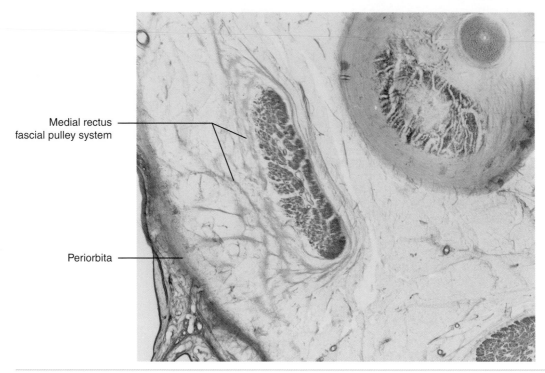

Figure 10-73 Medial rectus suspensory and pulley system at the level of the posterior globe.

Medial rectus
fascial pulley system

Periorbita

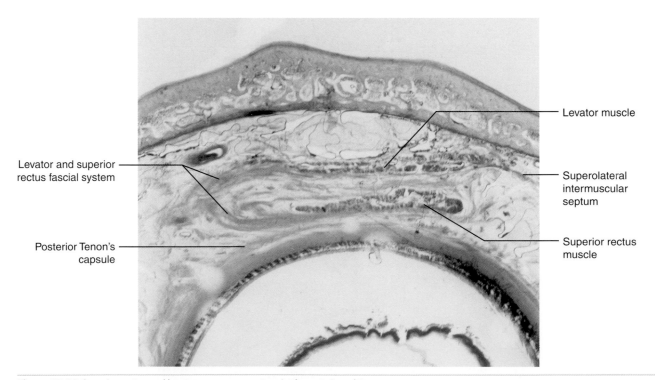

Figure 10-74 Superior rectus and levator suspensory system in the anterior orbit.

Levator and superior
rectus fascial system

Posterior Tenon's
capsule

Levator muscle

Superolateral
intermuscular
septum

Superior rectus
muscle

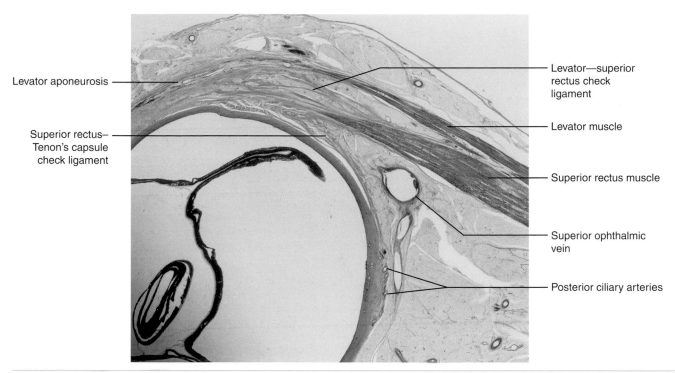

Levator aponeurosis

Superior rectus–
Tenon's capsule
check ligament

Levator—superior
rectus check
ligament

Levator muscle

Superior rectus muscle

Superior ophthalmic
vein

Posterior ciliary arteries

Figure 10-75 Sagittal section through the superior rectus and levator muscles and their suspensory systems, with posterior Tenon's capsule and the check ligaments.

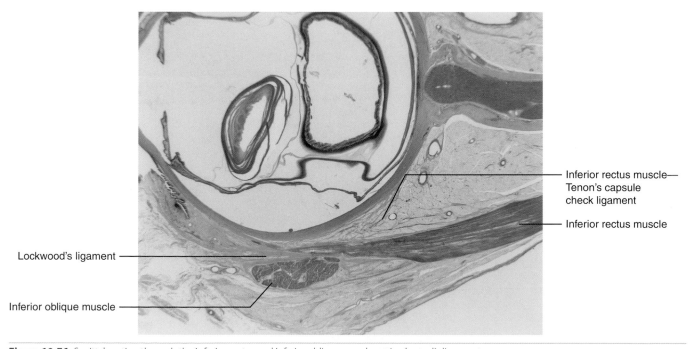

Inferior rectus muscle—
Tenon's capsule
check ligament

Inferior rectus muscle

Lockwood's ligament

Inferior oblique muscle

Figure 10-76 Sagittal section through the inferior rectus and inferior oblique muscles at Lockwood's ligament.

Medial and lateral canthal ligaments

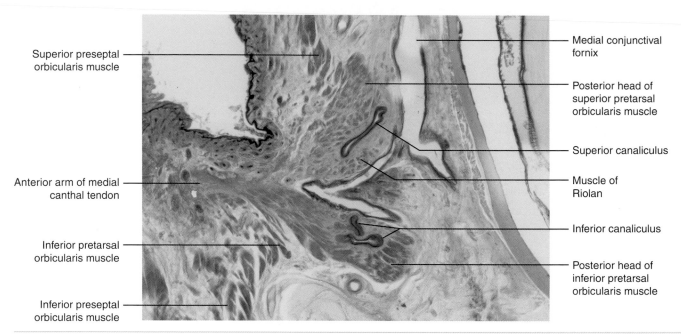

Superior preseptal orbicularis muscle

Anterior arm of medial canthal tendon

Inferior pretarsal orbicularis muscle

Inferior preseptal orbicularis muscle

Medial conjunctival fornix

Posterior head of superior pretarsal orbicularis muscle

Superior canaliculus

Muscle of Riolan

Inferior canaliculus

Posterior head of inferior pretarsal orbicularis muscle

Figure 10-77 Anterior surface of the medial canthal ligament and the muscles of Riolan.

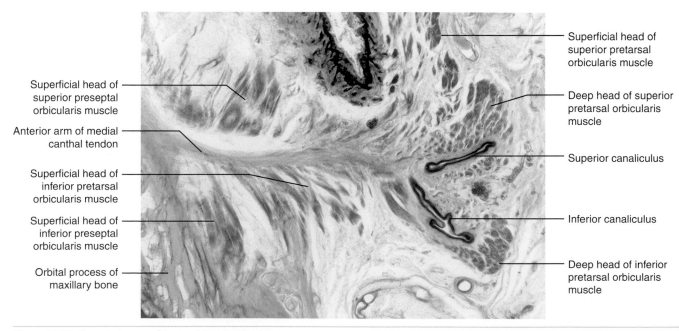

Superficial head of superior preseptal orbicularis muscle

Anterior arm of medial canthal tendon

Superficial head of inferior pretarsal orbicularis muscle

Superficial head of inferior preseptal orbicularis muscle

Orbital process of maxillary bone

Superficial head of superior pretarsal orbicularis muscle

Deep head of superior pretarsal orbicularis muscle

Superior canaliculus

Inferior canaliculus

Deep head of inferior pretarsal orbicularis muscle

Figure 10-78 The anterior arm of the medial canthal ligament.

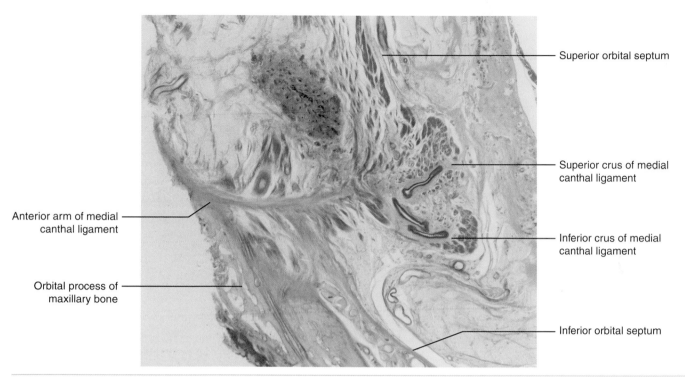

Superior orbital septum

Superior crus of medial canthal ligament

Inferior crus of medial canthal ligament

Anterior arm of medial canthal ligament

Orbital process of maxillary bone

Inferior orbital septum

Figure 10-79 Medial canthal ligament and the deep head of the preseptal orbicularis muscle.

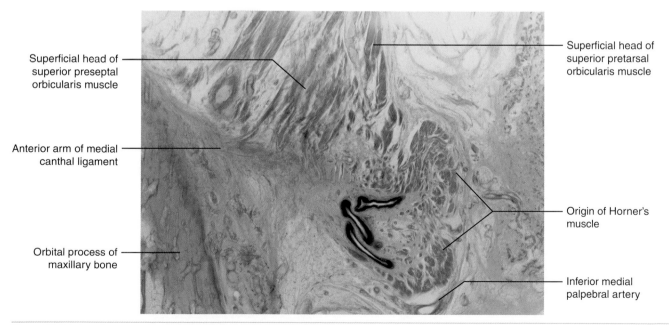

Superficial head of superior pretarsal orbicularis muscle

Superficial head of superior preseptal orbicularis muscle

Anterior arm of medial canthal ligament

Origin of Horner's muscle

Orbital process of maxillary bone

Inferior medial palpebral artery

Figure 10-80 Anterior arm and superior limb of the medial canthal ligament.

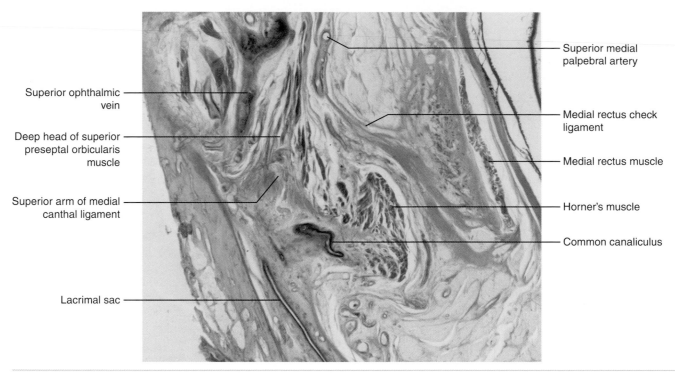

Superior ophthalmic vein

Deep head of superior preseptal orbicularis muscle

Superior arm of medial canthal ligament

Lacrimal sac

Superior medial palpebral artery

Medial rectus check ligament

Medial rectus muscle

Horner's muscle

Common canaliculus

Figure 10-81 Superior limb of the medial canthal ligament at the fascia of the lacrimal sac.

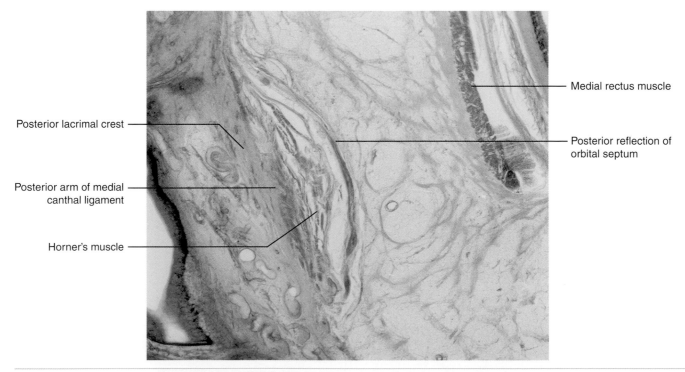

Posterior lacrimal crest

Posterior arm of medial canthal ligament

Horner's muscle

Medial rectus muscle

Posterior reflection of orbital septum

Figure 10-82 Horner's muscle and the posterior arm of the medial canthal ligament at the posterior lacrimal crest.

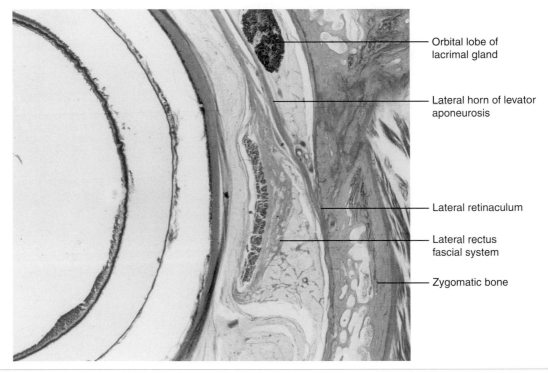

Figure 10-83 The lateral canthal ligament and lateral rectus check ligament at the lateral retinaculum.

- Orbital lobe of lacrimal gland
- Lateral horn of levator aponeurosis
- Lateral retinaculum
- Lateral rectus fascial system
- Zygomatic bone

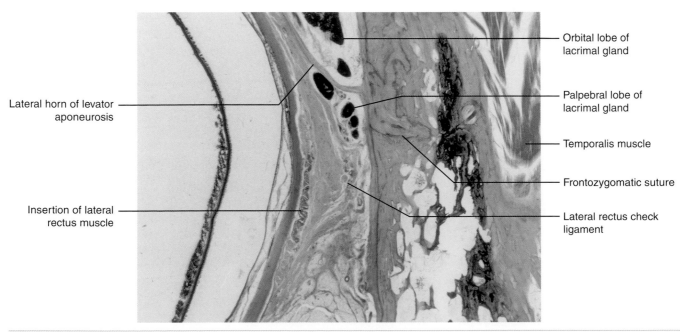

Figure 10-84 The posterior extent of the lateral retinaculum at the insertion of Whitnall's ligament.

- Lateral horn of levator aponeurosis
- Insertion of lateral rectus muscle
- Orbital lobe of lacrimal gland
- Palpebral lobe of lacrimal gland
- Temporalis muscle
- Frontozygomatic suture
- Lateral rectus check ligament

Eyelids

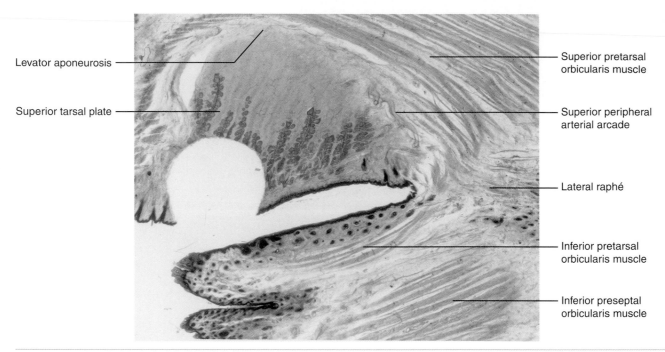

Levator aponeurosis

Superior tarsal plate

Superior pretarsal orbicularis muscle

Superior peripheral arterial arcade

Lateral raphé

Inferior pretarsal orbicularis muscle

Inferior preseptal orbicularis muscle

Figure 10-85 Tangential section through the upper and lower eyelid at the level of the orbicularis muscle and tarsal plate.

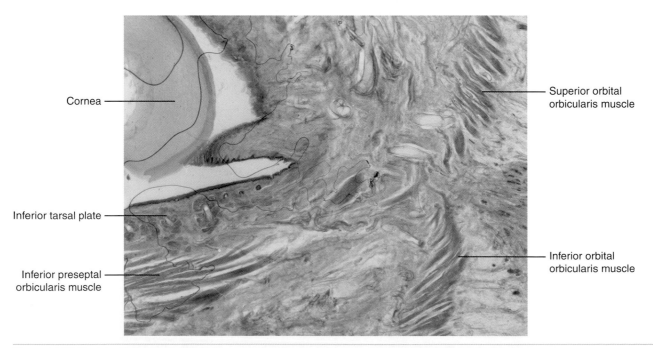

Cornea

Inferior tarsal plate

Inferior preseptal orbicularis muscle

Superior orbital orbicularis muscle

Inferior orbital orbicularis muscle

Figure 10-86 The lateral horizontal raphé.

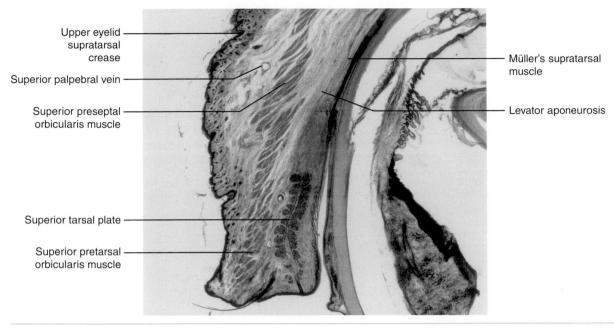

Upper eyelid supratarsal crease

Superior palpebral vein

Superior preseptal orbicularis muscle

Superior tarsal plate

Superior pretarsal orbicularis muscle

Müller's supratarsal muscle

Levator aponeurosis

Figure 10-87 Sagittal section through the upper eyelid.

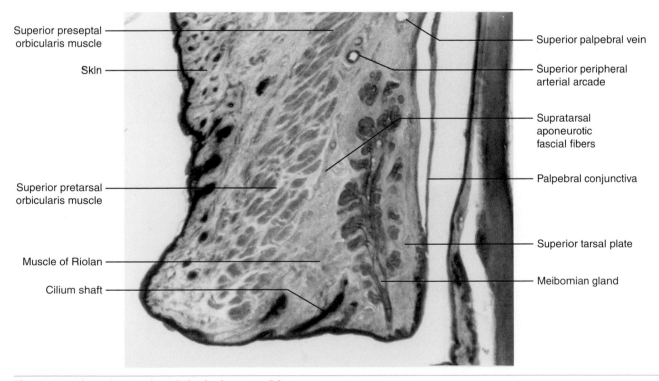

Superior preseptal orbicularis muscle

Skin

Superior pretarsal orbicularis muscle

Muscle of Riolan

Cilium shaft

Superior palpebral vein

Superior peripheral arterial arcade

Supratarsal aponeurotic fascial fibers

Palpebral conjunctiva

Superior tarsal plate

Meibomian gland

Figure 10-88 Sagittal section through the distal upper eyelid.

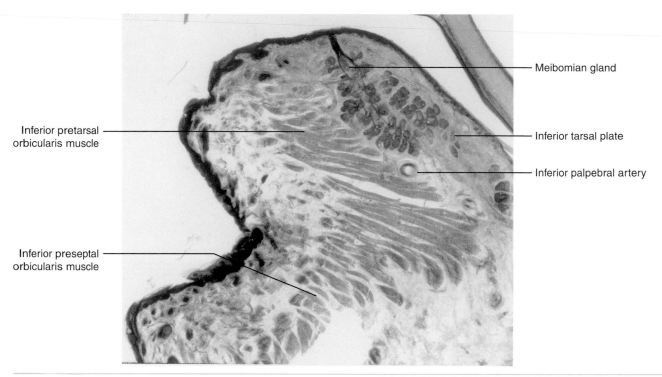

Meibomian gland

Inferior pretarsal
orbicularis muscle

Inferior tarsal plate

Inferior palpebral artery

Inferior preseptal
orbicularis muscle

Figure 10-89 Sagittal section through the lower eyelid.

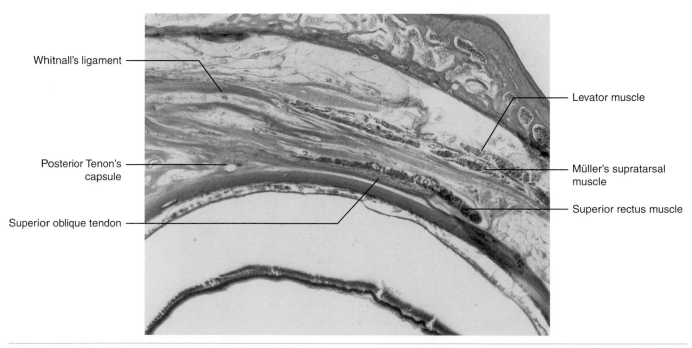

Whitnall's ligament

Levator muscle

Posterior Tenon's
capsule

Müller's supratarsal
muscle

Superior oblique tendon

Superior rectus muscle

Figure 10-90 Whitnall's ligament.

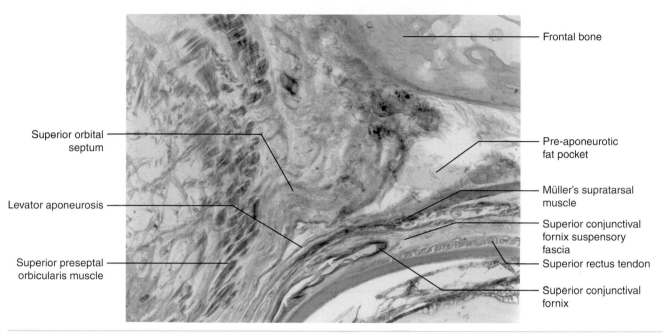

Superior orbital septum

Levator aponeurosis

Superior preseptal orbicularis muscle

Frontal bone

Pre-aponeurotic fat pocket

Müller's supratarsal muscle

Superior conjunctival fornix suspensory fascia

Superior rectus tendon

Superior conjunctival fornix

Figure 10-91 Sagittal section through the orbital septum at the superior arcus marginalis.

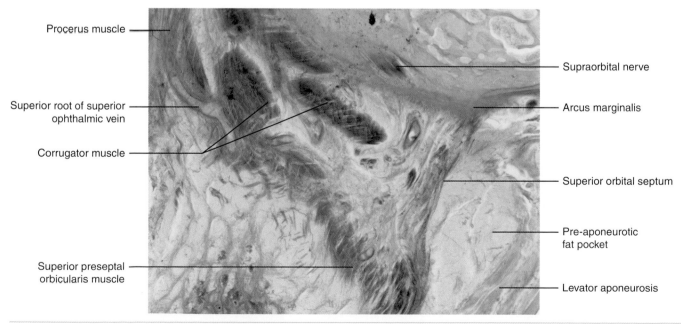

Procerus muscle

Superior root of superior ophthalmic vein

Corrugator muscle

Superior preseptal orbicularis muscle

Supraorbital nerve

Arcus marginalis

Superior orbital septum

Pre-aponeurotic fat pocket

Levator aponeurosis

Figure 10-92 Sagittal section through the corrugator muscle.

Lacrimal systems

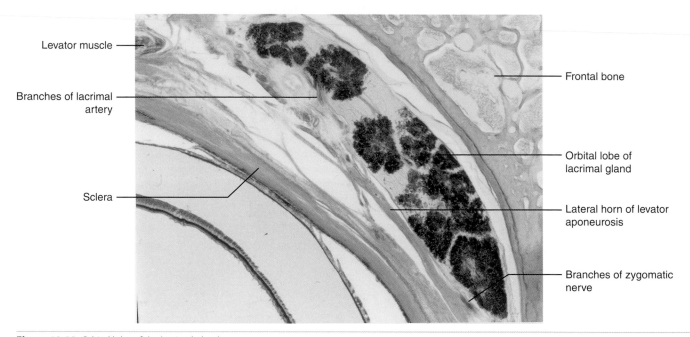

Levator muscle

Branches of lacrimal artery

Sclera

Frontal bone

Orbital lobe of lacrimal gland

Lateral horn of levator aponeurosis

Branches of zygomatic nerve

Figure 10-93 Orbital lobe of the lacrimal gland.

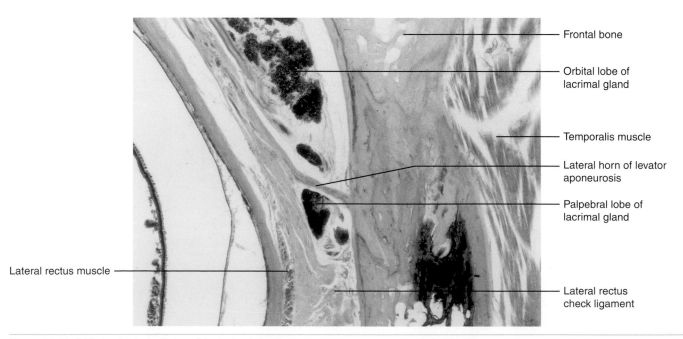

Frontal bone

Orbital lobe of lacrimal gland

Temporalis muscle

Lateral horn of levator aponeurosis

Palpebral lobe of lacrimal gland

Lateral rectus muscle

Lateral rectus check ligament

Figure 10-94 Orbital and palpebral lobes of the lacrimal gland.

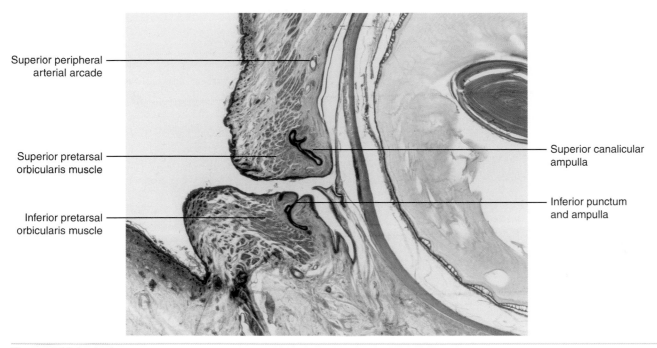

Superior peripheral arterial arcade

Superior pretarsal orbicularis muscle

Inferior pretarsal orbicularis muscle

Superior canalicular ampulla

Inferior punctum and ampulla

Figure 10-95 Lacrimal puncta.

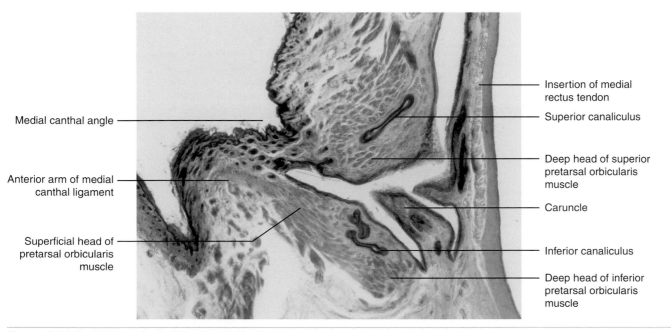

Medial canthal angle

Anterior arm of medial canthal ligament

Superficial head of pretarsal orbicularis muscle

Insertion of medial rectus tendon

Superior canaliculus

Deep head of superior pretarsal orbicularis muscle

Caruncle

Inferior canaliculus

Deep head of inferior pretarsal orbicularis muscle

Figure 10-96 Canaliculi near the medial conjunctival fornix.

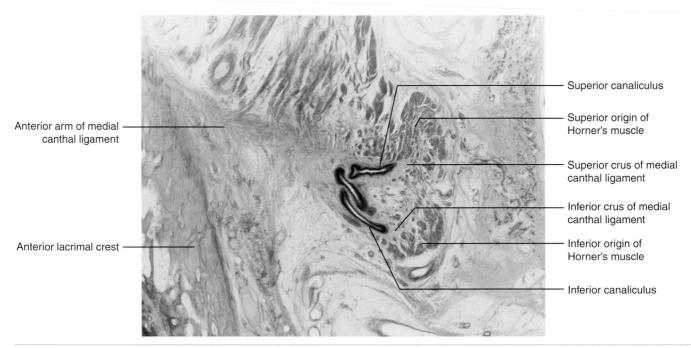

Superior canaliculus

Superior origin of Horner's muscle

Superior crus of medial canthal ligament

Inferior crus of medial canthal ligament

Inferior origin of Horner's muscle

Inferior canaliculus

Anterior arm of medial canthal ligament

Anterior lacrimal crest

Figure 10-97 Canaliculi within the medial canthal ligament.

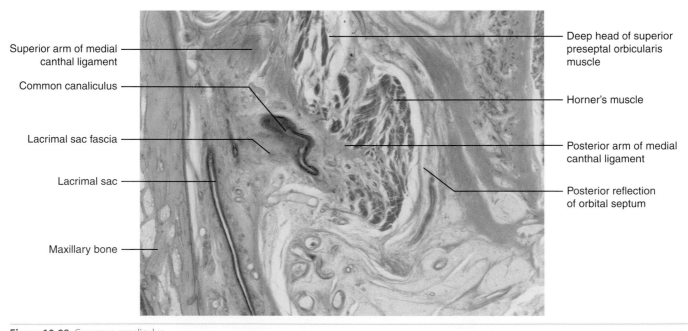

Superior arm of medial canthal ligament

Common canaliculus

Lacrimal sac fascia

Lacrimal sac

Maxillary bone

Deep head of superior preseptal orbicularis muscle

Horner's muscle

Posterior arm of medial canthal ligament

Posterior reflection of orbital septum

Figure 10-98 Common canaliculus.

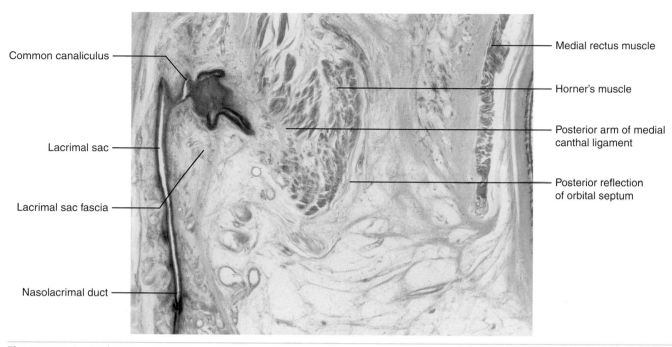

Common canaliculus

Lacrimal sac

Lacrimal sac fascia

Nasolacrimal duct

Medial rectus muscle

Horner's muscle

Posterior arm of medial canthal ligament

Posterior reflection of orbital septum

Figure 10-99 Lacrimal sac.

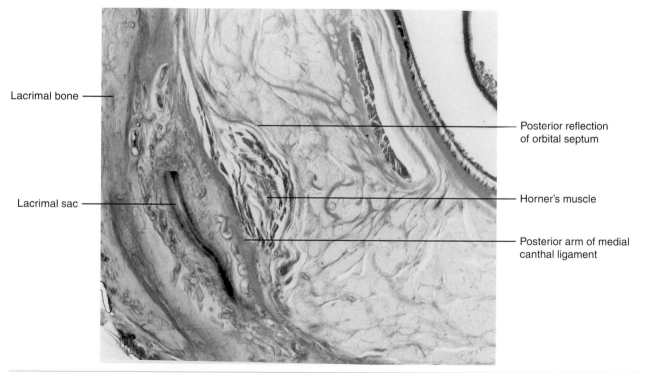

Lacrimal bone

Lacrimal sac

Posterior reflection of orbital septum

Horner's muscle

Posterior arm of medial canthal ligament

Figure 10-100 Lacrimal sac fascia and the posterior arm of the medial canthal tendon.

CHAPTER 11

Radiographic Correlations

Radiographic examination is an essential part in the evaluation of all patients with suspected orbital disease. Not only can this contribute to a specific diagnosis, but may also guide the physician in planning the most appropriate medical therapy or surgical approach. Although the plain orbital series may provide useful information on bony structure, and can often suggest soft tissue pathology, its use in evaluation of the orbit has largely been replaced by more sophisticated computerized tomographic and magnetic resonance imaging (MRI) techniques.[15,19] Advanced imaging techniques now allow the evaluation of an increasing number of normal anatomic structures,[2,5] as well as and pathologic processes in the orbit.[3,5]

Computerized tomography of the orbit

Thin-section, high-resolution computerized tomography (CT) has revolutionized the study of orbital pathology. It allows simultaneous examination of bony structures and associated soft tissue. This technique has proven to be superior to the plain orbital series for most orbital pathology, with a high level of diagnostic accuracy.[11,16,18,27,37,38] CT is considerd the initial imaging procedure of choice for evaluating orbital trauma.[21,35]

Computerized tomography utilizes thin collumated X-ray beams that pass through tissue along the rows and columns of an intersecting matrix. The area of intersection of any two beams is referred to as the pixel, and is analogous to a single gray dot in a newspaper photograph. Because the X-ray beam has a certain thickness, the area of beam intersection actually defines a volumetric space, with surface area equal to the pixel size, and depth equal to the beam width or slice thickness. This volumetric space is referred to as the voxel. As the X-ray beams traverse the body, they are attenuated according to the density of the tissues through which they pass. These attenuated beams are transmitted to a series of radiation detectors on the opposite side of the patient. The degree of attenuation of any two beams emerging from the tissue allows calculation of the mean attenuation value for all the tissues included in the area of intersection of the beams, or voxel. All tissues within the voxel are averaged together to yield a single attenuation value. The smaller the pixel and thinner the tissue slice thickness, the smaller the volume of the voxel, the less tissue included within it, and the higher the resolution of the final image.

In modern generation scanning machines the the detectors are arranged in a stationary ring surrounding the patient. The X-ray tube emits a fan beam which is read by various groups of detectors as the beam rotates. The slice thickness is generally between 1.0–1.5 mm, and the volume of the voxel may be less than 0.375 mm^3.[27] Such high degrees of spatial resolution, plus newer software capabilities that allow multiplanar transformations of axial scans to coronal, sagittal and oblique orientations, allow a high level of diagnostic and localizing accuracy.

Each voxel is assigned an attenuation value by the computer based on the mean attenuation of the X-ray beams passing through it. These values are designated in Houndsfield units, a 2000-unit scale from −1000 to +1000. By arbitrary convention, the density of air is assigned a value of −1000, the density of water is 0, and the density of bone is +1000. For visualization by the human eye, this scale is reduced to 32–64 gray levels between black and white on the X-ray film or computer screen. Thus, air appears black on the film, and bone appears white. All densities greater than bone, such as a metallic foreign body, also appear white.

For examination of specific anatomic detail, the image may be manipulated by setting windows. The window level refers to the Houndsfield unit on which a small range of units is to be centered. The window range is the number of Houndsfield units above and below this level that are to be expanded into the black to white scale for imaging. In examination of a soft-tissue lesion, for example, the window level may be set to +50, the density of muscle, and the window range to plus (+) and minus (−) 200 units. With these window settings muscle is depicted as medium grey, −150 on the scale appears black, and +250 appears white. All attenuation values below −150 also appear black, and there is no detail visible in the orbital fat. Similarly, all those values above +250 appear white, and there is no detail seen in bone. For examination of subtle bony changes, the window level must be adjusted upward to around +800 with a range of about +600 to +1000.

Iodinated intravenous contrast agents are frequently utilized to improve contrast by increasing the Houndsfield number of vessels or of highly vascularized tissues. Such agents may help outline normal anatomy, and can more clearly define pathologic processes.

Orbital computerized tomography should routinely include scans in both the axial and coronal planes. Special transformations in the sagittal and oblique orientations may be useful for some lesions. Contrast enhancement is generally less useful than for brain studies because of the lack of a blood-orbital barrier, but often provides valuable information on the nature of particular types of lesions. Unless otherwise contraindicated, contrasted studies should be included in all orbital scans. Where possible bony involvement is suspected, bone windows should be included.

Magnetic resonance imaging

Magnetic resonance imaging (MRI) offers several advantages over CT. It is superior for tissue differentiation and is the imaging procedure of choice for the evaluation of non-traumatic orbit pathology.[6,38] Because of the low signal generated from bone, soft tissue visualization in the region of the orbital apex, optic canal, and cavernous sinus is not degraded as in CT scans.[4,8,10,11,13,14,19] The manipulation of extrinsic parameters for weighting T1 and T2 signals provides contrast variability and tissue differentiation unobtainable with X-ray techniques.[9] With the introduction of small surface coil technology resulting in improved signal-to-noise ratios, the anatomic quality of orbital images is now equal or superior to that of computerized tomography.[26,29,30,31,33] Techniques for suppressing the high fat signals have further improved visualization of orbital lesions.[1,23,32] Additional new technologies allow dynamic MR angiography similar to CT angiography without the risks of iodinated contrast agents and ionizing radiation.[20] MRI has become a particularly important modality for imaging of the optic pathways.[34]

The generation of a magnetic resonance signal depends upon the presence of magnetic isotopes of common elements in biological tissues. The atom most frequently imaged is the ubiquitous hydrogen nucleus, or proton.[10,17] Like all atomic nuclei, the proton is normally in a state of axial spin. This spinning charged particle generates a magnetic field, with north and south poles analogous to a bar magnet. Under normal conditions, all the nuclei in a given volume of tissue are randomly oriented, with no net magnetic vector. When placed within a strong external magnetic field, the individual protons align with the external magnetic direction, either parallel or antiparallel. Because of the slight preponderance of alignments parallel to the magnetic field direction, the tissue assumes a mean magnetic moment in the same orientation. Most of the axes of individual protons are not perfectly aligned with the magnetic direction, but lie at various small angles to this mean magnetic moment. Also, these deviations are equally distributed 360° around it. Like spinning tops, these inclined axes wobble, with one pole remaining stationary and the other revolving, or precessing, around the mean magnetic direction. The rotating axes, therefore, describe a conical surface. The angular velocity of precession is determined by the strength of the external magnetic field, and by an intrinsic property of the particular atomic nucleus, called the gyromagnetic ratio, which is proportional to its magnetic moment.[19,29] The relationship between these factors is defined by the Larmor equation, and the resultant angular velocity is the resonant or Larmor frequency.

When this system is exposed to a radiofrequency (RF) pulse at the Larmor frequency, energy is absorbed by the atomic nuclei. As the spinning nuclei move into higher energy levels, the angular orientation of their axes to the external magnetic direction increases. Also, an induced magnetic field perpendicular to the radiofrequency pulse direction realigns the individual atomic axes to one side of the external magnetic direction. When the RF signal is turned off, the spinning nuclei return to equilibrium by giving up energy to the environment, again at the Larmor frequency. Return to equilibrium occurs by two simultaneous decay, or relaxation, processes.

During the T1 relaxation, the individual nuclear axes realign parallel to the external magnetic direction. In the process, they give up their absorbed energy which is detected as a resonance signal. The time required for this process is the T1, or spin-lattice relaxation time. It is influenced by the interaction of the proton to other atoms within the molecular lattice, and by temperature and viscosity of the tissue. A high T1 relaxation time yields maximum energy release per unit time, and therefore a higher resonance signal and brighter image on the final scan.

Immediately following the RF pulse signal, while the atomic nuclei are still grouped on one side of the mean magnetic axis, they generate a radiofrequency signal. This results from the tipped net magnetic vector of the spinning protons constantly cutting across the lines of force of the external magnetic direction, thus generating a small alternating current voltage. During the T2 relaxation, the atomic nuclei redistribute themselves evenly 360° around the external magnetic field direction, and as they do so the strength of this signal decreases due to canceling vectors. The time for complete decay of this RF signal is the T2, or spin-spin relaxation time. It is influenced by the induced magnetic fields generated around adjacent spinning nuclei. As with the T1 times, biochemical differences between tissues confer slightly different T2 relaxation times to their protons. Because it is the T1 and T2 signal strengths that determine the contrast intensity, these biochemical differences result in contrast differentiation on the final MR image. Since small differences in T1 and T2 relaxation can easily be detected, contrast differentiation between adjacent tissues on MRI is considerably better than with CT.

The T1 and T2 signals are measured by radiofrequency detectors. They will detect in mass fashion all similar signals at the Larmor frequency, regardless of their specific location within the tissue. Spatial encoding of resonant signals from particular small blocks of tissue is necessary for the creation of a visually meaningful two-dimensional image. This is achieved by deformation of the external magnetic field using gradient coils, such that the protons in every small volume of examined tissue (voxel) has a unique magnetic field strength, and therefore a unique Larmor frequency. Each unique frequency, therefore, will identify the precise location of the signal, and a topographically mapped image can be created.

The final MR image is determined by the proton density, and by variations in the T1 and T2 decay times of tissue components. The radiofrequency energy can be manipulated by application of various pulsed sequences, thus altering the way the T1 and T2 resonance signals are collected. The MR image can therefore be weighted in favor of the T1 or the T2 information. Also, the influence of both can be minimized, so that the final image more nearly represents only proton density.

The major component of the MRI system is the magnet which provides the primary polarizing field. This is usually a set of coils of superconducting wire suspended in liquid helium. The quality of the MRI image generally increases with the field strength measured in Tesla units (1 T = 10000 Gauss). Most systems operate at 0.5–1.5 T. Located within the bore of the magnet are the gradient coils which provide the spatial localization information during the imaging process. Within the gradient coils are the RF antennae ("coils") which transmit the RF energy to the tissues and receive the resonance signals. The use of smaller surface coils placed immediately over the are of interest increases the signal strength from these areas, and minimizes signals from outside this region, thus significantly improving the surface-to-noise ratio. These permit the acquisition of high resolution images of 0.5 mm pixels at 3 mm slice thickness. However, such coils are limited to the depth of penetration they can image, and they are associated with significant artifact.

Gadolinium is a rare earth element with paramagnetic properties. In the presence of an external magnetic influence its paramagnetic moment preferentially aligns with the field. The magnetic moment of gadolinium is 1000 times greater than that of a hydrogen nucleus, and its presence in tissues shortens the T1 relaxation time resulting in a marked increase in signal intensity.[19] This enhancing effect of gadolinium may result in decreased contrast in the orbit due to the intense signal from adjacent retrobulbar fat on routine T1 weighted sequences. Various fat-suppression techniques are now available that permit the evaluation of gadolinium enhanced tissues within the orbital fat.

Normal orbital anatomy in the axial plane

Axial section through the inferior orbit

The orbital floor reaches its lowest level about 1 cm behind the orbital rim, and from this point it rises upward toward the orbital apex. Therefore, in axial sections through the lowermost portion of the orbit, only the anterolateral part of the orbital cavity is seen. The orbital floor appears as a thin oblique density running from anteromedial to posterolateral, separating the orbit above from the maxillary sinus below. Since the floor gradually slopes backward and upward, it is cut in successively more posterior cross-sections on axial scan sequences from inferior to superior. In the midportion of the floor is an oval of moderate density. This is the infraorbital canal containing the infraorbital neurovascular bundle.

The anterior of the orbital cavity may be closed by the infraorbital rim which lies slightly higher than the floor. In slightly higher sections, the rim is incomplete so that the orbit appears as a triangle open anteriorly. The orbital space is bounded medially by the anterior lacrimal crest and lacrimal bone, and laterally by the lateral rim of the zygomatic bone. A thin line is seen arching across the orbital opening from the medial to the lateral bony rims. This represents structures in the lower eyelid, most notably the tarsal plate, orbicularis muscle, and orbital septum.

Depending upon the level of the cut, the orbital cavity may appear empty due to the presence of inferior extraconal orbital fat, or it may contain a rounded density representing the sclera cut tangentially (Figure 11-1). The inferior oblique muscle is seen as an oblique triangular band of medium-density tissue originating from the anterior lacrimal crest and running laterally and posteriorly across the globe. Laterally, the insertion of the inferior oblique muscle forms an elevated bulge on the scleral outline. The inferior rectus muscle appears as a band-like density running posteriorly from the globe to the bony floor. Because the inferior rectus is oriented upward and backward along the floor, it is cut in oblique cross-section, and is not usually represented along its entire length. The branch of the oculomotor nerve to the inferior oblique muscle may sometimes be seen along the lateral edge of the inferior rectus muscle.

Within the nasal cavity the nasal septum is seen anteriorly as a plate-like structure in the mid-sagittal plane terminating posteriorly at the vomer. On either side of the nasal septum, are the nasal bones. In the extreme anteromedial wall of the maxillary sinus is a small rounded lucency, the nasolacrimal canal. It is separated both from the sinus and the nasal cavity by thin lamina of bone. The density within the duct varies from black to gray depending upon whether it contains air or mucus.[28]

On either side of the nasal septum is the air-filled nasal cavity. Within it the inferior turbinate appears as a soft-tissue ridge that may be lying free in the nasal vestibule. These run along the entire medial wall of the maxillary sinus.

Immediately outside the lateral wall of the orbit is the temporal fossa. The density filling the fossa is the temporalis muscle. Just behind this, extending from the pterygoid plate to the ramus of the jaw is the lateral pterygoid muscle. More posteriorly the foramen magnum and structures of the basicranium may be visualized.[16]

Axial section through the lower orbit

In axial sections through the lower orbit neither the orbital floor nor the maxillary sinus are seen. The medial wall is formed by the thin lamina papyracea of the ethmoid sinus which usually bows into the orbit as a gentle curve (Figure 11-2). The lateral wall is considerably thicker and is formed by the zygomatic bone anteriorly and the greater wing of the sphenoid posteriorly. In slightly higher sections a small gap in the lateral wall posteriorly represents the superior orbital fissure.

Anteriorly the nasal bones and orbital process of the maxillary bones lie on either side of the nasal vestibule. In the anteromedial corner of the orbit the lacrimal sac fossa is seen as a depression or a lucency in the orbital process of the maxillary bone. Anterior and posterior to the sac, the crura of the medial canthal ligament may be visualized. A linear density extending across the anterior orbital space from the anterior lacrimal crest to the lateral orbital rim is the eyelid shadow, representing the orbital septum.

Within the anterior orbital space the globe appears as a rounded density. The sclera, choroid and retina appear as a single unit on CT, but may be seen as two layers on MRI. The darker central area is the vitreous cavity. Since the vitreous is primarily aqueous, it appears as low density on CT. On MRI scans the vitreous appears dark on T1 weighted sequences, and bright on T2 sequences. Liquefied vitreous will image slightly brighter than vitreous gel due to its shorter T1 relaxation time.[16]

Just posterior to the globe, the inferior rectus muscle appears as a band-like density in the central orbit that is not in contact with the globe, but extends back into the orbital apex. When this is enlarged, as in patients with thyroid orbitopathy, it may easily be mistaken for an orbital mass. The inferior medial vortex vein may be seen as a small vessel crossing the orbit from medial to lateral between the globe and the inferior rectus muscle. The inferior lateral vortex vein appears as a linear density parallel to the lateral rectus muscle. The medial ophthalmic vein is occasionally visible along the lamina papyracea extending from the region of the lacrimal sac to the superior orbital fissure. In the posterior orbit, a small vessel may be seen passing into the inferior orbital fissure, just anterior to the greater wing of the sphenoid. This is the inferior ophthalmic vein. The lower border of the medial and lateral rectus muscles may be seen in slightly higher sections, and lie along the orbital walls as thin densities that extend forward to contact the sclera.

Anteriorly, spanning the orbit from lateral rim to anterior lacrimal crest, are one or two lines. These represent the tarsus, orbicularis muscle, or orbital septum.

Axial section through the mid-orbit

On axial scans through the mid-orbit the globe is seen in horizontal equatorial section. Anteriorly the lens appears as an oval density. On MR sections, the ciliary body can be distinguished on either side of the lens (Figure 11-3). Behind the globe the optic nerve emerges from the posterior sclera and runs toward the orbital apex. Because the optic nerve describes a sinusoidal path through the orbit it is usually not seen in its entire length. Rather, the nerve may appear as several discontinuous segments of variable width.[36]

In the posterior third of the orbit the second portion of the ophthalmic artery is seen as a gently curved line that crosses the optic nerve from lateral to medial. Several linear densities may be seen running anteroposteriorly along the optic nerve. These are the posterior ciliary arteries and nerves, and they may appear irregular due to their undulating course. Small segments of the vortex veins may also be seen on some sections adjacent to the globe or free within the orbit. Along the lateral and medial orbital walls are the lateral and medial rectus muscles. At slightly higher levels, both the medial rectus and superior oblique muscles are often seen together.

The lacrimal sac is usually not seen at this level, its place being taken by the thickened frontal process of the maxillary bone. The medial and lateral canthal ligaments can usually be seen as densities near the medial and lateral orbital rims respectively.

Axial section through the upper orbit

At this level the orbital contour is narrower and terminates posteriorly in a rounded angle above the level of the optic canal. The uppermost portion of the superior orbital fissure may still be visible. Within the orbital outline the globe is represented in cross-section above the level of the lens, and on MRI the ciliary body is still seen (Figure 11-4). Along the medial wall the lower border of the superior oblique muscle and trochlea may be visualized. In lower mid-orbital sections the superior rectus muscle appears near the orbital apex as a broad band of tissue directed toward the globe.

The immediate retrobulbar portion of the optic nerve is visible adjacent to the posterior sclera. More posteriorly, the nerve is usually obscured by the superior rectus muscle. The superior ophthalmic vein is a curvilinear enhancing structure that crosses the orbit between the optic nerve and superior rectus muscle from anteromedial to posterolateral (Figure 11-5). Posteriorly, it is directed toward its exit through the superior orbital fissure. The lacrimal vein may be seen running along the lateral orbital wall, and just above it is the lacrimal artery. The superior vortex veins appear as thin linear densities at the scleral rim and free within the orbit.

Axial section through the orbital roof

In axial sections through the orbital roof the posterior limit of the orbit is seen further forward. This represents the frontal bone cut in oblique section. Medially, the frontal sinus is seen as a paired lucency on either side of the midline. The rectus gyri of the frontal lobes lie just medial to the orbits.

The superior rectus and levator muscle complex is seen as a broad band extending from the globe backward along the roof (Figure 11-6). Medially, the superior oblique muscle may still be visible, and the trochlea is clearly seen at the superomedial rim. The superior oblique tendon turns laterally and fans out over the globe toward its insertion.

The lacrimal gland is see in the superiolateral orbit between the globe and the orbital rim, and the lacrimal artry or vein may still be visible at this level. Just anterior to the globe and bridging across the anterior orbit is the upper eyelid, represented by the orbicularis muscle.

Normal orbital anatomy in the coronal plane

Coronal section through the orbital apex

At this level the orbit is seen as a small rounded space open inferiorly to the pterygopalatine fossa. Laterally the orbit is bounded by the greater wing of the sphenoid, and medially by the body of the sphenoid adjacent to the sphenoid sinus. Superolaterally in more posterior sections the orbit opens into the middle cranial fossa through the superior orbital fissure.

Within the orbital space, individual structures may be difficult to distinguish clearly. The rectus muscles merge into the annulus of Zinn which appears as a thickened ring that may be incomplete laterally (Figure 11-7). More anteriorly, the individual muscles become better defined and separated from one another. The optic nerve is a central density within the medial portion of the oculomotor foramen. The superior ophthalmic vein is a large rounded structure superolaterally between the superior rectus and lateral rectus muscles. The ophthalmic artery varies in position depending upon the level of the section. It begins inferior to the optic nerve, but then passes around the lateral edge of the nerve and crosses the orbit between the nerve and the superior rectus muscle. Slightly more anterior to the annulus of Zinn the origins of the levator and superior oblique muscles become visible.

More posteriorly, on T1 MRI sections through the level of the cavernous sinus, small foci of high-intensity signals can be seen in the lateral wall that correspond to cranial nerves III, V1, V2, and VI. Adjacent flowing blood produces negligible signals.[27] Cranial nerve IV cannot usually be identified because of its small size.

Coronal section through the posterior orbit

In the posterior orbit the bony contour widens to a triangular shape, with the apex directed toward the inferior orbital fissure and infratemporal fossa. Medially, the orbital wall is formed by the lamina papyracea of the ethmoid bone, and inferiorly the maxillary bone separates the orbit from the maxillary sinus. The orbital roof is formed by the frontal bone, and makes an undulating contour on the intracranial surface reflecting the gyri and sulci of the overlying frontal lobe.

Within the orbit the optic nerve lies centrally. The six extraocular muscles are clearly seen against the orbital walls (Figure 11-8). The superior ophthalmic vein has moved further laterally to a position beneath the lateral superior rectus muscle. Just above the optic nerve the ophthalmic artery seen as it continues its medial course over the nerve. The inferior ophthalmic vein is seen in the lateral orbit, between the inferior and lateral rectus muscles. The medial and lateral posterior ciliary arteries and nerves may be seen on either side of the optic nerve.

Coronal section through the central orbit

On coronal sections in the central orbit just behind the globe the medial orbital wall is a thin vertical plate formed by the lamina papyracea. Medial to this is the ethmoid sinus. Within the nose the middle turbinate forms a vertical plate that hangs from the nasal roof. The lateral orbital wall consists of the greater wing of the sphenoid bone. The floor appears as on previous sections as a thin plate sloping downward from medial to lateral, and separating the orbit from the maxillary sinus. Within the floor is the infraorbital canal and neurovascular bundle. Superiorly in the midline, the floor of the anterior cranial fossa extends below the level of the orbital roof, and the cribriform plates are seen on either side of the central crista galli.

Within the orbit the central space is occupied by the round optic nerve cut in cross-section. The central nerve can sometimes be distinguished from the nerve sheaths, and the two are separated by the clear subarachnoid space (Figure 11-9). The four rectus muscles, cut across their midbellies, are seen near their respective orbital walls. The levator muscle may be distinguished as a separate thin strap just above and medial to the superior rectus muscle. Above the medial rectus muscle, along the superomedial corner or the orbit, is the superior oblique muscle. Elements of the fascial connective tissue system can be seen associated with some of the extraocular muscles.

The superior ophthalmic vein appears as a round density between the optic nerve and the superior rectus muscle, as it crosses the orbit from medial to lateral. The smaller ophthalmic artery is usually situated near the superior oblique muscle, and may be difficult to distinguish from it. Along the orbital roof just above the medial edge of the levator muscle is the frontal nerve. The nasociliary nerve can often be seen between the optic nerve and the upper pole of the medial rectus muscle. On high-resolution CT and MRI scans numerous other small neurovascular elements can be differentiated.[22,31] These include the posterior ciliary arteries and nerves, the vortex veins, the lacrimal artery and vein, and the inferior ophthalmic vein.

Coronal section through the posterior globe

Coronal sections cut through the level of the posterior globe show the bony contour of the orbit similar to that of the central orbit, but somewhat more rounded. At this level the orbital roof exhibits an undulating upper surface reflecting the sulci and gyri of the overlying frontal lobes. In the midline the crista galli and cribriform plate are still easily visible. The nasal septum extends downward in the midline between the ethmoid labyrinths.

Centrally the globe is seen filling much of the orbital space. Superiorly the thin superior rectus and levator muscles lie just above the globe, and can usually be distinguished from each other (Figure 11-10). Medially the flattened medial rectus muscle lies within the orbital fat between the lamina papyracea and the globe. Just below the eye is the inferior rectus muscle, and laterally is the lateral rectus muscle, both becoming flat as they approach their respective tendons of insertion. In the superomedial corner a small round to oval shadow is the superior oblique muscle. In some sections the inferior oblique muscle may be seen along the sclera inferolaterally. A prominent shadow is seen connecting the levator and the lateral rectus muscles. This represents part of the superior and lateral fascial suspensory system. The lacrimal artery and nerve may be seen just above this structure in the superolateral orbit.

Numerous neurovascular elements can be seen at this level. Along the roof near the midline is the frontal nerve, and near it may be seen the frontal artery. The superior ophthalmic vein has moved further medially and is now located at the medial edge of the superior rectus-levator muscle complex. The terminal branch of the ophthalmic artery is seen below the superior oblique muscle along the medial orbital wall.

Coronal section through the mid globe

In coronal sections at the level of the mid globe the orbit assumes a nearly circular outline, and the eye fills most of the central portion. The rectus muscles have become narrow bands as they approach their tendons of insertion on the sclera. The levator muscle is well visualized. The superolateral intermuscular septum appears as a dense line running from the lateral edge of the levator to the lateral rectus muscle (Figure 11-11). In the superomedial orbit, the superior oblique tendon is seen as it narrows into a small rounded structure. The inferior oblique is seen as a crescentic shadow just lateral to the inferior rectus muscle.

Immediately below the superior oblique tendon the small terminal branch of the ophthalmic artery may be seen near the medial orbital wall. The superior ophthalmic vein is a larger round structure between the levator muscle and the superior oblique tendon. Superiorly, between the globe and orbital roof, the frontal artery and nerve can be seen as small rounded densities passing forward to the supraorbital notch. In more anterior sections, the posterior pole of the lacrimal gland may be visible in the superolateral orbit.

Coronal section through the anterior globe

In anterior orbital coronal sections the orbital contour is incomplete laterally where the rim lies in a more posterior plane (Figure 11-12). In the midline the frontal sinus is seen extending laterally into the orbital roof. In the inferomedial corner, on more anterior sections the lacrimal canal can be seen between the nasal cavity and the maxillary sinus.

Within the orbit the globe is seen centrally. In very anterior sections the lens and cornea may be appreciated within the globe. The rectus muscle tendons are seen only as flat elevations on the scleral surface. The inferior oblique muscle extends from the inferolateral globe to the orbital floor just lateral to the lacrimal canal. The superior oblique tendon and trochlea lie on the superomedial wall. The levator muscle is now broader in horizontal extent, and still shows prominent fascial connections to the lateral rectus system and to the lateral retinaculum. The lacrimal gland forms a prominent density between this shadow and the orbital wall.

The superior ophthalmic vein continues to run forward between the levator muscle and the superior oblique tendon. Terminal branches of the ophthalmic artery may be seen along the medial wall as the dorsal nasal or palpebral arteries. Elements of the extensive anterior fascial systems occur as fine irregular lines between the muscles.

Axial sections through the orbit

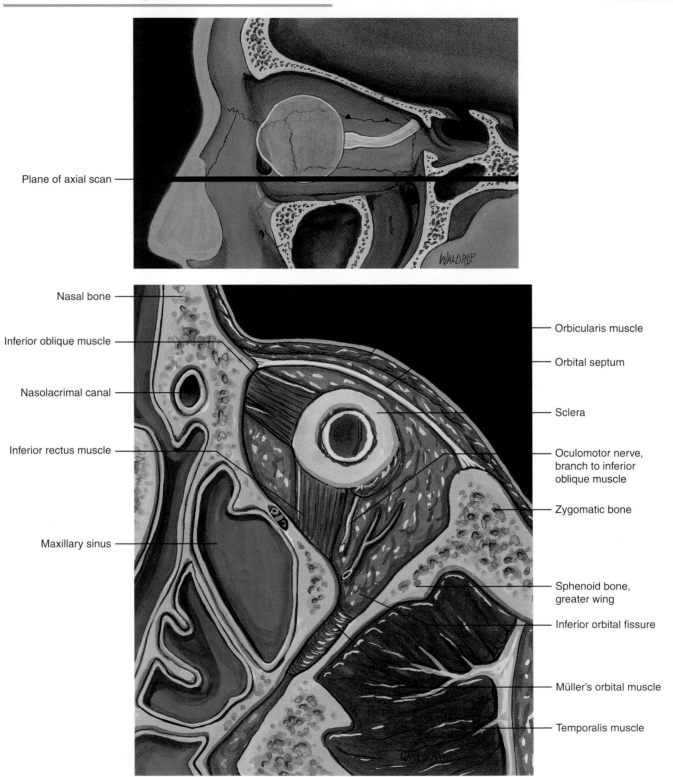

Plane of axial scan

Nasal bone

Inferior oblique muscle

Nasolacrimal canal

Inferior rectus muscle

Maxillary sinus

Orbicularis muscle

Orbital septum

Sclera

Oculomotor nerve, branch to inferior oblique muscle

Zygomatic bone

Sphenoid bone, greater wing

Inferior orbital fissure

Müller's orbital muscle

Temporalis muscle

Figure 11-1 Axial section through the inferior orbit, tangential to the sclera at the level of the inferior oblique muscle. The inferior rectus muscle is seen extending along the orbital floor.

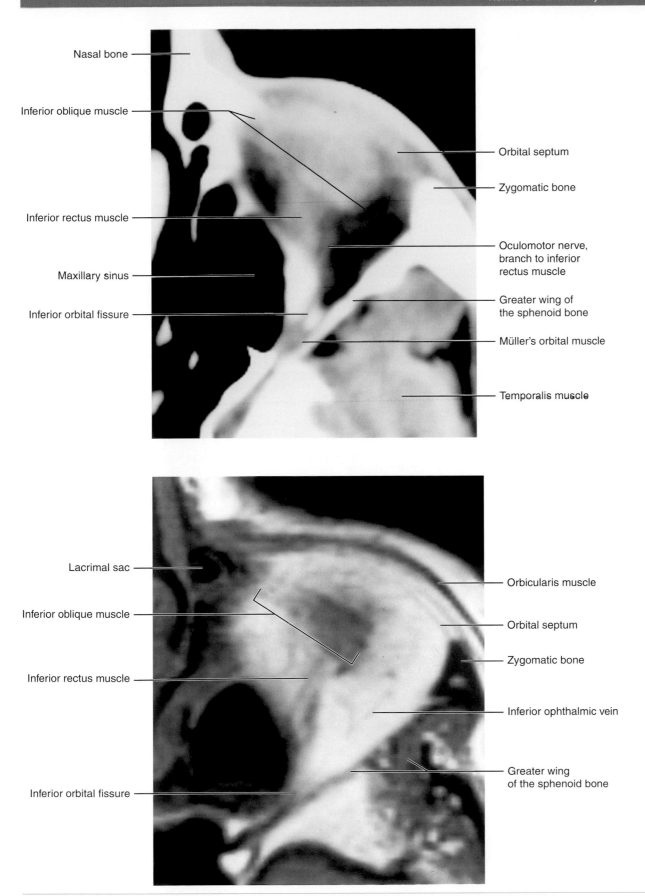

Nasal bone

Inferior oblique muscle

Inferior rectus muscle

Maxillary sinus

Inferior orbital fissure

Orbital septum

Zygomatic bone

Oculomotor nerve,
branch to inferior
rectus muscle

Greater wing of
the sphenoid bone

Müller's orbital muscle

Temporalis muscle

Lacrimal sac

Inferior oblique muscle

Inferior rectus muscle

Inferior orbital fissure

Orbicularis muscle

Orbital septum

Zygomatic bone

Inferior ophthalmic vein

Greater wing
of the sphenoid bone

Figure 11-1 cont'd

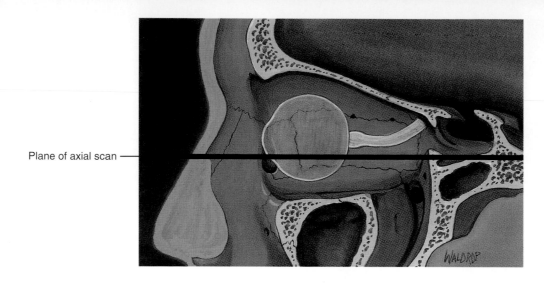

Plane of axial scan —

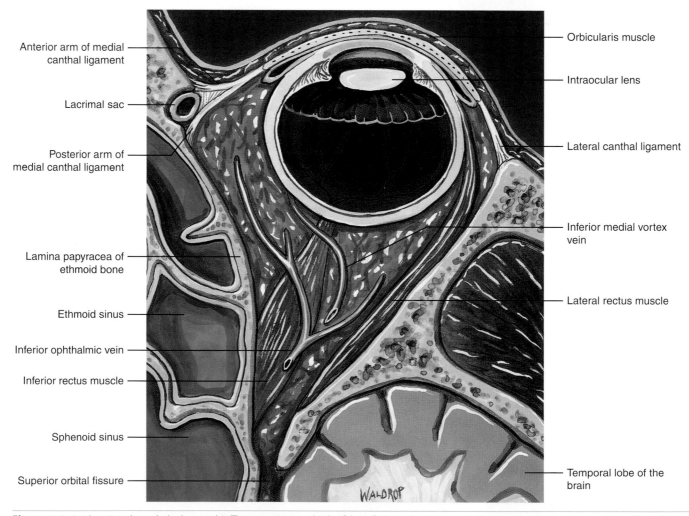

Anterior arm of medial canthal ligament —

Lacrimal sac —

Posterior arm of medial canthal ligament —

Lamina papyracea of ethmoid bone —

Ethmoid sinus —

Inferior ophthalmic vein —

Inferior rectus muscle —

Sphenoid sinus —

Superior orbital fissure —

— Orbicularis muscle

— Intraocular lens

— Lateral canthal ligament

— Inferior medial vortex vein

— Lateral rectus muscle

— Temporal lobe of the brain

Figure 11-2 Axial section through the lower orbit. The posterior two-thirds of the inferior rectus is seen, as is the lower portions of the medial and lateral rectus muscles.

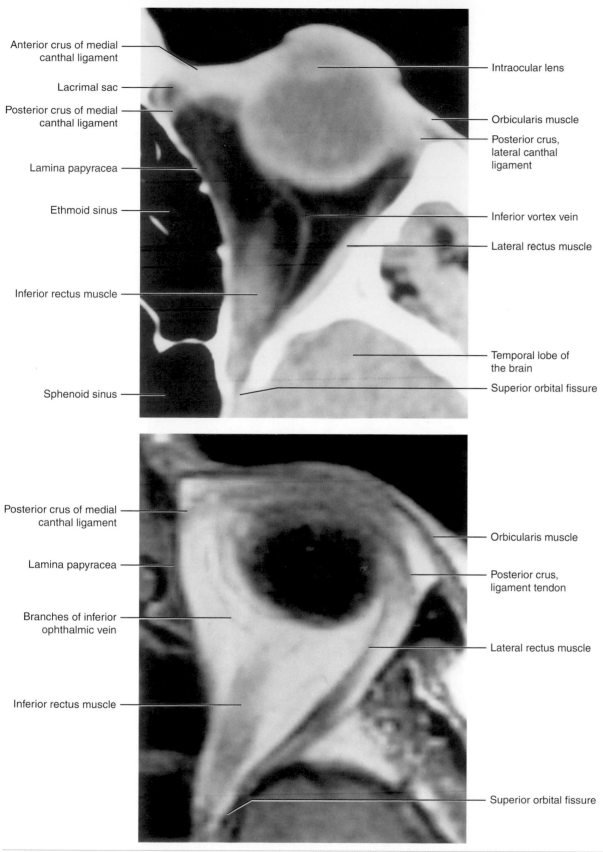

Anterior crus of medial canthal ligament

Lacrimal sac

Posterior crus of medial canthal ligament

Lamina papyracea

Ethmoid sinus

Inferior rectus muscle

Sphenoid sinus

Intraocular lens

Orbicularis muscle

Posterior crus, lateral canthal ligament

Inferior vortex vein

Lateral rectus muscle

Temporal lobe of the brain

Superior orbital fissure

Posterior crus of medial canthal ligament

Lamina papyracea

Branches of inferior ophthalmic vein

Inferior rectus muscle

Orbicularis muscle

Posterior crus, ligament tendon

Lateral rectus muscle

Superior orbital fissure

Figure 11-2 cont'd

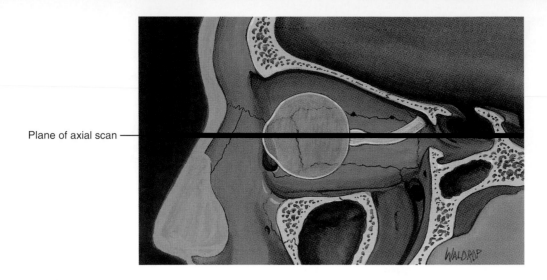

Plane of axial scan

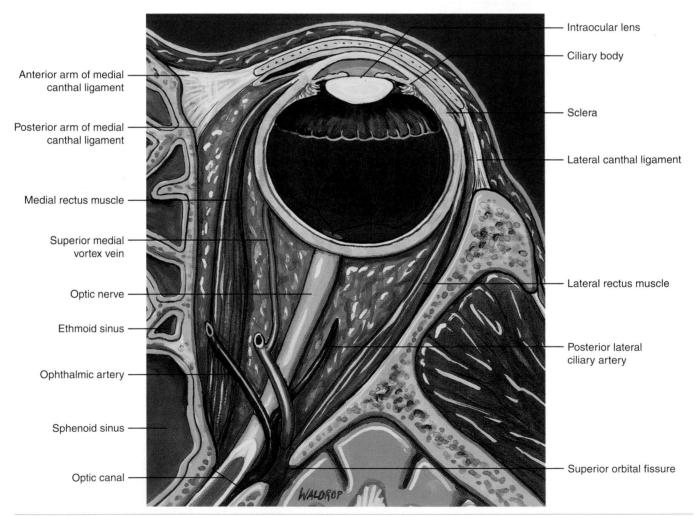

Intraocular lens

Ciliary body

Anterior arm of medial
canthal ligament

Posterior arm of medial
canthal ligament

Sclera

Lateral canthal ligament

Medial rectus muscle

Superior medial
vortex vein

Optic nerve

Lateral rectus muscle

Ethmoid sinus

Ophthalmic artery

Posterior lateral
ciliary artery

Sphenoid sinus

Optic canal

Superior orbital fissure

Figure 11-3 Axial section through the mid-orbit at the level of the optic nerve. The third portion of the ophthalmic artery is seen crossing the nerve in the posterior orbit.

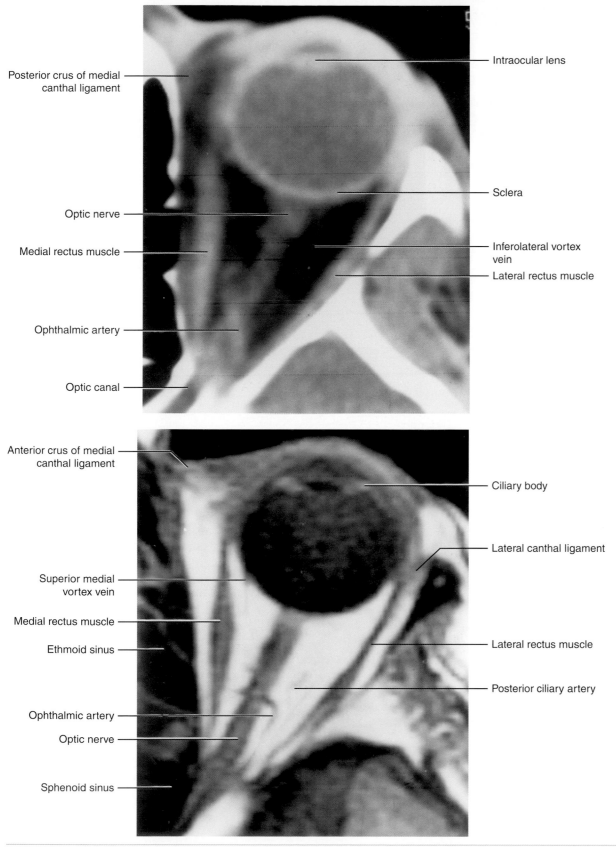

Posterior crus of medial canthal ligament

Intraocular lens

Optic nerve

Sclera

Medial rectus muscle

Inferolateral vortex vein

Lateral rectus muscle

Ophthalmic artery

Optic canal

Anterior crus of medial canthal ligament

Ciliary body

Superior medial vortex vein

Lateral canthal ligament

Medial rectus muscle

Ethmoid sinus

Lateral rectus muscle

Ophthalmic artery

Posterior ciliary artery

Optic nerve

Sphenoid sinus

Figure 11-3 cont'd

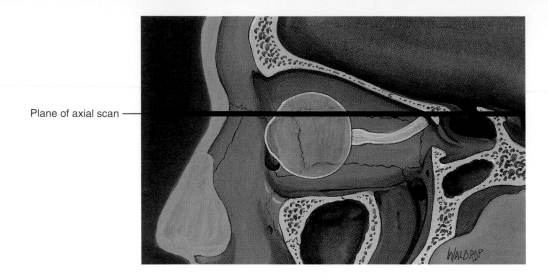

Plane of axial scan ——

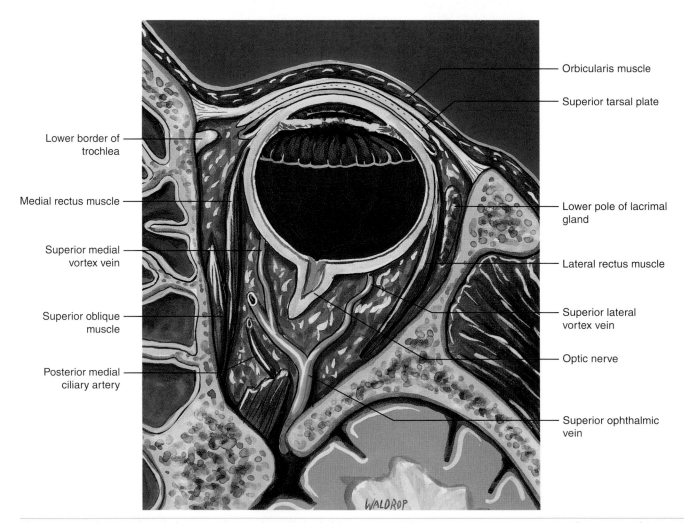

Orbicularis muscle

Superior tarsal plate

Lower border of trochlea ——

Medial rectus muscle ——

Lower pole of lacrimal gland

Superior medial vortex vein ——

Lateral rectus muscle

Superior oblique muscle ——

Superior lateral vortex vein

Posterior medial ciliary artery ——

Optic nerve

Superior ophthalmic vein

Figure 11-4 Axial section through the upper orbit just above the level of the optic nerve. The superior vortex veins are seen as well as portions of the superior ophthalmic vein.

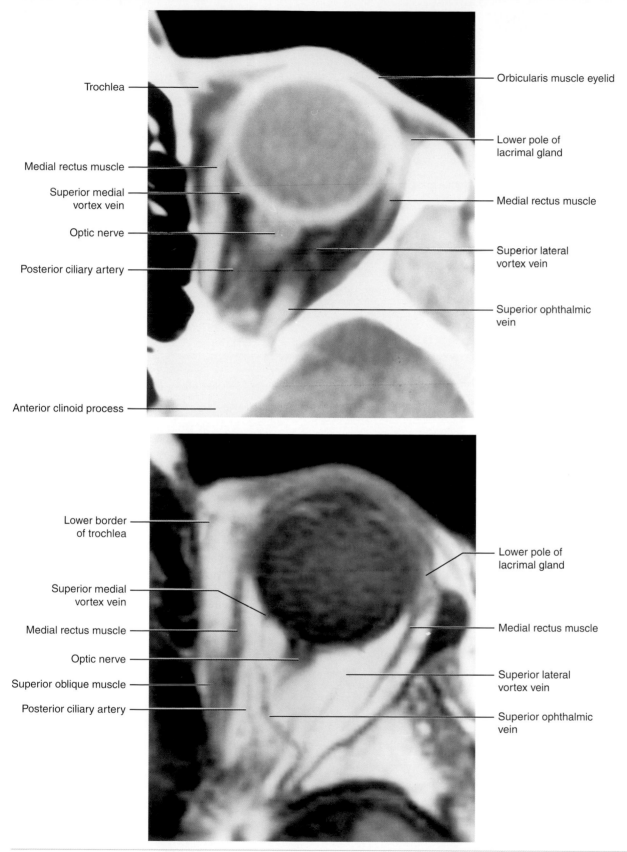

Trochlea

Orbicularis muscle eyelid

Lower pole of
lacrimal gland

Medial rectus muscle

Superior medial
vortex vein

Medial rectus muscle

Optic nerve

Superior lateral
vortex vein

Posterior ciliary artery

Superior ophthalmic
vein

Anterior clinoid process

Lower border
of trochlea

Lower pole of
lacrimal gland

Superior medial
vortex vein

Medial rectus muscle

Medial rectus muscle

Optic nerve

Superior lateral
vortex vein

Superior oblique muscle

Posterior ciliary artery

Superior ophthalmic
vein

Figure 11-4 cont'd

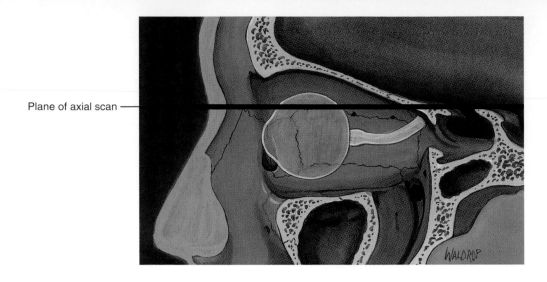

Plane of axial scan —

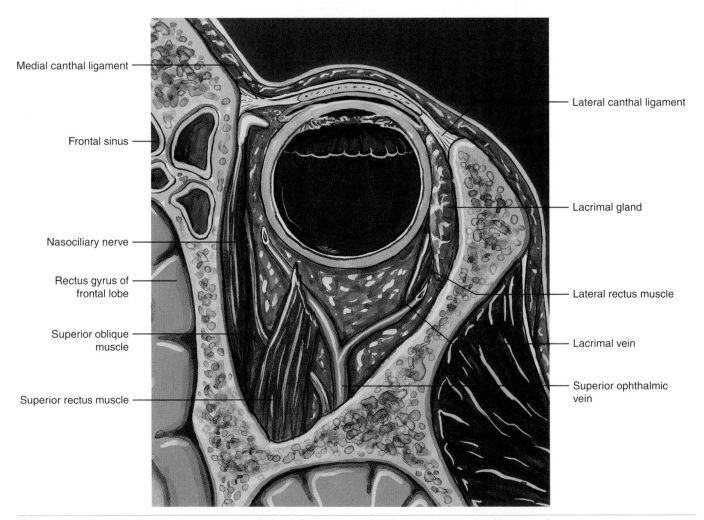

Medial canthal ligament —

Frontal sinus —

Nasociliary nerve —

Rectus gyrus of
frontal lobe —

Superior oblique
muscle —

Superior rectus muscle —

— Lateral canthal ligament

— Lacrimal gland

— Lateral rectus muscle

— Lacrimal vein

— Superior ophthalmic
vein

Figure 11-5 Axial section through the superior orbit at the level of the superior ophthalmic vein and superior oblique muscle.

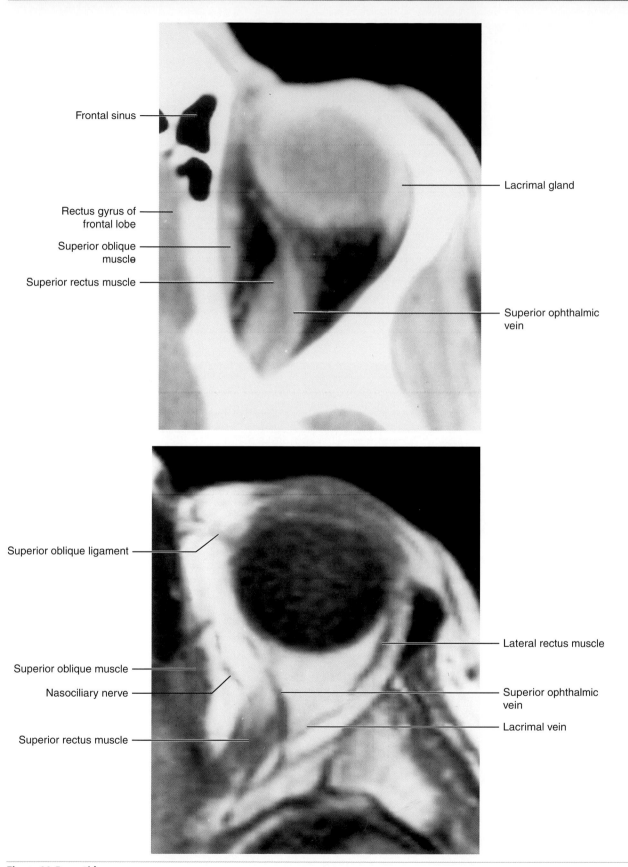

Frontal sinus

Rectus gyrus of frontal lobe

Superior oblique muscle

Superior rectus muscle

Lacrimal gland

Superior ophthalmic vein

Superior oblique ligament

Superior oblique muscle

Nasociliary nerve

Superior rectus muscle

Lateral rectus muscle

Superior ophthalmic vein

Lacrimal vein

Figure 11-5 cont'd

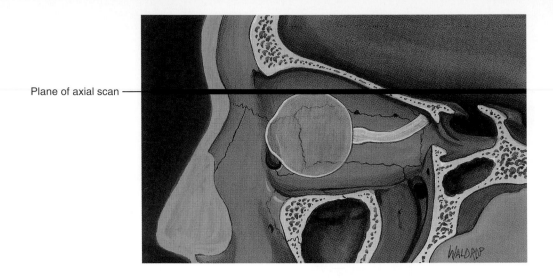

Plane of axial scan

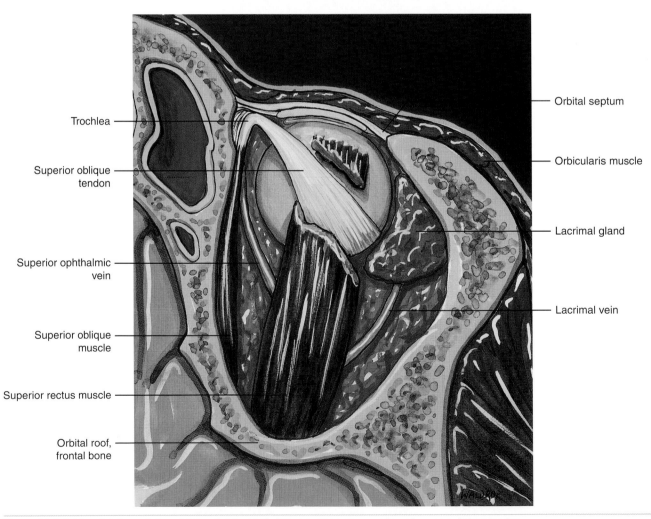

Trochlea

Superior oblique tendon

Superior ophthalmic vein

Superior oblique muscle

Superior rectus muscle

Orbital roof, frontal bone

Orbital septum

Orbicularis muscle

Lacrimal gland

Lacrimal vein

Figure 11-6 Axial section through the orbital roof at the level of the superior rectus muscle and superior oblique tendon.

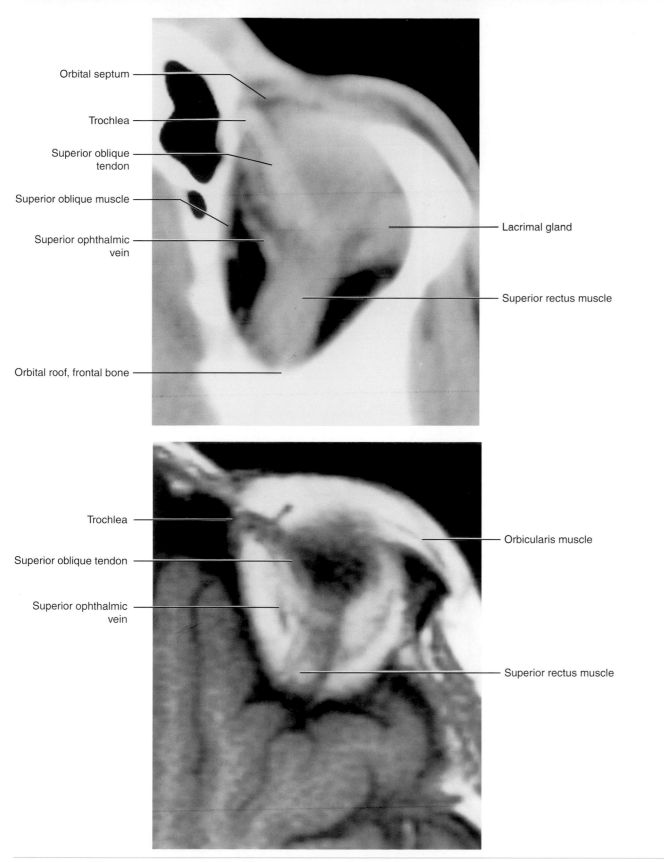

Orbital septum

Trochlea

Superior oblique
tendon

Superior oblique muscle

Superior ophthalmic
vein

Orbital roof, frontal bone

Lacrimal gland

Superior rectus muscle

Trochlea

Superior oblique tendon

Superior ophthalmic
vein

Orbicularis muscle

Superior rectus muscle

Figure 11-6 cont'd

Coronal sections through the orbit

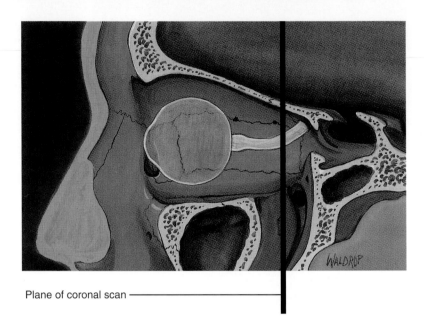

Plane of coronal scan ──────────────

Levator palpebrae superioris muscle

Ophthalmic artery

Superior oblique muscle

Sphenoid sinus

Medial rectus muscle

Inferior rectus muscle

Supraorbital nerve

Superior rectus muscle

Superior ophthalmic vein

Optic nerve

Lateral rectus muscle

Inferior ophthalmic vein

Müller's orbital muscle

Maxillary sinus

Figure 11-7 Coronal section through the orbital apex at the level of the annulus of Zinn.

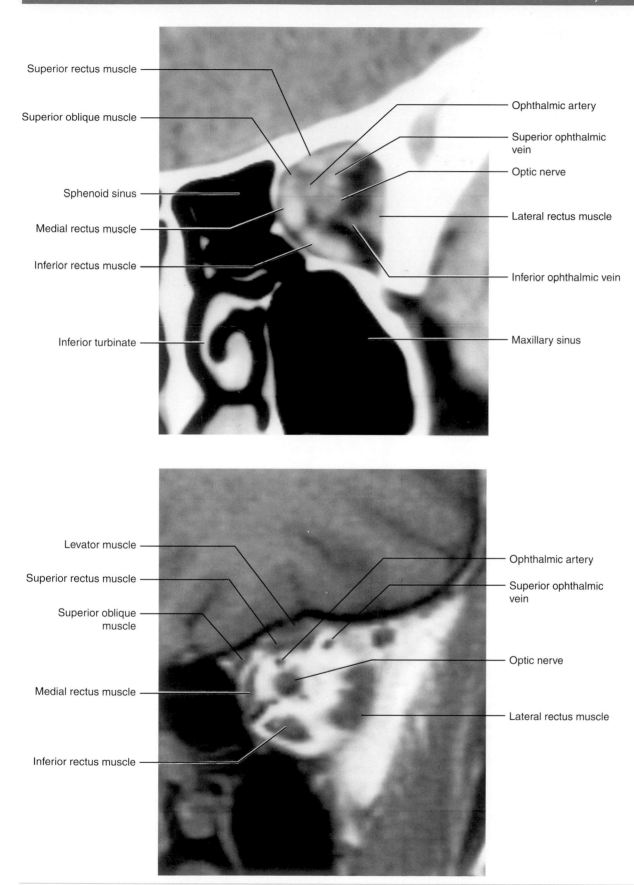

Superior rectus muscle

Superior oblique muscle

Sphenoid sinus

Medial rectus muscle

Inferior rectus muscle

Inferior turbinate

Ophthalmic artery

Superior ophthalmic vein

Optic nerve

Lateral rectus muscle

Inferior ophthalmic vein

Maxillary sinus

Levator muscle

Superior rectus muscle

Superior oblique muscle

Medial rectus muscle

Inferior rectus muscle

Ophthalmic artery

Superior ophthalmic vein

Optic nerve

Lateral rectus muscle

Figure 11-7 cont'd

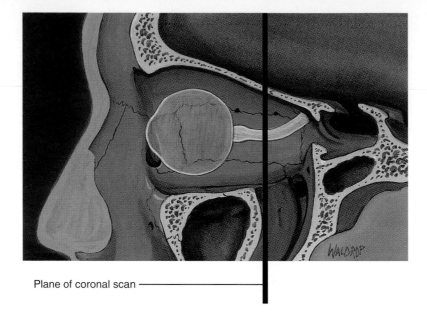

Plane of coronal scan ———————

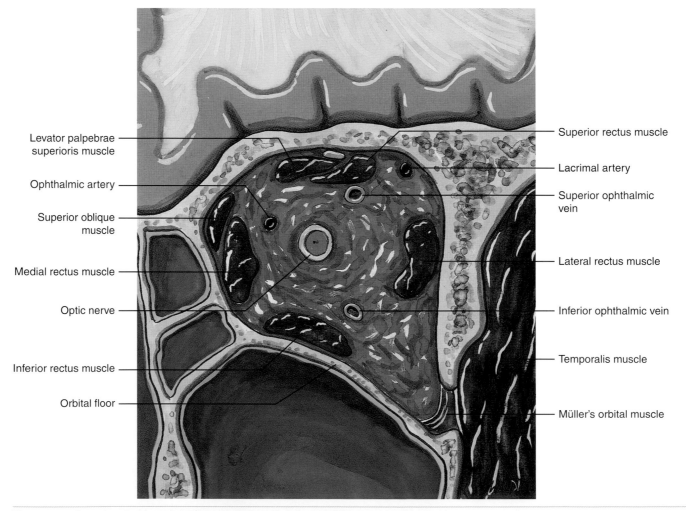

Levator palpebrae superioris muscle

Ophthalmic artery

Superior oblique muscle

Medial rectus muscle

Optic nerve

Inferior rectus muscle

Orbital floor

Superior rectus muscle

Lacrimal artery

Superior ophthalmic vein

Lateral rectus muscle

Inferior ophthalmic vein

Temporalis muscle

Müller's orbital muscle

Figure 11-8 Coronal section through the posterior orbit and inferior orbital fissure.

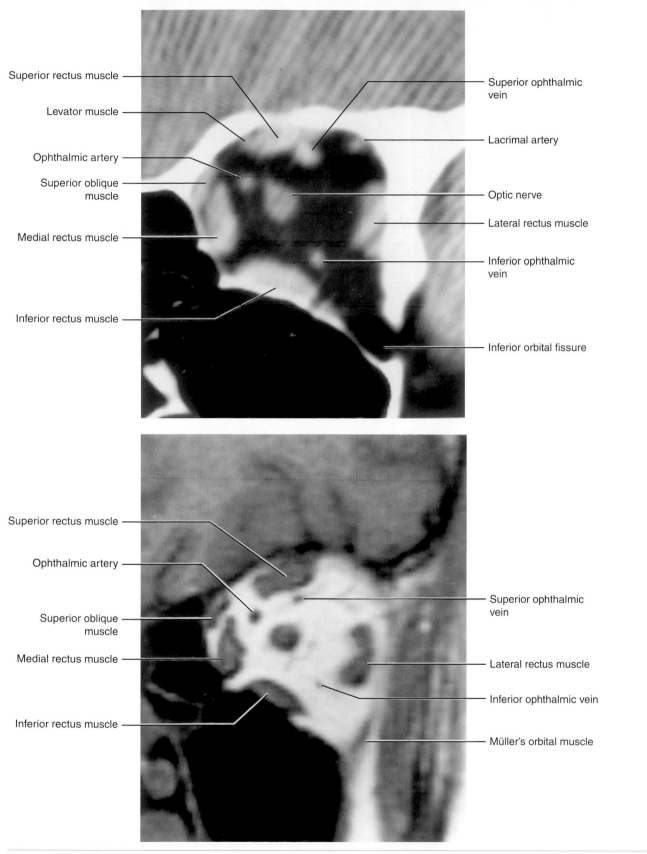

Superior rectus muscle

Levator muscle

Ophthalmic artery

Superior oblique
muscle

Medial rectus muscle

Inferior rectus muscle

Superior ophthalmic
vein

Lacrimal artery

Optic nerve

Lateral rectus muscle

Inferior ophthalmic
vein

Inferior orbital fissure

Superior rectus muscle

Ophthalmic artery

Superior oblique
muscle

Medial rectus muscle

Inferior rectus muscle

Superior ophthalmic
vein

Lateral rectus muscle

Inferior ophthalmic
vein

Müller's orbital muscle

Figure 11-8 cont'd

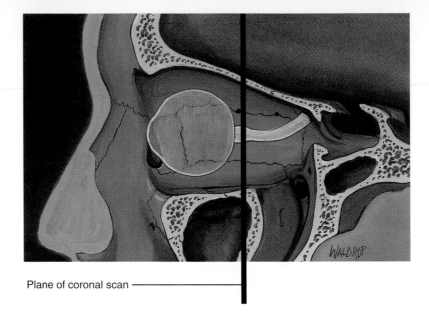

Plane of coronal scan

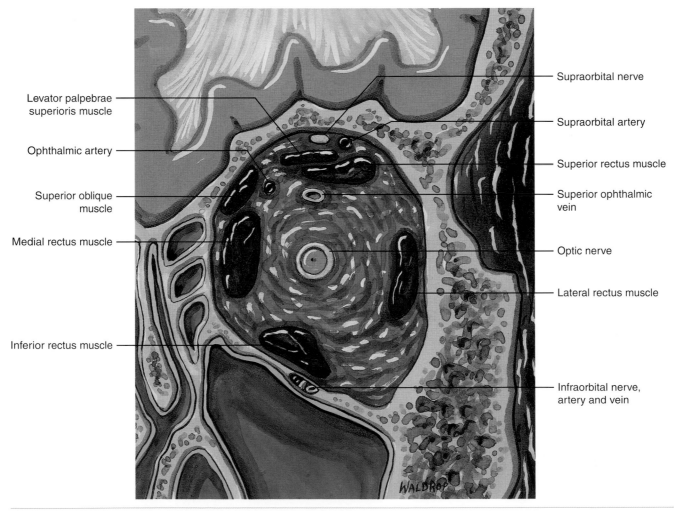

Levator palpebrae superioris muscle

Ophthalmic artery

Superior oblique muscle

Medial rectus muscle

Inferior rectus muscle

Supraorbital nerve

Supraorbital artery

Superior rectus muscle

Superior ophthalmic vein

Optic nerve

Lateral rectus muscle

Infraorbital nerve, artery and vein

Figure 11-9 Coronal section through the central orbit just posterior to the globe.

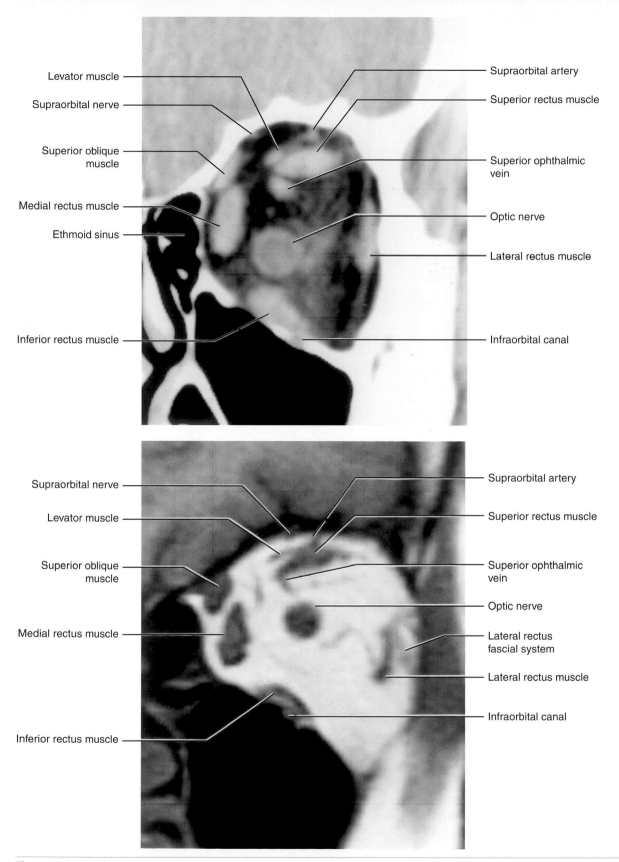

Levator muscle

Supraorbital nerve

Superior oblique muscle

Medial rectus muscle

Ethmoid sinus

Inferior rectus muscle

Supraorbital artery

Superior rectus muscle

Superior ophthalmic vein

Optic nerve

Lateral rectus muscle

Infraorbital canal

Supraorbital nerve

Levator muscle

Superior oblique muscle

Medial rectus muscle

Inferior rectus muscle

Supraorbital artery

Superior rectus muscle

Superior ophthalmic vein

Optic nerve

Lateral rectus fascial system

Lateral rectus muscle

Infraorbital canal

Figure 11-9 cont'd

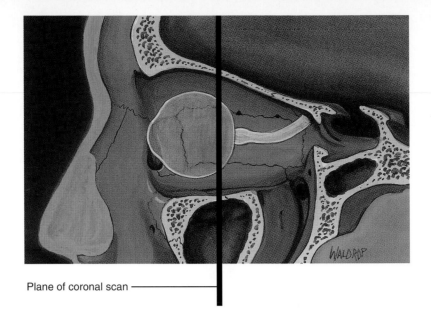

Plane of coronal scan ——————

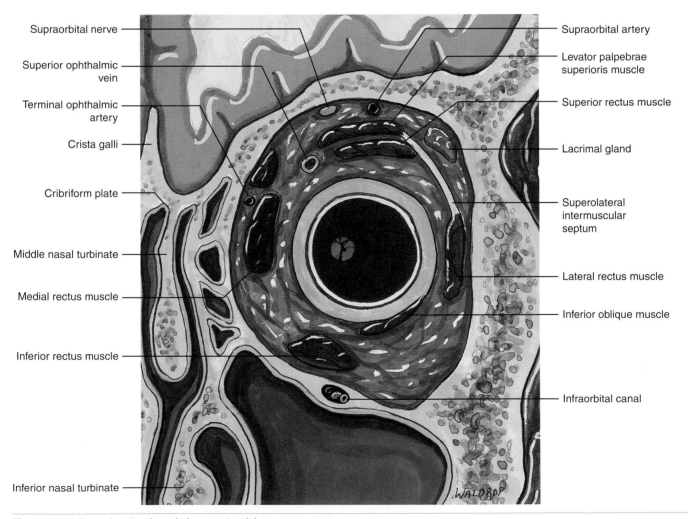

Supraorbital nerve ——————

Superior ophthalmic vein ——————

Terminal ophthalmic artery ——————

Crista galli ——————

Cribriform plate ——————

Middle nasal turbinate ——————

Medial rectus muscle ——————

Inferior rectus muscle ——————

Inferior nasal turbinate ——————

—————— Supraorbital artery

—————— Levator palpebrae superioris muscle

—————— Superior rectus muscle

—————— Lacrimal gland

—————— Superolateral intermuscular septum

—————— Lateral rectus muscle

—————— Inferior oblique muscle

—————— Infraorbital canal

Figure 11-10 Coronal section through the posterior globe.

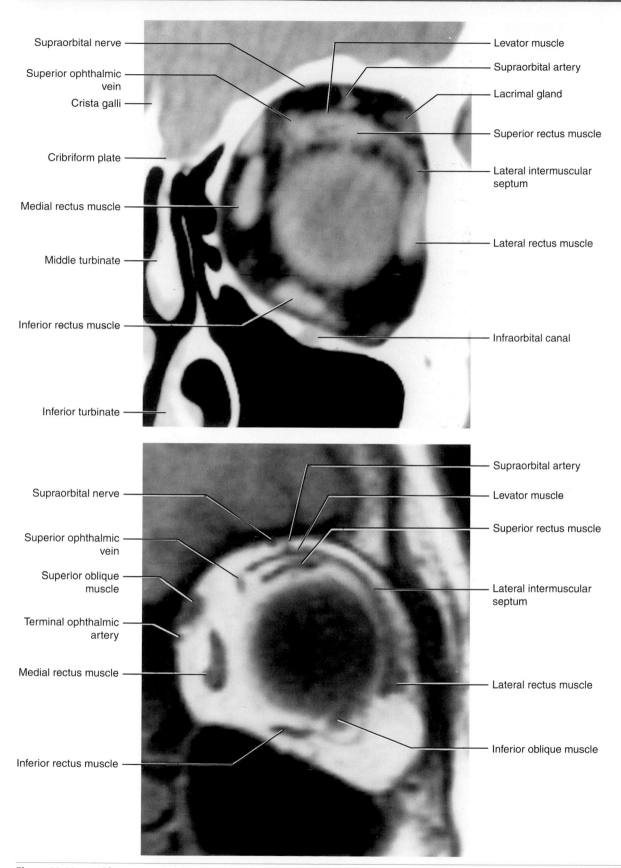

Supraorbital nerve

Superior ophthalmic vein

Crista galli

Cribriform plate

Medial rectus muscle

Middle turbinate

Inferior rectus muscle

Inferior turbinate

Levator muscle

Supraorbital artery

Lacrimal gland

Superior rectus muscle

Lateral intermuscular septum

Lateral rectus muscle

Infraorbital canal

Supraorbital nerve

Superior ophthalmic vein

Superior oblique muscle

Terminal ophthalmic artery

Medial rectus muscle

Inferior rectus muscle

Supraorbital artery

Levator muscle

Superior rectus muscle

Lateral intermuscular septum

Lateral rectus muscle

Inferior oblique muscle

Figure 11-10 cont'd

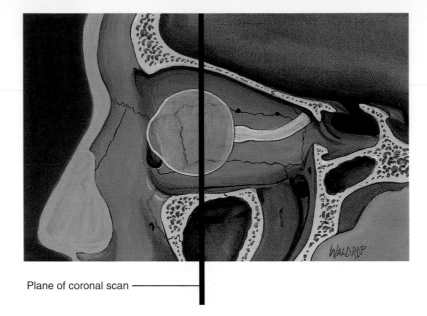

Plane of coronal scan ——

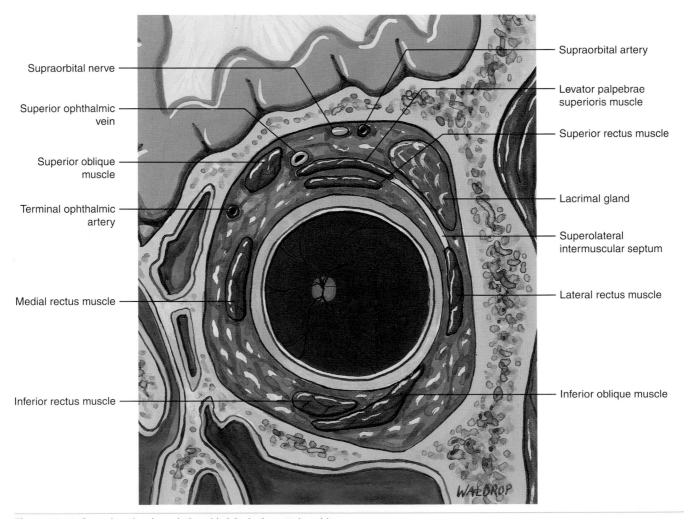

Supraorbital nerve ——

Superior ophthalmic vein ——

Superior oblique muscle ——

Terminal ophthalmic artery ——

Medial rectus muscle ——

Inferior rectus muscle ——

—— Supraorbital artery

—— Levator palpebrae superioris muscle

—— Superior rectus muscle

—— Lacrimal gland

—— Superolateral intermuscular septum

—— Lateral rectus muscle

—— Inferior oblique muscle

Figure 11-11 Coronal section through the mid globe in the anterior orbit.

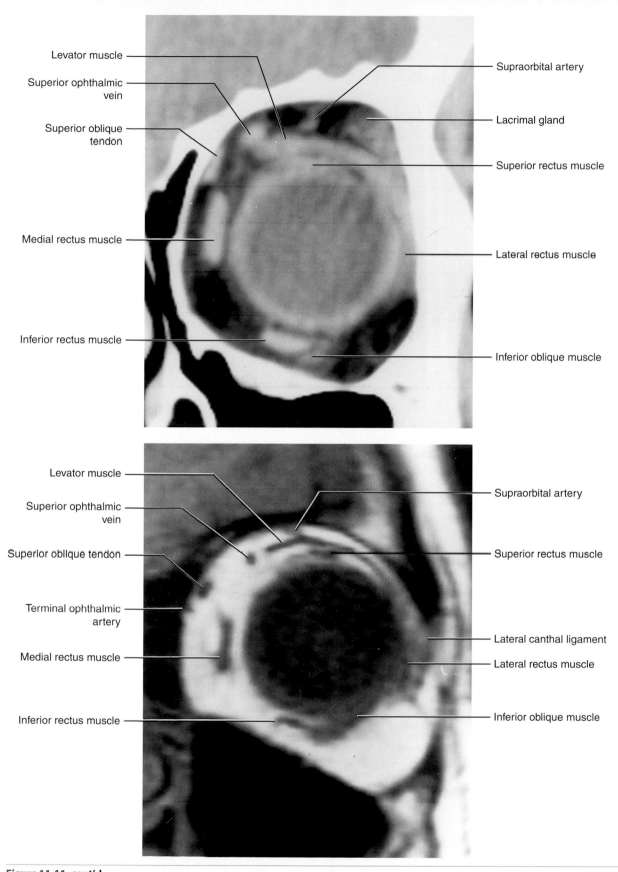

Levator muscle

Superior ophthalmic vein

Superior oblique tendon

Medial rectus muscle

Inferior rectus muscle

Supraorbital artery

Lacrimal gland

Superior rectus muscle

Lateral rectus muscle

Inferior oblique muscle

Levator muscle

Superior ophthalmic vein

Superior oblique tendon

Terminal ophthalmic artery

Medial rectus muscle

Inferior rectus muscle

Supraorbital artery

Superior rectus muscle

Lateral canthal ligament

Lateral rectus muscle

Inferior oblique muscle

Figure 11-11 cont'd

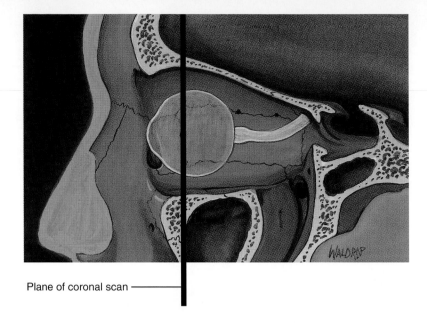

Plane of coronal scan ———

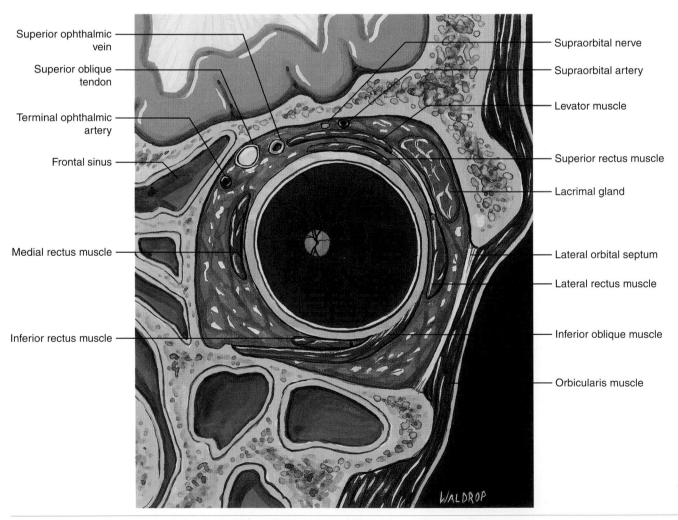

Superior ophthalmic vein

Superior oblique tendon

Terminal ophthalmic artery

Frontal sinus

Medial rectus muscle

Inferior rectus muscle

Supraorbital nerve

Supraorbital artery

Levator muscle

Superior rectus muscle

Lacrimal gland

Lateral orbital septum

Lateral rectus muscle

Inferior oblique muscle

Orbicularis muscle

Figure 11-12 Coronal section through the anterior globe and orbit at the level of the inferior oblique muscle.

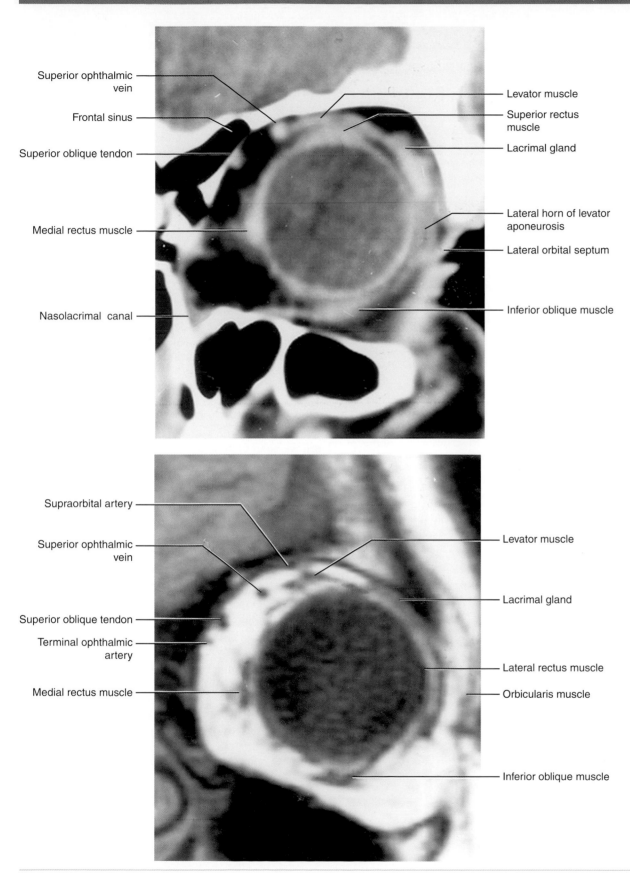

Superior ophthalmic vein

Frontal sinus

Superior oblique tendon

Medial rectus muscle

Nasolacrimal canal

Levator muscle

Superior rectus muscle

Lacrimal gland

Lateral horn of levator aponeurosis

Lateral orbital septum

Inferior oblique muscle

Supraorbital artery

Superior ophthalmic vein

Superior oblique tendon

Terminal ophthalmic artery

Medial rectus muscle

Levator muscle

Lacrimal gland

Lateral rectus muscle

Orbicularis muscle

Inferior oblique muscle

Figure 11-12 cont'd

References

1. Atlas SW, Grossman RI, Hackney HI, et al: STIR MR imaging of the orbit. *Am J Roentgenol* 151:1025, 1988.

2. Aviv RI, Casselman J: Orbital imaging: Part 1. Normal anatomy. *Clin Radiol* 60:279, 2005.

3. Aviv RI, Miszkiel K: Orbital imaging: Part 2. Intraorbital pathology. *Clin Radiol* 60(3):288, 2005.

4. Beyer-Enke SA, Tiedemann K, Görich J: Gamroth. Thin section computerized tomography of the skull base. *Radiologe* 27:483, 1987.

5. Braffman BH, Naidich TP, Chaneles M: Imaging anatomy of the normal orbit. *Semin Ultrasound CT MR* 18:403, 1997.

6. Conneely MF, Hacein-Bay L, Jay WM: Magnetic resonance imaging of the orbit. *Semin Ophthalmol* 23:179, 2008.

7. Daniels DL, Pech P, Mark L, et al: Magnetic resonance imaging of the cavernous sinus. *Am J Roentgenol* 144:1009, 1985.

8. Daniels DL, Yu S, Pech P, Haughton VM: Computed tomography and magnetic resonance imaging of the orbital apex. *Radiol Clin North Amer* 25:803, 1987.

9. Dortzbach RK, Kronish JW, Gentry LR: Magnetic resonance imaging of the orbit. Part I. Physical principles. *Ophthalm Plast Reconstr Surg* 5:151, 1989.

10. Dortzbach RK, Kronish JW, Gentry LR: Magnetic resonance imaging of the orbit. Part II. Clinical applications. *Ophthalm Plast Reconstr Surg* 5:160, 1989.

11. Dutton JJ, Klingele TG, Burde RM, Gado M: Evaluation of the suprasellar cistern by computed tomography. *Ophthalmology* 89:1220, 1982.

12. Dutton JJ: *Radiology of the Orbit and Visual Pathways.* London, Saunders/Elsevier, 2010.

13. Ettl A, Zwrtek K, Daxer A, Salomonowitz E: Anatomy of the orbital apex and cavernous sinus on high-resolution magnetic resonance images. *Surv Ophthalmol* 44:303, 2000.

14. Ettl AR, Salomonowitz E, Koornneef L: Magnetic resonance imaging of the orbit. Basic principles and anatomy. *Orbit* 19:211, 2000.

15. Goh PS, Gi MT, Charlton A, et al: Review of orbital imaging. *Eur J Radiol* 66:387, 2008.

16. Gonzalez RG, Cheng H-M, Barnett P, et al: Nuclear magnetic resonance of the vitreous body. *Science* 223:399, 1984.

17. Gore JC, Emery EW, Orr JS, Doyle FH: Medical nuclear magnetic resonance imaging: I. Physical principles. *Invest Radiol* 16:269, 1981.

18. Gyldensted C, Lester J, Fledelius H: Computed tomography of orbital lesions. *Neuroradiology* 13:141, 1977.

19. Hammerschlag SB, O'Reilly GVA, Naheedy MH: Computed tomography of the optic canals. *AJNR* 2:593, 1981.

20. Ivancevic MK, Geerts L, Weadock WJ, et al: Technical principles of MR angiography methods. *Magn Reson Imaging Clin N Am* 17:1, 2009.

21. Kubal WS: Imaging of orbital trauma. *Radiographics* 28:1729, 2008.

22. Langer BG, Mafee MF, Pollock S, et al: MRI of the normal orbit and optic pathway. *Radiol Clin N Am* 25:429, 1987.

23. Lee AG, Brazis PW, Garrity JA, White M: Imaging for neuro-ophthalmic and orbital disease. *Am J Ophthalmol* 138:852, 2004.

24. Lee AG, Johnson MC, Policeni BA, Smoker WR: Imaging for neuro-ophthalmic and orbital disease—a review. *Clin Exp Ophthalmol* 37:30, 2008.

25. Lee HJ, Jilani M, Frohman L, Baker S: CT of orbital trauma. *Emerg Radiol* 10:168, 2004.

26. Macoviski A: MRI: a charmed past and an exciting future. *J Magn Reson Imaging* 30:919, 2009.

27. Niloskelainen E, Enzmann DR, Sogg RL, Rosenthal AR: Computerized tomography of the orbits. *Acta Ophthalmol* 55:885, 1977.

28. Russell EJ, Czervionke L, Huckman M, et al: CT of the inferomedial orbit and the lacrimal drainage apparatus: normal and pathologic anatomy. *AJNR* 145:1147, 1985.

29. Sassani JW, Osbakken MD: Anatomic features of the eye disclosed with nuclear magnetic resonance imaging. *Arch Ophthalmol* 102:541, 1984.

30. Schenck JF, Hart HR, Foster TH, et al: High resolution magnetic resonance imaging using surface coils. In: Kressel HY (ed): *Magnetic Resonance Annual 1986.* New York, Raven, 1986, p 123.

31. Schenck JF, Hart HR, Foster TH, et al: Improved imaging of the orbit at 1.5T with surface coils. *Am J Roenthenol* 144:1033, 1985.

32. Simon J, Szumowski J, Totterman S, et al: Fat-suppression MR imaging of the orbit. *AJNR* 9:961, 1988.

33. Sullivan JA, Harms SE: Characterization of orbital lesions by surface coil MR imaging. *Radiographics* 7:9, 1987.

34. Tamiraz JC, Outin-Tamiraz C, Saban R: MR imaging anatomy of the optic pathways. *Radiol Clin N Am* 37:1, 1988.

35. Tonini M, Krainik A, Bessou P, et al: How helical CT helps the surgeon in oculo-orbital trauma. *J Neuroraiol* 36:185, 2009.

36. Unsöld R, DeGroot J, Newton TH: Images of the optic nerve: anatomic-CT correlation. *Am J Roentgenol* 135:767, 1980.

37. Wende S, Aulich A, Nover A, et al: Computed tomography of orbital lesions. A comparative study of 210 cases. *Neuroradiology* 13:123, 1977.

38. Wippold FJ II: Head and neck imaging: the role of CT and MRI. *J Magn Reson Imaging* 25:453, 2007.

Note: Page numbers followed by *f* indicate figures.